293
Current Topics in Microbiology and Immunology

Editors

R.W. Compans, Atlanta/Georgia
M.D. Cooper, Birmingham/Alabama
T. Honjo, Kyoto · H. Koprowski, Philadelphia/Pennsylvania
F. Melchers, Basel · M.B.A. Oldstone, La Jolla/California
S. Olsnes, Oslo · M. Potter, Bethesda/Maryland
P.K. Vogt, La Jolla/California · H. Wagner, Munich

B. Kyewski and E. Suri-Payer (Eds.)

CD4⁺CD25⁺ Regulatory T Cells: Origin, Function and Therapeutic Potential

With 22 Figures and 9 Tables

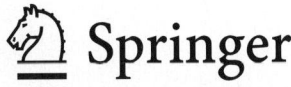

Professor Dr. Bruno Kyewski
Deutsches Krebsforschungszentrum
Forschungsschwerpunkt
Tumorimmunologie
Abteilung Entwicklungsimmunologie
Im Neuenheimer Feld 280
69120 Heidelberg
Germany

e-mail: B.Kyewski@dkfz-heidelberg.de

Dr. Elisabeth Suri-Payer
Deutsches Krebsforschungszentrum
Forschungsschwerpunkt
Tumorimmunologie
Abteilung Immungenetik
Im Neuenheimer Feld 280
69120 Heidelberg
Germany

e-mail: E.Suri-Payer@dkfz-heidelberg.de

Cover figures by S. K. Tung

Library of Congress Catalog Number 72-152360

ISSN 0070-217X
ISBN-10 3-540-24444-1 Springer Berlin Heidelberg New York
ISBN-13 978-3-540-24444-8 Springer Berlin Heidelberg New York

This work is subject to copyright. All rights reserved, whether the whole or part of the material is concerned, specifically the rights of translation, reprinting, reuse of illustrations, recitation, broadcasting, reproduction on microfilm or in any other way, and storage in data banks. Duplication of this publication or parts thereof is permitted only under the provisions of the German Copyright Law of September, 9, 1965, in its current version, and permission for use must always be obtained from Springer-Verlag. Violations are liable for prosecution under the German Copyright Law.

Springer is a part of Springer Science+Business Media
springeronline.com
© Springer-Verlag Berlin Heidelberg 2005
Printed in Germany

The use of general descriptive names, registered names, trademarks, etc. in this publication does not imply, even in the absence of a specific statement, that such names are exempt from the relevant protective laws and regulations and therefore free for general use.
Product liability: The publisher cannot guarantee the accuracy of any information about dosage and application contained in this book. In every individual case the user must check such information by consulting the relevant literature.

Editor: Dr. Paul Roos, Heidelberg
Desk editor: Anne Clauss, Heidelberg
Production editor: Nadja Kroke, Leipzig
Cover design: design & production GmbH, Heidelberg
Typesetting: LE-TeX Jelonek, Schmidt & Vöckler GbR, Leipzig
Printed on acid-free paper   SPIN 11019459   21/3150/YL – 5 4 3 2 1 0

Preface

The vertebrate immune system defends the organism against invading pathogens while at the same time being self-tolerant to the body's own constituents thus preserving its integrity. Multiple mechanisms act in concert to ensure self-tolerance. During intrathymic development, the nascent T cell repertoire is purged from autoreactive T cells via negative selection, a process also known as recessive tolerance. Ridding of self-reactivity, however, is not complete, as attested by the presence of self-reactive T cells in the peripheral T cell repertoire. Hence, additional tolerance mechanisms, collectively referred to as dominant tolerance, have been postulated on theoretical grounds (see the chapter by A. Coutinho et al. in this volume) and experimental proof for their existence had been repeatedly claimed in the past 40 years. While some of these claims, largely based on in vitro experiments, later fell into disrepute (i.e., the infamous CD8 suppressor cells expressing I-J molecules), concurrent, but less well publicized strings of research, provided unremitting evidence for dominant tolerance mechanisms. These include the postnatal thymectomy model pioneered by Nishizuka and Sakakura in 1969, the dominant tolerance model in chicken and quail chimeras introduced by le Douarin and colleagues, and studies on infectious tolerance by the Waldmann laboratory. A breakthrough in this field was achieved by the identification and isolation by Sakaguchi's and Shevach's groups of a $CD4^+CD25^+$ T cell subset exerting suppression on effector T cells both in vitro and in vivo. This instigated an avalanche of publications on suppressor T cells. While largely overlooked for so many years, there is now hardly any aspect of immunity that does not seem to be affected by suppressor T cells. This volume will hardly be more than a snapshot in this fast-moving field, yet we hope that it will offer inspiration and orientation to the scientist who would like to enter this field.

To date, many different cells have been described that can suppress other cells of the immune system: $CD4^+CD25^+$ regulatory T cells (Treg), $CD4^+CD25^-$ regulatory T cells, T regulatory 1 cells (Tr1), T-helper 3 cells (Th3), $CD8^+CD28^-$ T cells, NKT cells, as well as tolerogenic dendritic cells. Suppressive CD4 T cells fall at least into two categories. So called natural

CD4$^+$CD25$^+$ Treg form part of the intra-thymically selected T cell repertoire and apparently constitute a distinct lineage. In contrast, "adaptive" regulatory T cells are instructed in the periphery to become suppressive cells, they form a more heterogeneous group including CD4$^+$ CD25$^+$ Treg, Tr1, and Th3 cells.

As natural Treg are so far the best characterized entity, the first three contributions of this volume (C. Cozzo et al., C.-S. Hsieh et al., and L. Klein et al.) will trace these cells from their origin in the thymus to their site of action in peripheral lymphoid organs and tissues. Thymocytes recognizing self-peptides at an affinity range, just below the threshold for negative selection, seem to be "instructed" into the Treg lineage, though the parameters specifying Treg lineage commitment are not known. The repertoire of Treg is clearly biased towards recognition of self-antigens including tissue-restricted antigens (see the chapter by C.-S. Hsie et al.), thereby potentially preventing organ-specific autoimmune diseases such as gastritis (see the chapter by R.S. McHugh) and oophoritis (see the chapter by K.S.K. Tung et al.).

Bearing in mind that many tumor-associated antigens, including those currently selected for clinical trials of immunotherapy, are un-mutated self-antigens, Treg may also interfere with spontaneous and induced anti-tumor immune responses (see the chapter by T. Nomura and S. Sakaguchi).

It has recently become clear that suppressor T cells not only contain autoreactivity, but also regulate immune reactions towards foreign antigens encoded by infectious agents, dietary proteins, allergens, and transplantation antigens (see the chapter by L.S. Taams and A.N. Akbar, and by H. Waldmann et al.). It is agreed that Treg need to be activated via the TCR by cognate antigen and then exert their suppression in an antigen nonspecific manner, allowing for "bystander suppression." It remains presently unclear whether suppression of immunity against foreign antigens involves Treg of corresponding specificity or entails bystander suppression by self-reactive Treg. It is also conceivable that natural, self-reactive Treg may instruct naïve CD4 T cells of different specificity into a regulatory network, a process termed "infectious tolerance" (see the chapters by A. Coutinho et al. and H. Waldmann et al.). Furthermore, CD4$^+$CD25$^+$ cells, IL-10-producing Tr1 cells, and other regulatory CD4 cells may be induced via other tolerogenic signals in the periphery, e.g., tolerogenic DC, IL-10, TGFβ (see the chapters by C. Cozzo et al., L. Klein et al., M.K. Levings and M.G. Roncarolo, K. Mahnke and A.H. Enk, and L.S. Taams and A.N. Akbar). In all cases, the action of Treg, be it on effector T cell function or the instruction of a second wave of Treg, requires presumably close cell–cell contact as provided by T cell–DC clusters in secondary lymphoid organs. T cells recognizing antigen(s) presented by the same APC would thus come under each other's influence, and suppression would be confined to such microenvironments (see the chapter by J. Huehn et al.).

The issue of the target range of suppressor T cells is closely linked to the question of how suppressor T cells mediate their function. After discovering the role of Treg in preventing autoimmune diseases, *in vitro* assay systems have been developed in order to dissect their mode of action. While there is consensus that suppression *in vitro* is dependent on direct cell contact between Treg and effector T cell, with some reports implying a role for membrane-bound TGFβ, the molecular mechanisms involved are still unknown (see the chapters by R.S. McHugh, and M.K. Levings and M.G. Roncarolo). There is even more uncertainty concerning the effector mode of various suppressor cell subsets *in vivo*. Depending on the disease model, a variety of cytokines have been implicated, pointing to the complexity of dominant tolerance. Likewise, it is not yet clear whether suppression is a direct event between Treg and effector T cells or whether it involves antigen-presenting cells as intermediaries (see the chapters by R.S. McHugh, M. Gad, and L.S. Taams and A.N. Akbar).

Part of our difficulties in answering these open questions stem from a lack of unambiguous markers which allow the identification and isolation of the various regulatory cells. Even the identification of the well-studied "natural" Treg still relies on the expression of the general activation marker CD25. While the transcriptional repressor Foxp3 now serves as a useful lineage marker for natural Treg at the population level, its expression cannot be analyzed at the single cell level. This shortcoming has now been remedied by inserting a marker gene into the Foxp3 locus. Because of this caveat, $CD25^+$ cells may encompass a mixture of different types of regulatory cells that suppress via different mechanisms, as well as recently activated effector T cells. The situation is even less satisfactory for Tr1 cells for which we lack any reliable marker. These problems still hamper the analysis of Treg function in humans, and their dys-regulation in autoimmune diseases and cancer (see the chapters by M.K. Levings and M.G. Roncarolo, and T. Nomura and S. Sakaguchi).

The phenomenon of dominant tolerance, not at all novel, is by now firmly established. It will offer new conceptual insights and hopefully new tools for the successful treatment of autoimmune diseases, improved cancer immunotherapy, and transplant survival. The fulfillment of these high expectations will, however, require the unambiguous identification of Treg, their successful in vitro propagation, and a better understanding of their mode of action.

Heidelberg, April 2005   Bruno Kyewski and Elisabeth Suri-Payer

List of Contents

Part I. Origin and Generation

Selection of CD4$^+$CD25$^+$ Regulatory T Cells by Self-Peptides 3
C. Cozzo, M. A. Lerman, A. Boesteanu, J. Larkin III, M. S. Jordan,
and A. J. Caton

The Role of TCR Specificity in Naturally Arising
CD25$^+$ CD4$^+$ Regulatory T Cell Biology 25
C.-S. Hsieh and A. Y. Rudensky

Thymic Commitment of Regulatory T Cells Is a Pathway
of TCR-Dependent Selection That Isolates Repertoires
Undergoing Positive or Negative Selection 43
A. Coutinho, I. Caramalho, E. Seixas, and J. Demengeot

Selection and Behavior of CD4$^+$ CD25$^+$ T Cells In Vivo:
Lessons from T Cell Receptor Transgenic Models 73
L. Klein, J. Emmerich, L. d'Cruz, K. Aschenbrenner, and K. Khazaie

Migration Rules: Functional Properties of Naive and Effector/Memory-Like
Regulatory T Cell Subsets 89
J. Huehn, K. Siegmund, and A. Hamann

Peripheral Generation and Function of CD4$^+$CD25$^+$ Regulatory T Cells 115
L. S. Taams and A. N. Akbar

Dendritic Cells: Key Cells for the Induction of Regulatory T Cells? 133
K. Mahnke and A. H. Enk

Part II. Involvement of Disease Models

Autoimmune Gastritis Is a Well-Defined Autoimmune Disease Model
for the Study of $CD4^+CD25^+$ T Cell-Mediated Suppression 153
R. S. McHugh

Regulatory T Cells in Experimental Colitis 179
M. Gad

Autoimmune Ovarian Disease in Day 3-Thymectomized Mice:
The Neonatal Time Window, Antigen Specificity of Disease Suppression,
and Genetic Control 209
K. S. K. Tung, Y. Y. Setiady, E. T. Samy, J. Lewis, and C. Teuscher

Regulatory T Cells in Transplantation Tolerance 249
H. Waldmann, L. Graca, E. Adams, P. Fairchild, and S. Cobbold

$CD4^+CD25^+$ Regulatory T Cells in Hematopoietic Stem Cell Transplantation . . . 265
P. Hoffmann, J. Ermann, and M. Edinger

Naturally Arising $CD25^+CD4^+$ Regulatory T Cells in Tumor Immunity 287
T. Nomura and S. Sakaguchi

Phenotypic and Functional Differences
Between Human $CD4^+CD25^+$ and Type 1 Regulatory T Cells 303
M. K. Levings and M. G. Roncarolo

Subject Index 327

List of Contributors

(Addresses stated at the beginning of respective chapters)

Adams, E.   249
Akbar, A. N.   115
Aschenbrenner, K.   73

Boesteanu, A.   3

Caramalho, I.   43
Caton, A. J.   3
Cobbold, S.   249
Coutinho, A.   43
Cozzo, C.   3

d'Cruz, L.   73
Demengeot, J.   43

Edinger, M.   265
Emmerich, J.   73
Enk, A. H.   133
Ermann, J.   265

Fairchild, P.   249

Gad, M.   179
Graca, L.   249

Hamann, A.   89
Hoffmann, P.   265
Hsieh, C.-S.   25
Huehn, J.   89

Jordan, M. S.   3

Khazaie, K.   73
Klein, L.   73

Larkin III, J.   3
Lerman, M. A.   3
Levings, M. K.   303
Lewis, J.   209

Mahnke, K.   133
McHugh, R. S.   153

Nomura, T.   287

Roncarolo, M. G.   303
Rudensky, A. Y.   25

Sakaguchi, S.   287
Samy, E. T.   209
Seixas, E.   43
Setiady, Y. Y.   209
Siegmund, K.   89

Taams, L. S.   115
Teuscher, C.   209
Tung, K. S. K.   209

Waldmann, H.   249

Part I
Origin and Generation

Grids and Datafication

Selection of CD4⁺CD25⁺ Regulatory T Cells by Self-Peptides

C. Cozzo[1] · M. A. Lerman[1] · A. Boesteanu[1] · J. Larkin III[1] · M. S. Jordan[2] · A. J. Caton[1] (✉)

[1]The Wistar Institute, 3601 Spruce Street, Philadelphia, PA 19104, USA
caton@wistar.upenn.edu

[2]Signal Transduction Laboratory, Abrahamson Family Cancer Research Institute, University of Pennsylvania, Philadelphia, PA 19104, USA

1	Introduction	4
2	**CD4⁺CD25⁺ Regulatory T Cell Selection in the Thymus**	4
2.1	CD4⁺CD25⁺ Regulatory T Cells Develop Intrathymically	5
2.2	Self-Peptides Can Direct CD4⁺CD25⁺ Thymocyte Selection	6
2.3	Thymocytes Can Undergo Both Deletion and CD4⁺CD25⁺ Regulatory T Cell Selection in Response to an Agonist Peptide	8
2.4	Role of TCR Specificity in Thymic CD4⁺CD25⁺ Regulatory T Cell Selection	10
2.5	Role of Thymic Epithelium in CD4⁺CD25⁺ Regulatory T Cell Selection	11
3	**Role of the Periphery in CD4⁺CD25⁺ Regulatory T Cell Repertoire Formation**	12
3.1	Self-Peptides Drive CD4⁺CD25⁺ Regulatory T Cell Expansion in the Periphery	13
3.2	CD4⁺CD25⁺ Regulatory T Cell Accumulation and Survival	15
3.3	Peripheral Generation of CD4⁺CD25⁺ Regulatory T Cells	16
4	**Conclusions and Future Directions**	17
	References	19

Abstract Regulatory T cells have been shown to prevent the development of autoimmune disease, and can modulate immune responses during infections or following tissue transplantation. Recently, the processes by which CD4⁺CD25⁺ regulatory T cells are produced during immune repertoire formation have begun to be elucidated. This review focuses on the role of self-peptides in mediating CD4⁺CD25⁺ regulatory T cell selection in the thymus. How self-peptides continue to have an important influence on the accumulation of CD4⁺CD25⁺ regulatory T cells in the periphery is also discussed.

1
Introduction

A singular characteristic of the immune system is its ability to identify and eradicate a multitude of pathogens, while at the same time existing in and remaining tolerant of an environment that possesses a comparable diversity of self-antigens. The healthy organism will maintain this characteristic, or will otherwise become susceptible to infection or autoimmunity. For cells of the adaptive immune system, the capacity to distinguish between self and foreign antigens is acquired during B and T lymphocyte development and maintained in the periphery. Autoreactive T and B cells can undergo deletion if they encounter their antigen during development (Sprent and Kishimoto 2002; Starr et al. 2003). Yet there is evidence that potentially self-reactive clones of T and B cells are present in healthy, non-autoimmune individuals (Wekerle et al. 1996). Thus, the immune system has developed additional mechanisms to establish self-tolerance. One of these is the production of regulatory cells, which can suppress the activity of potentially autoreactive cells (Shevach 2000).

Although several types of regulatory cells are likely to exist, a well-characterized population comprises approximately 5%–10% of the peripheral CD4$^+$ T cell repertoire in mice and humans and is identified by the constitutive expression of the IL-2Rα chain (CD25) (Maloy and Powrie 2001; Shevach 2000). CD4$^+$CD25$^+$ regulatory T cells have been shown to prevent the development of several autoimmune diseases, and can also modulate immune responses to infections and in transplantation settings (Maloy and Powrie 2001; Sakaguchi 2004). CD4$^+$CD25$^+$ regulatory T cells are hypoproliferative in response to TCR stimulation in vitro; however, once stimulated via the TCR, they can suppress the function of responder cells (Piccirillo and Shevach 2001; Takahashi et al. 1998; Thornton and Shevach 1998). This review will describe studies aimed at determining how CD4$^+$CD25$^+$ regulatory T cells are generated during CD4$^+$ T cell repertoire formation in the thymus based on their interactions with self-peptides. How ongoing interactions with self-peptides in the periphery contribute to the development of a repertoire that effectively prevents autoimmune disease, while not compromising the ability to respond to infectious agents, will also be described.

2
CD4$^+$CD25$^+$ Regulatory T Cell Selection in the Thymus

T cell development begins in the thymus, where developing thymocytes rearrange their TCR genes. Positive selection rescues thymocytes from programmed cell death based on the ability of the TCR to react with host MHC molecules, which are mostly occupied by self-peptides (Starr et al. 2003). This ensures that only thymocytes expressing TCRs that have the capacity to recognize the host's MHC molecules when they are displaying foreign peptides will be exported to the periphery. However, since an additional outcome of gene rearrangement is the production of autoreactive TCRs, thymocytes must also survive negative selection. Negative selection can eliminate or functionally inactivate those thymocytes with autoreactive TCR specificities, and, like positive selection, must also be guided by the reactivity of TCRs toward MHC molecules expressing self-peptides (Sprent and Kishimoto 2002). How do interactions between the TCR of developing thymocytes and the repertoire of self-peptides that are presented by MHC molecules influence positive and/or negative selection? Perhaps the most popular model is one in which the probability of selection is based on the strength of the signal received through the TCR; thymocytes survive to maturity if they receive a signal that is strong enough to indicate MHC restriction, yet weak enough to ensure non-self-specificity. This avidity model proposes that a window of signal strength from peptide:MHC-TCR interactions exists in which DP thymocytes must fall in order to be positively selected and avoid negative selection (Sprent and Kishimoto 2002; Starr et al. 2003). However, it is also possible that different thymic cell types may specialize in promoting these different outcomes; for example, cortical epithelium appears to be efficient at inducing positive selection (Laufer et al. 1999; Lo and Sprent 1986; Vukmanovic et al. 1992). More recently, the formation of CD4$^+$CD25$^+$ regulatory T cells has been found to represent another thymic selection event that is based on the reactivity that thymocytes exhibit toward self-peptides presented by MHC molecules (Jordan et al. 2001), although the cues that cause these processes to differ from positive or negative selection remain to be defined.

2.1
CD4$^+$CD25$^+$ Regulatory T Cells Develop Intrathymically

Early studies showing that CD4$^+$CD25$^+$ T cells possess important regulatory activities pointed to thymic processes in their formation. In these studies, thymectomy of 3-day-old neonatal mice (d3Tx) led to the development of organ-specific autoimmune diseases unless mice were given unfractionated CD4$^+$ T cells, or just the CD4$^+$CD25$^+$ subset of T cells, within 2 weeks of thymectomy (Shevach 2000). Sakaguchi's group went on to show that approximately 3%–5% of CD4SP thymocytes also express CD25, and that these CD4SP CD25$^+$ thymocytes are as suppressive as peripheral CD4$^+$CD25$^+$ regulatory T cells in in vitro suppression assays (Itoh et al. 1999). Furthermore, 1 week after Thy1.2 CD4CD8 DP BALB/c thymocytes were injected intrathymically into Thy1.1 BALB/c recipients, a significant fraction of CD4SP CD25$^+$ cells were Thy1.2$^+$, providing evidence that CD4$^+$CD25$^+$ T cells could develop intrathymically from CD4CD8 DP thymocytes (Itoh et al. 1999). CD4$^+$CD25$^+$ cells are also present in the thymus when no CD4$^+$ T cells are detectable in the spleen, and BrdU-labeling studies showed that CD4$^+$CD25$^+$ thymocytes acquire label before CD4$^+$ T cells in the periphery (Asano et al. 1996; Jordan et al. 2001). Collectively, these studies indicated that CD4$^+$CD25$^+$ regulatory T cells could be formed intrathymically, diminishing the possibility that the detection of CD4$^+$CD25$^+$ thymocytes was due to the formation of these cells in the periphery and their subsequent recirculation to the thymus.

2.2
Self-Peptides Can Direct CD4$^+$CD25$^+$ Thymocyte Selection

Studies aimed at defining how TCR specificity guides T cell development in many cases rely on the use of TCR transgenic mice. TCR transgenic mice were used to develop the avidity model of thymocyte development, for example, and have the practical advantage of simplifying the enormously diverse repertoire of TCRs that would otherwise be expressed by thymocytes and mature T cells. Of course, this approach has limitations; it creates mice containing unusually high proportions of T cells with a particular specificity, and the TCR transgenes may be expressed at unusual stages of thymocyte development that may affect selection events. In addition, co-expression of endogenous non-transgene-encoded TCRs (particularly TCR α-chains, which are not subjected to efficient allelic exclusion even in non-transgenic T cells (Heath and Miller 1993; Heath et al. 1995; Zal et al. 1996)) can exert a significant impact on the specificity of the T cells under study.

Indeed, early clues that regulatory T cells were important in preventing autoimmune disease came in studies in which mice expressing an encephalatogenic CD4$^+$ TCR as a transgene were protected against the development of autoimmune encephalitis when maintained on a background that permitted endogenous TCR gene rearrangement (termed T/R$^+$ mice). However, T/R$^-$ mice (generated by mating with RAG–/– mice to ensure exclusive expression of the transgenic TCR) developed severe encephalitis (Olivares-Villagomez et al. 1998; Van de Keere and Tonegawa 1998). Transfer of unfractionated CD4$^+$ T cells from non-transgenic mice into T/R$^-$ mice was sufficient to prevent disease, and an interpretation of these data was that CD4$^+$ regulatory T cells were playing a role in disease prevention (Olivares-Villagomez et al. 1998; Van de Keere and Tonegawa 1998). Subsequent studies showed that in T/R$^+$ mice, CD4$^+$CD25$^+$ regulatory T cells only develop among T cells that co-express endogenous TCR chains in addition to the transgenic TCR; CD4$^+$CD25$^+$ regulatory T cells do not develop in RAG-deficient T/R$^-$ mice (which could not express endogenous TCR chains) (Hori et al. 2002).

In this model, restricting CD4$^+$ T cells to expression of the transgenic TCR prevented the formation of an effective regulatory T cell repertoire, and allowed CD4$^+$ T cells expressing the transgenic TCR to induce disease. Indeed, the development of CD4$^+$CD25$^+$ regulatory T cells depended on the co-expression of endogenous TCR chains, and the transgenic TCR appeared incapable of undergoing CD4$^+$CD25$^+$ T cell selection. These studies suggested that TCR specificity could play a role in directing CD4$^+$CD25$^+$ regulatory T cell formation, although the exact mechanism was not discernable.

We developed a transgenic mouse system in which specific interactions between a TCR and a single self-peptide could be shown to provide the basis for CD4$^+$CD25$^+$ regulatory T cell selection. TS1 mice express a transgenic TCR from a CD4$^+$ T cell clone that had been isolated from an influenza virus PR8-infected BALB/c mouse. The TS1 TCR recognizes the S1 determinant of the PR8 hemagglutinin (HA) presented in the context of the MHCII I-E^d, and can be detected with the anti-clonotypic monoclonal antibody 6.5 (Kirberg et al. 1994). The 6.5$^+$CD4$^+$ T cells that develop in TS1 mice are largely CD25$^-$ T cells; however, approximately 5%–10% are CD25$^+$ regulatory T cells (Jordan et al. 2000, 2001; Thornton and Shevach 2000). In contrast, 6.5$^+$CD4$^+$CD25$^+$ T cells are undetectable in TS1.RAG$^{-/-}$ mice (which are incapable of endogenous TCR gene rearrangement) (Jordan et al. 2001). Thus, as was observed in T/R$^+$ mice, the development of CD4$^+$CD25$^+$ regulatory T cells in TS1 mice depends on the expression of endogenous TCR α-chains.

However, a crucial observation was made when TS1 mice were mated with HA28 mice, which express HA as a neo-self-antigen under the control of the SV40 early region promoter/enhancer. In TS1xHA28 mice, 6.5$^+$CD4$^+$ T cells develop in similar numbers to TS1 mice (that lack the HA transgene), but in TS1xHA28 mice approximately half of these 6.5$^+$CD4$^+$ T cells are CD25$^+$ regulatory T cells (Jordan et al. 2000; Jordan et al. 2001). These studies showed that interactions with a single self-peptide (S1) induced thymocytes expressing the 6.5 TCR to undergo selection to become CD4$^+$CD25$^+$ regulatory T cells. Moreover, when TS1.RAG$^{-/-}$ bone marrow, which could not rearrange endogenous TCR genes, was given to HA28 recipients, 6.5$^+$CD4$^+$CD25$^+$ regulatory T cells developed as efficiently as in TS1xHA28 mice (Jordan et al. 2001). Thus, thymocytes that can only express the 6.5 TCR cannot undergo CD4$^+$CD25$^+$ T cell selection in response to the self-peptides that are presented by thymic MHC molecules in TS1 mice. However, they do so abundantly when a single additional peptide (S1) is presented in the diverse milieu of self-peptides in TS1xHA28 mice.

Similar processes guiding CD4$^+$CD25$^+$ regulatory T cell development have also been described using another transgenic system. In DO11.10 TCR transgenic mice, a small fraction (5%–10%) of the CD4$^+$ T cells expressing the clonotypic KJ-126 TCR are CD25$^+$ regulatory T cells when the mice are on a RAG-sufficient background, but KJ-126$^+$CD4$^+$CD25$^+$ T cells are undetectable in DO11.10 RAG$^{-/-}$ mice (Itoh et al. 1999). As was observed in TS1 (and T/R$^+$) mice, the KJ-126 TCR lacks a ligand in BALB/c mice that can induce selection of CD4$^+$CD25$^+$ regulatory T cells; the CD4$^+$CD25$^+$ regulatory T cell selection that occurs in a RAG-sufficient background is most likely mediated by endogenous TCR chains interacting with self-peptide:MHC complexes (Itoh et al. 1999; Suto et al. 2002). However, when DO11.1 TCR transgenic mice were mated with mice expressing ovalbumin either as a nuclear antigen or under the control of a rat insulin promoter, KJ-126$^+$CD4$^+$CD25$^+$ regulatory T cells were formed in increased numbers compared to DO11.10 mice (Kawahata et al. 2002; Walker et al. 2003). KJ-126$^+$CD4$^+$CD25$^+$ regulatory T cells were also formed in mice lacking RAG expression and co-expressing the OVA peptide, again showing that introduction of a single peptide into the milieu of thymic self-peptides can provide a ligand that promotes CD4$^+$CD25$^+$ regulatory T cell formation (in this case of the KJ-126 TCR) (Kawahata et al. 2002; Walker et al. 2003). It seems likely, based on these transgenic models, that CD4$^+$CD25$^+$ regulatory T cell formation in non-transgenic mice (and humans) similarly involves thymic selection events driven by TCR recognition of self-peptide:MHC complexes.

2.3
Thymocytes Can Undergo Both Deletion and CD4$^+$CD25$^+$ Regulatory T Cell Selection in Response to an Agonist Peptide

One of the most prominent features of the findings in TS1xHA28 mice was the high frequency of 6.5$^+$CD4$^+$ T cells (both CD25$^+$ and CD25$^-$) that were present. Indeed, 6.5$^+$CD4$^+$ T cells were as abundant in the LNs and spleens of TS1xHA28 mice as they were in TS1 mice (that lack S1 peptide); however, in TS1xHA28 mice, approximately half of the 6.5$^+$CD4$^+$ T cells were CD25$^+$ (Jordan et al. 2000). The minimal deletion of 6.5$^+$CD4$^+$ T cells in TS1xHA28 mice was also in sharp contrast to findings in other lineages of mice we had examined (termed TS1xHA12 and TS1xHA104), in which HA expression is also driven by the SV40 early region promoter/enhancer (Riley et al. 2000). Thymocytes expressing the 6.5 TCR are subject to much more extensive deletion in TS1xHA12 and TS1xHA104 mice than in TS1xHA28 mice (Jordan et al. 2001; Riley et al. 2000). The findings in these lineages showed that thymocytes bearing TCRs with identical specificities for a self-peptide could undergo either overt deletion or abundant CD4⁺CD25⁺ regulatory T cell formation as processes of tolerance induction. Moreover, differences in the expression of S1 peptide between these lineages (induced by differences in their transgene integration sites) must play a decisive role in directing these different outcomes, since the same TCR could be subjected to these differing fates.

To extend these findings, we have generated additional lineages of HA transgenic mice, in part to better understand the relationship between CD4⁺CD25⁺ regulatory T selection and deletion of autoreactive thymocytes. We were also interested in determining how idiosyncratic TS1xHA28 mice might be, and whether the development of such large numbers of 6.5⁺CD4⁺CD25⁺ T cells might be dependent on some aspect of the presentation of the S1 peptide that could be unique to this lineage. We used the β-globin locus control region to target transgene expression to erythroid lineage cells in PevHA mice (Antoniou and Grosveld 1990; Yeoman and Mellor 1992), and the β-myosin heavy chain promoter to target HA expression to cardiac and skeletal muscle in β-myoHA mice (Rindt et al. 1993). We found that HA mRNA could be detected in the thymus of each lineage; similar findings have been made with other transgenic mice, using ostensibly tissue-specific promoters, that promiscuous expression by thymic epithelial cells may make a significant contribution to establishing CD4⁺ T cell tolerance to tissue-specific self-antigens (Derbinski et al. 2001; Klein et al. 1998).

There was a striking similarity in 6.5⁺CD4⁺ T cell development between TS1xHA28 and TS1xPevHA mice. Similar total numbers of 6.5⁺ CD4SP thymocytes and 6.5⁺CD4⁺ LN cells are generated in each lineage, and among these the percentages that were CD25⁺ were also very similar (Lerman et al. 2004). Smaller percentages of CD4SP and CD4⁺ cells were 6.5⁺ in TS1xβ-myoHA mice than in TS1xHA28 and TS1xPevHA mice, indicating that more extensive deletion of 6.5⁺ cells occurs. Nevertheless, large fractions of the 6.5⁺CD4SP thymocytes and 6.5⁺CD4⁺ T cells in TS1xβ-myoHA mice were CD25⁺ regulatory cells, as is the case in TS1xHA28 and TS1xPevHA mice (Lerman et al. 2004). Similar studies have been carried out in mice expressing HA under the control of an Igκ promoter; in this case too, substantially fewer 6.5⁺CD4⁺CD25⁺ T cells were present in the periphery than in TS1xHA28 mice, although they again existed as mixtures of CD25⁺ and CD25⁻ T cells (Apostolou et al. 2002). These studies show that the 6.5 TCR can be subjected to substantial deletion by the S1 peptide; however, even under these conditions of extreme deletion some CD4⁺CD25⁺ regulatory T cell formation can occur. However, in other cases, the peptide is presented in a way that imposes much less deletion; instead, it induces the selection of the 6.5 TCR into CD4⁺CD25⁺

regulatory T cells at frequencies near those directing positive selection of the 6.5 TCR into the CD4$^+$ T cell repertoire of BALB/c mice.

2.4
Role of TCR Specificity in Thymic CD4$^+$CD25$^+$ Regulatory T Cell Selection

These studies using TCR transgenic mice have provided evidence that the generation of CD4$^+$CD25$^+$ T cells can occur through a thymic selection process that has characteristics of positive selection (e.g., upregulation of CD69 and CD5 among 6.5$^+$ DP thymocytes [Azzam et al. 1998; Dutz et al. 1995; Jordan et al. 2001; Merkenschlager et al. 1997]). However, CD4$^+$CD25$^+$ regulatory T cell selection is different from conventional positive selection in that it is associated with increased CD25 expression and the acquisition of unique phenotypic and functional characteristics (i.e., regulatory activity). Thymic selection of CD4$^+$CD25$^+$ regulatory T cells also appears to differ from positive selection with respect to the specificity requirements for recognition of self-peptide(s). An elegant series of studies compared the peptides that could promote the positive selection of thymocytes expressing a MHC class I-restricted TCR in FTOC with the agonist peptide that was known to promote full activation of mature CD8$^+$ T cells expressing this TCR (Ashton-Rickardt et al. 1994; Hogquist et al. 1994; Sebzda et al. 1994). Peptides bearing minimal sequence identity with and reactivity relative to the agonist peptide could promote positive selection of the transgenic TCR (Hogquist et al. 1994, 1997). Positive selection appears then to be based on low-level reactivity with self-peptides that are presented by thymic MHC molecules. By contrast, the studies in both the HA and OVA systems showed that introducing a peptide that is a known agonist for the transgenic TCR could promote thymic CD4$^+$CD25$^+$ regulatory T cell selection, and as outlined above, the endogenous pool of self-peptides is incapable of promoting this selection.

To begin to examine the specificity with which thymocytes and CD4$^+$ T cells must react with self-peptides to undergo CD4$^+$CD25$^+$ regulatory T cell selection, we generated an additional TCR transgenic mouse, termed TS1(SW), using TCR genes from a CD4$^+$ T cell hybridoma that recognizes a homologue of the S1 peptide, termed S1(SW), which differs from the S1 determinant by two amino acid substitutions. The TS1(SW) TCR is roughly 100-fold less reactive toward the S1 peptide than is the 6.5 TCR (Jordan et al. 2001). CD4$^+$CD25$^+$ T cells expressing the TS1(SW) TCR were no more abundant in TS1(SW)xHA28 mice than in TS1(SW) mice, unlike the findings in TS1xHA28 mice where 6.5$^+$CD4$^+$CD25$^+$ T cells were increased relative to 6.5$^+$CD4$^+$CD25$^+$ T cells in TS1 mice. In addition, TS1(SW) mice were mated with the HA12 and HA104 lineages, which induce overt deletion of the 6.5 TCR, as well as with an additional lineage (termed HACII mice), which expresses PR8 HA under control of a MHC class II-promoter and induces extreme deletion of 6.5^+ thymocytes. Although the TS1(SW) TCR could undergo deletion in response to the S1 peptide (particularly in TS1(SW)xHACII mice), in none of the mice did it undergo increased selection to become $CD25^+$ (Jordan et al. 2001). These findings provide evidence that $CD4^+CD25^+$ regulatory T cell selection may require a high intrinsic affinity of an autoreactive TCR for a selecting peptide, although it remains possible that some unknown properties of the TS1(SW) TCR contribute to an inability to undergo $CD4^+CD25^+$ selection. This issue can be examined more closely by generating additional transgenic mouse lineages that express the S1(SW) peptide and by determining whether S1(SW) expression induces the TS1(SW) TCR to undergo $CD4^+CD25^+$ regulatory T cell selection. The evidence to date suggests that the thymic selection of $CD4^+CD25^+$ regulatory T cells is exquisitely sensitive to, and dependent upon, interactions between thymocytes and individual self-peptides against which the TCR is highly reactive.

2.5
Role of Thymic Epithelium in $CD4^+CD25^+$ Regulatory T Cell Selection

The production of regulatory T cells by thymic epithelium was first suggested by studies in which allogeneic thymic epithelium from strain A mice was engrafted into athymic strain B mice. Low numbers of $CD4^+$ cells from these engrafted animals would induce autoimmune disease when transferred into additional athymic strain A mice, but this did not occur when larger numbers of cells were transferred (Modigliani et al. 1996). These results were interpreted to indicate that thymic epithelium normally generates mixed populations of autoreactive and regulatory T cells with overlapping specificities, and that insufficient regulatory T cells had been introduced to prevent autoimmunity when low doses of cells were transferred. In bone marrow chimera studies, $6.5^+CD4^+CD25^+$ regulatory T cells only developed when HA was expressed on radioresistant cell types, and in this setting $6.5^+CD4^+CD25^+$ T cell selection closely resembled that of intact TS1xHA28, TS1xPevHA, and TS1xβ-myoHA mice (Jordan et al. 2001; Lerman et al. 2004). Radioresistant thymic epithelial cells (TECs) were also shown to direct $6.5^+CD4^+CD25^+$ regulatory T cell selection in Igκ-HA mice (Apostolou et al. 2002). Moreover, in a different system, $CD4^+CD25^+$ regulatory T cells were able to develop in transgenic mice in which expression of MHCII is largely restricted to cortical TEC (cTEC) (Bensinger et al. 2001).

Work from several groups has demonstrated that TECs express mRNA transcripts for proteins that are otherwise generally restricted to differentiated peripheral tissues (Anderson et al. 2002; Derbinski et al. 2001). More recently, the transcription factor AIRE was found to direct expression of mRNA transcripts of "peripheral" antigens in thymic epithelial cells (principally medullary TECs [mTECs]) (Anderson et al. 2002; Liston et al. 2003). However, it appears that disruption of the AIRE gene may affect deletion of autoreactive thymocytes to a greater degree than it affects $CD4^+CD25^+$ regulatory T cell formation (Anderson et al. 2002; Liston et al. 2003). Nevertheless, "promiscuous" expression of peripheral antigens, perhaps selectively by cTECs and perhaps under the control of some other as yet unidentified transcription factor, may play an important role in directing formation of $CD4^+CD25^+$ regulatory T cells for tissue-specific antigens. In this respect, however, it is worth noting that the studies in T/R^+ and T/R^- mice suggest that peptides from some tissue-specific antigens might not be expressed in the thymus in a way that can induce either $CD4^+CD25^+$ regulatory T cell formation or substantial deletion of an encephalotogenic TCR. Yet, encephalotogenic T cell activity can nonetheless be prevented by $CD4^+CD25^+$ regulatory T cells either with distinct TCRs specific for the same self-peptide, or that more likely underwent selection in response to different self-peptides.

3
Role of the Periphery in $CD4^+CD25^+$ Regulatory T Cell Repertoire Formation

Although thymic development plays a major role, peripheral processes also significantly influence the composition of the $CD4^+$ T cell repertoire. Homeostatic mechanisms that affect lifespan and proliferation control the size and composition of the $CD4^+$ T cell compartment and are mediated by cytokine and TCR signals (Jameson 2002). Cytokines (particularly IL-7) are important in promoting the proliferation and survival of naïve $CD4^+$ T cells (Fry and Mackall 2001). In addition, TCR-derived signals can induce homeostatic proliferation of naïve $CD4^+$ T cells and may be important for their survival (Jameson 2002). In contrast to cytokine-mediated signals, those that result from $CD4^+$ T cells interacting with MHC may promote expansion or survival based on specificity for self-peptides. When naïve TCR transgenic T cells are adoptively transferred into lymphopenic recipients that do not express their cognate antigen, they can undergo homeostatic division, showing that in a lymphopenic environment they can divide in response to weak interactions with self-peptides:MHC complexes (Ernst et al. 1999; Goldrath and Bevan 1999). Moreover, there is evidence that the peptides mediating positive selection in the thymus can also be responsible for directing the homeostatic proliferation and survival of naïve T cells in the periphery (Ernst et al. 1999; Goldrath and Bevan 1999).

An initial indication that the presence of peripheral self-antigen may be required for the sustained persistence of CD4$^+$ regulatory T cells came from work done by Seddon and Mason (Seddon and Mason 1999). In this study, CD4SP thymocytes from athyroid rats did not induce thyroiditis upon transfer into thyroid-bearing recipients, whereas the peripheral CD4$^+$ T cells could induce thyroiditis while remaining protective against diabetes. The interpretation of these data was that thyroid tissue-specific regulatory cells could develop in the thymus of athyroid rats, but in order for those cells to persist in the periphery, the tissue expressing their self-antigen (the thyroid) had to be present. Similarly, studies using mice in which the ovaries had been removed showed that ovary-specific CD4$^+$CD25$^+$ regulatory T cells, which were present in normal mice, were not detectable (Garza et al. 2000; Sakaguchi et al. 1982; Tung et al. 2001). Thus, interactions with peripheral self-antigen appeared to play a critical role in the persistence of CD4$^+$ regulatory T cells, although how tissue-specific regulatory T cells were being maintained was not known.

3.1
Self-Peptides Drive CD4$^+$CD25$^+$ Regulatory T Cell Expansion in the Periphery

Even though a defining characteristic of CD4$^+$CD25$^+$ regulatory T cells is their hyporesponsiveness to TCR stimulation in vitro, adoptive transfer experiments have indicated that these cells can proliferate in vivo (Annacker et al. 2001; Fisson et al. 2003; Gavin et al. 2002; Klein et al. 2003; McHugh and Shevach 2002; Shevach 2000; Walker et al. 2003). Adoptive transfer of polyclonal CD4$^+$CD25$^+$ regulatory T cells into lymphopenic recipients induced several rounds of homeostatic division, and this division was comparable to the extent of CD4$^+$CD25$^-$ T cell division (McHugh and Shevach 2002). In this study, however, the specificity of the transferred CD4$^+$CD25$^+$ regulatory T cells was unknown. Furthermore, when interactions between transferred CD4$^+$CD25$^+$ regulatory T cells and MHCII were eliminated by transfer into MHCII-deficient hosts, homeostatic proliferation was greatly reduced (Gavin et al. 2002). Proliferation of monoclonal CD4$^+$CD25$^+$ regulatory T cells in response to cognate self-antigen has also been demonstrated in both the DO11.10/OVA and 6.5/HA transgenic systems. OVA-specific KJ-126$^+$CD4$^+$CD25$^+$ T cells proliferated when transferred into OVA-expressing recipients, although their proliferation was reduced compared to that of KJ-126$^+$CD4$^+$CD25$^-$ T cells (Walker et al. 2003). Similarly, HA-specific 6.5$^+$CD4$^+$CD25$^+$ regulatory T cells proliferated in response to stimulation when transferred into mice that had been immunized with S1 peptide (Klein et al. 2003). These studies showed that $CD4^+CD25^+$ regulatory T cells have the ability to proliferate in response to TCR stimulation in vivo, although how TCR- versus cytokine-derived signals might each contribute to their peripheral expansion under homeostatic conditions was not clear.

To examine this question we analyzed the ability of purified $CD4^+CD25^+$ regulatory T cells, and of $CD4^+CD25^-$ T cells, from TS1xHA28 mice to proliferate following transfer into HA28 or BALB/c mice that either had or had not been made lymphopenic by irradiation (Cozzo et al. 2003). We found that whereas $6.5^+CD4^+CD25^-$ T cells underwent division in response to lymphopenia in irradiated BALB/c mice, $6.5^+CD4^+CD25^+$ regulatory T cells did not divide under these conditions. Significantly, however, the $6.5^+CD4^+CD25^+$ regulatory T cells underwent division when transferred into HA28 mice, even in the absence of lymphopenia. The $6.5^+CD4^+CD25^-$ T cells also divided when transferred into HA28 mice, and the ability of $6.5^+CD4^+CD25^+$ versus $6.5^+CD4^+CD25^-$ T cells to divide in response to S1 peptide in vivo directly correlated with the differing abilities of these populations to proliferate in response to S1 peptide in vitro. The failure of $6.5^+CD4^+CD25^+$ regulatory T cells to proliferate in response to lymphopenia alone correlated with a reduced level of expression of the high affinity receptor for IL-7 (CD127) relative to conventional $CD4^+$ T cells (Cozzo et al. 2003; Gavin et al. 2002; Walker et al. 2003). Thus, the presence of self-antigen drives the expansion of $CD4^+CD25^+$ regulatory T cells, and signals derived from lymphopenia alone are insufficient to promote this proliferation.

It is interesting that $6.5^+CD4^+CD25^+$ regulatory T cells appear to be exquisitely dependent on the presence of S1 peptide for their proliferation in vivo, even under conditions of lymphopenia. As outlined above, thymic selection of $CD4^+CD25^+$ regulatory T cells appears only to occur in the presence of an agonist peptide for the TCR (that is presented in an amount or cell type that can induce selection), whereas positive selection of conventional $CD4^+$ T cells is promoted by interactions with weakly reactive peptide-MHC complexes. The $6.5^+CD4^+CD25^-$ T cells underwent homeostatic proliferation in mice that lack the S1 peptide (Cozzo et al. 2003), and studies in other systems have indicated that interactions with self-peptide MHC complexes are likely to contribute to this expansion (Ernst et al. 1999; Goldrath and Bevan 1999). In this respect, then, low specificity or degenerate recognition events contribute to both positive selection and homeostatic expansion of conventional $CD4^+$ T cells, whereas both selection and peripheral expansion of $CD4^+CD25^+$ regulatory T cells appear to require highly specific interactions with agonist self-peptides. It will be interesting in future experiments to determine whether lower affinity interactions (such as those that might occur between the TS1(SW) TCR and the S1 peptide) can allow for peripheral expansion of $CD4^+CD25^+$ regulatory T cells, even if they cannot support their thymic selection.

At this stage, the evidence suggests that the expansion of $CD4^+CD25^+$ regulatory T cells in the periphery may be driven by highly specific interactions with peptides that also induced their selection in the thymus. Their differing responsiveness to TCR- vs cytokine-mediated signals provides a mechanism by which the activity and expansion of $CD4^+CD25^+$ T cells specific for tissue-restricted self-antigens may be directed in a manner that promotes tolerance while maintaining immunity. The stringent specificity with which $CD4^+CD25^+$ regulatory T cells must interact with self-peptides during both thymic selection and homeostatic expansion may also play an important role in causing $CD4^+CD25^+$ regulatory T cells to accumulate selectively at sites of antigen expression, even under conditions of lymphopenia.

3.2
$CD4^+CD25^+$ Regulatory T Cell Accumulation and Survival

Studies showing that $CD4^+CD25^+$ regulatory T cells require stimulation with specific peptide:HC complexes to expand in the periphery do not exclude a possible role for cytokine signals in determining their relative survival in the periphery. Little is yet known about the lifespan and turnover of $CD4^+CD25^+$ regulatory T cells compared to that of naïve $CD4^+$ T cells. Signals mediated from IL-2/IL-2R and through CD28/B7 signaling seem to be necessary for the maintenance of $CD4^+CD25^+$ regulatory T cells (Nelson 2004; Salomon et al. 2000; Tang et al. 2003). Still, interactions between the TCR and self-peptide:MHC may also be important for $CD4^+CD25^+$ regulatory T cell survival, as is the case for conventional $CD4^+$ T cells. Transfer into MHCII-deficient recipients inhibited the homeostatic proliferation of $CD4^+CD25^+$ regulatory T cells, but also diminished recovery of these cells (Gavin et al. 2002). An interpretation of these results is that TCR-self-peptide:MHC signals promote $CD4^+CD25^+$ regulatory T cell longevity, although studies addressing the MHC requirement for T cell survival are often complicated by the difficulty in dissecting the contribution of (or lack of) lymphopenia-induced proliferation to the final recovery of cells (Dorfman and Germain 2002). So, given that $CD4^+CD25^+$ regulatory T cells expand in response to and are likely activated by self-antigens, it is likely that contact with cognate self-peptides is important for $CD4^+CD25^+$ regulatory T cell maintenance and survival. But whether this again depends on interactions with a specific peptide–MHC complex, or can be achieved by more degenerate cross-reactive recognition, is not known.

With respect to factors governing their survival in the periphery, it is worth noting that $CD4^+CD25^+$ regulatory T cells express an antigen-experienced phenotype that may affect their expression of survival factors and their lifespan relative to conventional naïve CD4$^+$ T cells (Read et al. 2000; Schluns et al. 2000; Shimizu et al. 2002; Takahashi et al. 2000; Xue et al. 2002). CD4$^+$CD25$^+$ regulatory T cells may, for example, have an enhanced ability to respond to small amounts of a trophic cytokine, IL-2, because their constitutive expression of CD25 permits them to respond to low levels that naïve CD4$^+$CD25$^-$ T cells would not detect. Although both CD4$^+$CD25$^-$ T cells and CD4$^+$CD25$^+$ regulatory T cells proliferate in response to interactions with peripheral peptide, whether these two cell types differ in sensitivity to antigen-induced cell death (AICD) as a consequence of peptide-induced proliferation is unknown. Recovery of transferred polyclonal CD4$^+$CD25$^-$ vs CD4$^+$CD25$^+$ (CD62L^{hi}) regulatory T cells in Thy1.1 congenic recipients demonstrated that although both populations initially increased in number, CD4$^+$CD25$^-$ T cell numbers quickly decreased, whereas numbers of CD4$^+$CD25$^+$(CD62L^{hi}) T cells remained steady for a longer time before decreasing (Fisson et al. 2003). Although the antigen specificity of the CD4$^+$CD25$^+$ regulatory T cells in these studies was not known, these data suggest that CD4$^+$CD25$^+$ regulatory T cells have a lower sensitivity to AICD in response to self-antigen than CD4$^+$CD25$^-$ T cells. In this regard, it is not yet known how the "activated" phenotype expressed by CD4$^+$CD25$^+$ regulatory T cells affects their patterns of recirculation in the lymphoid tissue, and whether the phenotype of these cells is dependent upon on-going interactions with the self-peptide in vivo. Insight into these processes will be important for a full understanding of the role peptide specificity plays in guiding the regional accumulation and activity of CD4$^+$CD25$^+$ regulatory T cells.

3.3
Peripheral Generation of CD4$^+$CD25$^+$ Regulatory T Cells

While there is clear evidence that CD4$^+$CD25$^+$ regulatory T cells are generated in the thymus and appear to be maintained as a distinct lineage, it remains possible that CD4$^+$CD25$^+$ regulatory T cells could be generated in the periphery from mature CD4$^+$CD25$^-$ T cells. In both the OVA and HA systems, the development of clonotype$^+$CD4$^+$CD25$^+$ regulatory T cells in the presence of an agonist peptide is accompanied by the development of an equivalent number of clonotype$^+$CD4$^+$ T cells that are CD25$^-$ (Apostolou et al. 2002; Jordan et al. 2000; Jordan et al. 2001; Lerman 2004; Walker et al. 2003). These clonotype$^+$CD4$^+$CD25$^-$ T cells are potentially autoreactive cells that likely also encounter cognate self-antigen. Therefore, one way to keep these cells from becoming pathogenic in response to antigen re-encounter may be to induce CD4$^+$CD25$^+$ regulatory T cell phenotype and function. Yet whether and how conversion from CD4⁺CD25⁻ T cells to a CD25⁺ regulatory T cell phenotype might take place is not yet understood.

To date, conversion of CD4⁺CD25⁻ T cells into CD4⁺CD25⁺ regulatory T cells has been demonstrated in several systems, both in vivo and in vitro. In one in vitro study, CD4⁺CD25⁺ regulatory T cells were induced from CD4⁺CD25⁻ T cells by combining TCR stimulation with TGF-β treatment (Chen et al. 2003). These TGF-β-induced CD4⁺CD25⁺ regulatory T cells could suppress the development of an induced allergic response. CD4⁺CD25⁺ regulatory T cells could also be induced by alloantigen treatment from a population of polyclonal CD4⁺CD25⁻ T cells in a thymus-independent process (Karim et al. 2004). Antigen-specific CD4⁺CD25⁺ regulatory T cells have been generated from transgenic CD4⁺CD25⁻ T cells via immunization with low doses of antigen, or by orally administered antigen (Thorstenson and Khoruts 2001). In these studies, though, the contribution of recirculation through the thymus to the conversion of CD4⁺CD25⁻ T cells into CD4⁺CD25⁺ regulatory T cells, and the possibility that peptide immunization was expanding rare populations of CD4⁺CD25⁺ regulatory T cells that had been generated intrathymically (perhaps via co-expression of endogenous TCR chains) could not be assessed. Recently, clear evidence emerged that 6.5⁺CD4⁺CD25⁻ T cells could undergo conversion to become CD25⁺ regulatory T cells in the periphery of BALB/c mice into which had been implanted osmotic pumps delivering low doses of S1 peptide (Apostolou and Boehmer 2004). The ability to generate CD4⁺CD25⁺ regulatory T cells with defined specificity in the periphery may have potential therapeutic benefits.

4
Conclusions and Future Directions

This review has described studies aimed at determining how specificity for self-peptides can guide the thymic selection and peripheral expansion of CD4⁺CD25⁺ regulatory T cells. We have presented evidence that both processes are exquisitely sensitive to and dependent on the ability of a TCR undergoing selection to recognize its selecting self-peptide as an agonist ligand. Many questions are raised by these findings and remain to be addressed. What factors determine whether an autoreactive thymocyte undergoes deletion vs CD4⁺CD25⁺ regulatory T cell formation in response to an agonist self-peptide? It is difficult to fit the data outlined here into a simple model in which the avidity with which a TCR reacts with self-peptide:MHC complexes plays a decisive role in directing these outcomes, because thymocytes expressing the 6.5 TCR undergo overt deletion or abundant CD4⁺CD25⁺ regulatory

T cell formation in response to variations in how the S1 peptide is expressed in different lineages. Perhaps expression in different thymic stromal cells (e.g., cTECs vs mTECs) is important, but it may also be that a combination of expression of a self-peptide under conditions of low overall avidity but high specificity, possibly by a particular cell type, provides a signal that promotes $CD4^+CD25^+$ regulatory T cell formation. For example, how might varying signals from peptide:MHC complexes affect the induction of the transcription factor FoxP3 in $CD4^+CD25^+$ regulatory T cell development? As described elsewhere in this volume, expression of FoxP3 is tightly linked with $CD4^+CD25^+$ regulatory T cell formation and activity (Fontenot et al. 2003; Hori et al. 2003; Khattri et al. 2003), and whether particular cues are provided by expression of self-peptides in certain amounts and/or cell types that induce its expression remains to be determined.

Finally, why do $CD4^+CD25^+$ regulatory T cells co-exist with $CD4^+CD25^-$ T cells expressing the same TCR in the transgenic systems that have been studied to date? Even in the context of varying degrees of deletion, $CD4^+CD25^+$ regulatory T cells expressing the transgenic TCR are typically present as mixtures with $CD4^+CD25^-$ T cells. Perhaps stochastic processes governing FoxP3 expression cause a subset of autoreactive thymocytes to develop along the $CD4^+CD25^+$ regulatory T cell pathway, while others do not. But in this model, the selection of $CD4^+CD25^+$ regulatory T cells appears to still depend on the ability of the thymocyte TCR to receive a signal from an agonist peptide ligand, and the processes that protect $CD4^+CD25^-$ thymocytes expressing the same TCR from deletion in these settings are not obvious. An intriguing possibility is that the thymus typically exports mixtures of clonally related $CD4^+CD25^+$ and $CD4^+CD25^-$ T cells; it is clear from the autoimmune diseases that can develop under conditions when $CD4^+CD25^+$ regulatory T cell are selectively eliminated that $CD4^+CD25^-$ T cells with the potential to exert pathologic autoreactivity exist in the normal immune repertoire, and that they can appear to react with the same target organs. The studies to date in TCR transgenic mice raise the notion that these autoreactive and regulatory T cells could possess identical specificities, even if this is difficult to understand on theoretical grounds. A future challenge will be to test these hypotheses in additional transgenic and non-transgenic systems, and doing so may aid in the application of regulatory T cells in therapeutic settings.

Acknowledgements This manuscript was supported by grants from the National Institutes of Health, by the Lupus Foundation of Southeastern Pennsylvania, and by the Commonwealth Universal Research Enhancement Program, Pennsylvania Department of Health.

References

Anderson MS, Venanzi ES, Klein L, Chen Z, Berzins SP, Turley SJ, von Boehmer H, Bronson R, Dierich A, Benoist C, Mathis D (2002) Projection of an immunological self shadow within the thymus by the aire protein. Science 298:1395–1401

Annacker O, Pimenta-Araujo R, Burlen-Defranoux O, Barbosa TC, Cumano A, Bandeira A (2001) CD25+ CD4+ T cells regulate the expansion of peripheral CD4 T cells through the production of IL-10. J Immunol 166:3008–3018

Antoniou M, Grosveld F (1990) Beta-globin dominant control region interacts differently with distal and proximal promoter elements. Genes Dev 4:1007–1013

Apostolou I, Sarukhan A, Klein L, von Boehmer H (2002) Origin of regulatory T cells with known specificity for antigen. Nat Immunol 3:756–763

Apostolou I, Von Boehmer, H (2004) In vivo instruction of suppressor commitment in naive T cells. J Exp Med 199:1401–1408

Asano M, Toda M, Sakaguchi N, Sakaguchi S (1996) Autoimmune disease as a consequence of developmental abnormality of a T cell subpopulation. J Exp Med 184:387–396

Ashton-Rickardt PG, Bandeira A, Delaney JR, Van Kaer L, Pircher HP, Zinkernagel RM, Tonegawa S (1994) Evidence for a differential avidity model of T cell selection in the thymus. Cell 76:651–663

Azzam HS, Grinberg A, Lui K, Shen H, Shores EW, Love PE (1998) CD5 expression is developmentally regulated by T cell receptor (TCR) signals and TCR avidity. J Exp Med 188:2301–2311

Bensinger SJ, Bandeira A, Jordan MS, Caton AJ, Laufer TM (2001) Major histocompatibility complex class II-positive cortical epithelium mediates the selection of CD4(+)25(+) immunoregulatory T cells. J Exp Med 194:427–438

Chen W, Jin W, Hardegen N, Lei KJ, Li L, Marinos N, McGrady G, Wahl SM (2003) Conversion of peripheral CD4+CD25- naive T Cells to CD4+CD25+ regulatory T cells by TGF-beta induction of transcription factor Foxp3. J Exp Med 198:1875–1886

Cozzo C, Larkin J, 3rd, Caton AJ (2003) Self-peptides drive the peripheral expansion of CD4+CD25+ regulatory T cells. J Immunol 171:5678–5682

Derbinski J, Schulte A, Kyewski B, Klein L (2001) Promiscuous gene expression in medullary thymic epithelial cells mirrors the peripheral self. Nat Immunol 2:1032–1039

Dorfman JR, Germain RN (2002) MHC-dependent survival of naive T cells? A complicated answer to a simple question. Microbes Infect 4:547–554

Dutz JP, Ong CJ, Marth J, Teh HS (1995) Distinct differentiative stages of CD4+CD8+ thymocyte development defined by the lack of coreceptor binding in positive selection. J Immunol 154:2588–2599

Ernst B, Lee DS, Chang JM, Sprent J, Surh CD (1999) The peptide ligands mediating positive selection in the thymus control T cell survival and homeostatic proliferation in the periphery. Immunity 11:173–181

Fisson S, Darrasse-Jeze G, Litvinova E, Septier F, Klatzmann D, Liblau R, Salomon BL (2003) Continuous activation of autoreactive CD4+ CD25+ regulatory T cells in the steady state. J Exp Med 198:737–746

Fontenot JD, Gavin MA, Rudensky AY (2003) Foxp3 programs the development and function of CD4+CD25+ regulatory T cells. Nat Immunol 4:330–336

Fry TJ, Mackall CL (2001) Interleukin-7: master regulator of peripheral T-cell homeostasis? Trends Immunol 22:564–571

Garza KM, Agersborg SS, Baker E, Tung KS (2000) Persistence of physiological self antigen is required for the regulation of self tolerance. J Immunol 164:3982–3989

Gavin MA, Clarke SR, Negrou E, Gallegos A, Rudensky A (2002) Homeostasis and anergy of CD4(+)CD25(+) suppressor T cells in vivo. Nat Immunol 3:33–41

Goldrath AW, Bevan MJ (1999) Low-affinity ligands for the TCR drive proliferation of mature CD8+ T cells in lymphopenic hosts. Immunity 11:183–190

Heath WR, Miller JF (1993) Expression of two alpha chains on the surface of T cells in T cell receptor transgenic mice. J Exp Med 178:1807–1811

Heath WR, Carbone FR, Bertolino P, Kelly J, Cose S, Miller JF (1995) Expression of two T cell receptor alpha chains on the surface of normal murine T cells. Eur J Immunol 25:1617–1623

Hogquist KA, Jameson SC, Heath WR, Howard JL, Bevan MJ, Carbone FR (1994) T cell receptor antagonist peptides induce positive selection. Cell 76:17–27

Hogquist KA, Tomlinson AJ, Kieper WC, McGargill MA, Hart MC, Naylor S, Jameson SC (1997) Identification of a naturally occurring ligand for thymic positive selection. Immunity 6:389–399

Hori S, Haury M, Coutinho A, Demengeot J (2002) Specificity requirements for selection and effector functions of CD25+4+ regulatory T cells in anti-myelin basic protein T cell receptor transgenic mice. Proc Natl Acad Sci U S A 99:8213–8218

Hori S, Nomura T, Sakaguchi S (2003) Control of regulatory T cell development by the transcription factor Foxp3. Science 299:1057–1061

Itoh M, Takahashi T, Sakaguchi N, Kuniyasu Y, Shimizu J, Otsuka F, Sakaguchi S (1999) Thymus and autoimmunity: production of CD25+CD4+ naturally anergic and suppressive T cells as a key function of the thymus in maintaining immunologic self-tolerance. J Immunol 162:5317–5326

Jameson SC (2002) Maintaining the norm: T-cell homeostasis. Nat Rev Immunol 2:547–556

Jordan MS, Riley MP, von Boehmer H, Caton AJ (2000) Anergy and suppression regulate CD4(+) T cell responses to a self peptide. Eur J Immunol 30:136–144

Jordan MS, Boesteanu A, Reed AJ, Petrone AL, Holenbeck AE, Lerman MA, Naji A, Caton AJ (2001) Thymic selection of CD4+CD25+ regulatory T cells induced by an agonist self-peptide. Nat Immunol 2:301–306

Karim M, Kingsley CI, Bushell AR, Sawitzki BS, Wood KJ () Alloantigen-induced CD25+CD4+ regulatory T cells can develop in vivo from CD25-CD4+ precursors in a thymus-independent process. J Immunol 172:923–928

Kawahata K, Misaki Y, Yamauchi M, Tsunekawa S, Setoguchi K, Miyazaki J, Yamamoto K (2002) Generation of CD4(+)CD25(+) regulatory T cells from autoreactive T cells simultaneously with their negative selection in the thymus and from nonautoreactive T cells by endogenous TCR expression. J Immunol 168:4399–4405

Khattri R, Cox T, Yasayko SA, Ramsdell F (2003) An essential role for Scurfin in CD4+CD25+ T regulatory cells. Nat Immunol 4:337–342

Kirberg J, Baron A, Jakob S, Rolink A, Karjalainen K, von Boehmer H (1994) Thymic selection of CD8+ single positive cells with a class II major histocompatibility complex-restricted receptor. J Exp Med 180:25–34

Klein L, Klein T, Ruther U, Kyewski B (1998) CD4 T cell tolerance to human C-reactive protein, an inducible serum protein, is mediated by medullary thymic epithelium. J Exp Med 188:5–16

Klein L, Khazaie K, von Boehmer H (2003) In vivo dynamics of antigen-specific regulatory T cells not predicted from behavior in vitro. Proc Natl Acad Sci U S A 100:8886–8891

Laufer TM, Glimcher LH, Lo D (1999) Using thymus anatomy to dissect T cell repertoire selection. Semin Immunol 11:65–70

Lerman MA, Larkin J 3rd, Cozzo, C, Jordan, MS, Caton, AJ (2004) CD4+CD25+ regulatory T cell repertoire formation in response to varying expression of a neo-self-antigen. J Immunol 173:236–244

Liston A, Lesage S, Wilson J, Peltonen L, Goodnow CC (2003) Aire regulates negative selection of organ-specific T cells. Nat Immunol 4:350–354

Lo D, Sprent J (1986) Identity of cells that imprint H-2-restricted T-cell specificity in the thymus. Nature 319:672–675

Maloy KJ, Powrie F (2001) Regulatory T cells in the control of immune pathology. Nat Immunol 2:816–822

McHugh RS, Shevach EM (2002) Cutting edge: depletion of CD4+CD25+ regulatory T cells is necessary, but not sufficient, for induction of organ-specific autoimmune disease. J Immunol 168:5979–5983

Merkenschlager M, Graf D, Lovatt M, Bommhardt U, Zamoyska R, Fisher AG (1997) How many thymocytes audition for selection? J Exp Med 186:1149–1158

Modigliani Y, Coutinho A, Pereira P, Le Douarin N, Thomas-Vaslin V, Burlen-Defranoux O, Salaun J, Bandeira A (1996) Establishment of tissue-specific tolerance is driven by regulatory T cells selected by thymic epithelium. Eur J Immunol 26:1807–1815

Nelson BH (2004) IL-2, regulatory T cells, and tolerance. J Immunol 172:3983–3988

Olivares-Villagomez D, Wang Y, Lafaille JJ (1998) Regulatory CD4(+) T cells expressing endogenous T cell receptor chains protect myelin basic protein-specific transgenic mice from spontaneous autoimmune encephalomyelitis. J Exp Med 188:1883–1894

Piccirillo CA, Shevach EM (2001) Cutting edge: control of CD8+ T cell activation by CD4+CD25+ immunoregulatory cells. J Immunol 167:1137–1140

Read S, Malmstrom V, Powrie F (2000) Cytotoxic T lymphocyte-associated antigen 4 plays an essential role in the function of CD25(+)CD4(+) regulatory cells that control intestinal inflammation. J Exp Med 192:295–302

Riley MP, Cerasoli DM, Jordan MS, Petrone AL, Shih FF, Caton AJ (2000) Graded deletion and virus-induced activation of autoreactive CD4+ T cells. J Immunol 165:4870–4876

Rindt H, Gulick J, Knotts S, Neumann J, Robbins J (1993) In vivo analysis of the murine beta-myosin heavy chain gene promoter. J Biol Chem 268:5332–5338

Sakaguchi S (2004) Naturally arising CD4+ regulatory T cells for immunologic self-tolerance and negative control of immune responses. Annu Rev Immunol 22:531–562

Sakaguchi S, Takahashi T, Nishizuka Y (1982) Study on cellular events in post-thymectomy autoimmune oophoritis in mice. II. Requirement of Lyt-1 cells in normal female mice for the prevention of oophoritis. J Exp Med 156:1577–1586

Salomon B, Lenschow DJ, Rhee L, Ashourian N, Singh B, Sharpe A, Bluestone JA (2000) B7/CD28 costimulation is essential for the homeostasis of the CD4+CD25+ immunoregulatory T cells that control autoimmune diabetes. Immunity 12:431–440

Schluns KS, Kieper WC, Jameson SC, Lefrancois L (2000) Interleukin-7 mediates the homeostasis of naive and memory CD8 T cells in vivo. Nat Immunol 1:426–432

Sebzda E, Wallace VA, Mayer J, Yeung RS, Mak TW, Ohashi PS (1994) Positive and negative thymocyte selection induced by different concentrations of a single peptide. Science 263:1615–1618

Seddon B, Mason D (1999) Peripheral autoantigen induces regulatory T cells that prevent autoimmunity. J Exp Med 189:877–882

Shevach EM (2000) Regulatory T cells in autoimmmunity. Annu Rev Immunol 18:423–449

Shimizu J, Yamazaki S, Takahashi T, Ishida Y, Sakaguchi S (2002) Stimulation of CD25(+)CD4(+) regulatory T cells through GITR breaks immunological self-tolerance. Nat Immunol 3:135–142

Sprent J, Kishimoto H (2002) The thymus and negative selection. Immunol Rev 185:126–135

Starr TK, Jameson SC, Hogquist KA (2003) Positive and negative selection of T cells. Annu Rev Immunol 21:139–176

Suto A, Nakajima H, Ikeda K, Kubo S, Nakayama T, Taniguchi M, Saito Y, Iwamoto I (2002) CD4(+)CD25(+) T-cell development is regulated by at least 2 distinct mechanisms. Blood 99:555–560

Takahashi T, Kuniyasu Y, Toda M, Sakaguchi N, Itoh M, Iwata M, Shimizu J, Sakaguchi S (1998) Immunologic self-tolerance maintained by CD25+CD4+ naturally anergic and suppressive T cells: induction of autoimmune disease by breaking their anergic/suppressive state. Int Immunol 10:1969–1980

Takahashi T, Tagami T, Yamazaki S, Uede T, Shimizu J, Sakaguchi N, Mak TW, Sakaguchi S (2000) Immunologic self-tolerance maintained by CD25(+)CD4(+) regulatory T cells constitutively expressing cytotoxic T lymphocyte-associated antigen 4. J Exp Med 192:303–310

Tang Q, Henriksen KJ, Boden EK, Tooley AJ, Ye J, Subudhi SK, Zheng XX, Strom TB, Bluestone JA (2003) Cutting edge: CD28 controls peripheral homeostasis of CD4+CD25+ regulatory T cells. J Immunol 171:3348–3352

Thornton AM, Shevach EM (1998) CD4+CD25+ immunoregulatory T cells suppress polyclonal T cell activation in vitro by inhibiting interleukin 2 production. J Exp Med 188:287–296

Thornton AM, Shevach EM (2000) Suppressor effector function of CD4+CD25+ immunoregulatory T cells is antigen nonspecific. J Immunol 164:183–190

Thorstenson KM, Khoruts A (2001) Generation of anergic and potentially immunoregulatory CD25+CD4 T cells in vivo after induction of peripheral tolerance with intravenous or oral antigen. J Immunol 167:188–195

Tung KS, Agersborg SS, Alard P, Garza KM, Lou YH (2001) Regulatory T-cell, endogenous antigen and neonatal environment in the prevention and induction of autoimmune disease. Immunol Rev 182:135–148

Van de Keere F, Tonegawa S (1998) CD4(+) T cells prevent spontaneous experimental autoimmune encephalomyelitis in anti-myelin basic protein T cell receptor transgenic mice. J Exp Med 188:1875–1882

Vukmanovic S, Grandea AG 3rd, Faas SJ, Knowles BB, Bevan MJ (1992) Positive selection of T-lymphocytes induced by intrathymic injection of a thymic epithelial cell line. Nature 359:729–732

Walker LS, Chodos A, Eggena M, Dooms H, Abbas AK (2003) Antigen-dependent proliferation of CD4+ CD25+ regulatory T cells in vivo. J Exp Med 198:249–258

Wekerle H, Bradl M, Linington C, Kaab G, Kojima K (1996) The shaping of the brain-specific T lymphocyte repertoire in the thymus. Immunol Rev 149:231–243

Xue HH, Kovanen PE, Pise-Masison CA, Berg M, Radovich MF, Brady JN, Leonard WJ (2002) IL-2 negatively regulates IL-7 receptor alpha chain expression in activated T lymphocytes. Proc Natl Acad Sci U S A 99:13759–13764

Yeoman H, Mellor AL (1992) Tolerance and MHC restriction in transgenic mice expressing a MHC class I gene in erythroid cells. Int Immunol 4:59–65

Zal T, Weiss S, Mellor A, Stockinger B (1996) Expression of a second receptor rescues self-specific T cells from thymic deletion and allows activation of autoreactive effector function. Proc Natl Acad Sci U S A 93:9102–9107

The Role of TCR Specificity in Naturally Arising $CD25^+$ $CD4^+$ Regulatory T Cell Biology

C.-S. Hsieh[1] (✉) · A. Y. Rudensky[2]

[1]Department of Medicine, Division of Rheumatology, University of Washington, Seattle, WA 98195, USA
cshsieh@u.washington.edu

[2]Howard Hughes Medical Institute and the Department of Immunology, University of Washington, Seattle, WA 98195, USA

1	Introduction	25
2	The Antigen Specificity of Naturally Arising T_R	26
3	Antigenic Specificity of Induced Regulatory T Cells	28
4	The Paradox of Foreign Antigen Recognition by Regulatory T Cells	30
5	T_R Appear to Have a Diverse TCR Repertoire That Is Different from the $CD25^-$ TCR Repertoire	33
6	A Large Proportion of Peripheral $CD25^+$ TCRs Have Greater Self-Reactivity than $CD25^-$ TCRs	34
7	What Is the Tissue Distribution of T_R Target Self-Antigens?	36
	References	40

Abstract $CD25^+$ $CD4^+$ T cells (T_R) are a naturally arising subset of regulatory T cells important for the preservation of self-tolerance and the prevention of autoimmunity. Although there is substantial data that TCR specificity is important for T_R development and function, relatively little is known about the antigen specificity of naturally arising T_R. Here, we will review the available evidence regarding naturally arising T_R TCR specificity in the context of T_R development, function, and homeostasis.

1
Introduction

A fundamental finding regarding the significance of T cell receptor specificity for the development of $CD25^+$ $CD4^+$ regulatory T cells (T_R) is that T_R are not observed in TCR transgenic mice lacking RAG genes (Hori et al. 2002; Itoh et al. 1999, Olivares-Villagomes et al. 1998). The presence of functional RAG genes does permit the development of $CD25^+$ T_R in TCR transgenic mice, presumably via expression of endogenously rearranged TCR chains. The likely explanation for the lack of $CD25^+$ T cell development in these monoclonal TCR transgenic mice is that the transgenic $CD4^+$ TCRs reported so far most likely originated from $CD25^-$ T cells. This is inferred from the well-known inability of T_R to proliferate or produce IL-2 in response to TCR engagement in vitro (Takahashi et al. 1998; Thornton and Shevach 1998), which would favor the use of TCRs in these transgenic mice from $CD25^-$, and not $CD25^+$, T cells expanded after in vivo immunization and in vitro re-stimulation. Thus, these data demonstrate that a particular TCR specificity is required to facilitate T_R development.

In addition to affecting T_R development, TCR specificity likely controls T_R function. In vitro studies using both polyclonal and TCR transgenic T_R clearly show that activation through the TCR is required for suppression of $CD25^-$ $CD4^+$ T cell proliferation via a contact-dependent mechanism (Takahashi et al. 1998; Thornton and Shevach 1998). Similar in vivo studies have been performed using T_R isolated from TCR transgenic mice (Apostolou et al. 2002; Walker et al. 2003a). In these experimental models, TCR transgenic T_R encounter with its cognate peptide ligand can be conveniently controlled, with the caveat that the transgenic TCR interaction with its cognate peptide may be of higher affinity than those interactions involving naturally arising T_R TCRs. Taken together, these data suggest that T_R may have antigen specificity different from conventional $CD25^-$ T cells, and that this TCR specificity is required for their development and function. In this review, we will discuss the currently available evidence for the antigen specificity of T_R and hypothesize how this specificity may direct T_R development and dictate the activation of T_R to suppress the immune response.

2
The Antigen Specificity of Naturally Arising T_R

The prevailing hypothesis regarding the TCR specificity of naturally arising regulatory T cells is that they recognize self-antigen, and that this interaction is important for T_R development and function to suppress autoimmunity. This model was originally prompted by two studies in the 1990s that indirectly suggested that naturally arising T_R recognize tissue-specific self-antigens. Initial studies by Taguchi and colleagues suggested that the functional maintenance of $CD4^+$ T cells capable of protection against prostatitis or oophoritis required the presence of the corresponding organ, as adoptive transfer of T cells from male mice were more effective at preventing neonatal thymectomy-induced autoimmune prostatitis than oophoritis, and vice versa for T cells from female mice (Taguchi et al. 1994). Studies from Mason's group extended this observation by demonstrating that ablation of the thyroid gland resulted in the selective functional loss of T cells within the $CD4^+$ population capable of preventing radiation-induced autoimmune thyroiditis, but not diabetes (Seddon and Mason 1999). Curiously, thyroid ablation did not result in the loss of protective thymic $CD4^+$ T cells. Although the $CD4^+$ T cell population was not fractionated in these studies to ensure that the suppressing cells were indeed $CD25^+$ T_R, these data support the hypothesis that tissue-specific antigen recognition by T_R is necessary for their survival, development, and/or expansion in the periphery, as the tissue-protective $CD4^+$ T cell population is functionally lost in the absence of the target organs studied.

Studies of TCR transgenic models offer additional support for the hypothesis that T_R may recognize self-antigen. These models rely on the expression of the cognate ligand for the transgenic TCR as a neo-self-antigen driven by another transgene (Jooss et al. 2001; Jordan et al. 2001; Walker et al. 2003a). In one well-characterized model, a high level of peptide expression resulted in the deletion of TCR transgenic T cells, whereas a moderate level resulted in partial deletion, with the development of $CD25^+$ cells resembling T_R in approximately 50% of the remaining cells (Jordan et al. 2001). Thus, these data serve as a direct demonstration that regulatory T cells could develop due to interactions with self-peptide:MHC complexes.

Where does this TCR interaction with antigen occur? Early reports suggested that $CD25^+$ T cells originate in the thymus, as animals thymectomized at day 3 of life develop spontaneous autoimmunity which could be rescued by the adoptive transfer of normal $CD25^+$ regulatory T cells (Sakaguchi et al. 1995). Thus, the development of autoreactive cells relative to T_R is favored under the conditions of early thymectomy, and these observations suggested that the cause of autoimmunity in day 3-thymectomized mice was the insufficient export of T_R from the thymus during the first few days ex utero. Further work directly demonstrated that regulatory T cells are indeed generated in the thymus, and that these thymic $CD25^+$ $CD4^+$ mature cells are capable of suppressor function as revealed by adoptive transfer experiments (Itoh et al. 1999; Seddon and Mason 2000). Consistent with these earlier reports, it was found in one of the TCR transgenic models described above that the expression of cognate peptide by radiation-resistant thymic stromal cells alone was sufficient for the generation of $CD25^+$ TCR transgenic T cells in bone marrow chimera studies (Jordan et al. 2001). Development of $CD25^+$ T cells with suppressor capabilities has also been observed in mice that express class II only on thymic epithelium and not bone marrow-derived cells (Bensinger et al. 2001). Thus, these data form the current paradigm for T_R development, which maintains that T_R develop due to an interaction with self-antigen in the thymus at an avidity range between positive and negative selection (reviewed in Maloy and Powrie 2001).

However, there are some data that suggest that a simple avidity threshold model does not satisfactorily explain T_R development. For example, it has been argued that regulatory T cell development depends on a high affinity interaction between TCR and peptide:MHC class II complexes. This was suggested based on the use of two transgenic TCRs with a 100-fold difference in the sensitivity of the response to the cognate hemagglutinin (HA) peptide as assessed by an in vitro proliferation assay (Jordan et al. 2001). As described above, enhanced $CD25^+$ T_R development was observed in transgenic mice expressing a higher affinity anti-HA TCR. In contrast, increased development of $CD25^+$ T cells was not observed in mice co-expressing a lower-affinity HA-specific transgenic TCR with several transgenic constructs driving varying levels of HA peptide expression, even though mild to marked deletion of T cells expressing this lower-affinity TCR was observed in the double transgenic mice. Although it remains possible that the transgenic mice utilized in this study were unable to express the HA-peptide at levels optimal for development of T_R expressing this lower-affinity TCR, these data do suggest that TCR engagement by a higher-affinity ligand may result in a qualitatively different signal required for regulatory T cell development. Thus, these results question a simple avidity model for T_R development.

Very recently, an alternative view of the role of TCR-ligand interactions in T_R development has been offered by the Mathis and Benoist group (van Santen et al. 2004). Using mice co-expressing a transgenic TCR (tgTCR) and its cognate peptide ligand encoded by a tet-inducible transgene, these investigators observed increasing percentages of $CD25^+$ $tgTCR^+$ T cells in the thymus corresponding to the level of the TCR ligand induced upon doxycycline treatment. However, there was a relatively small increase in the absolute numbers of thymic $CD25^+$ T cells, despite their significantly elevated frequency. This model implies that thymic T_R precursors are relatively insensitive to deletion (Fig. 1), which may be due to previously reported up-regulation of pro-survival factors, e.g., OX40, GITR, TNF-RII (Gavin et al. 2002; McHugh et al. 2002), and that the development of regulatory T cells is not instructed by TCR signals, but is determined either stochastically or influenced by non-TCR signals. Nevertheless, the existing data supporting this alternative stochastic-selective model of T_R development, in our opinion, do not dispute an essential role for TCR signaling in T_R development and cannot definitively rule out the original instructive model.

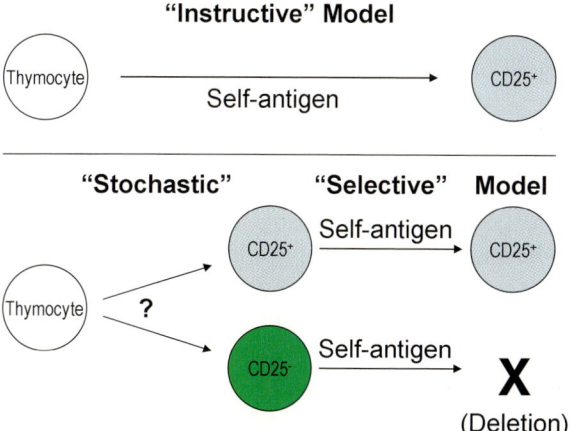

Fig. 1 Models for the role of TCR signals in regulatory T cell development in the thymus. The "instructive" model (*top*) suggests that regulatory T cell development results from specific TCR signals due to encounter with self ligands, whereas the "stochastic selective" model argues that regulatory T cell precursors develop due to stochastic expression of non-TCR signals, or factors such as Foxp3, affecting regulatory T cell commitment. Engagement of TCR by high-affinity ligands would result in a selective increase in the frequency of regulatory versus non-regulatory T cells of the same specificity due to preferential deletion of non-regulatory T cells upon encounter with self-ligands. Regulatory T cells would be relatively resistant to deletion in this model. However, a hybrid model based on "instructive" TCR signals for recruitment into the T_R phenotype coupled with preferential "selection" or survival of $CD25^+$ T cells may represent the most likely mechanism of thymic T_R development

3
Antigenic Specificity of Induced Regulatory T Cells

Our discussion so far has focused on studies addressing the role of TCR specificity in regulatory T cells that arise naturally in the absence of immune challenge. Other studies have examined the antigen specificity of regulatory T cells elicited under inflammatory conditions. Such T cells have been described as "adaptive" regulatory T cells (reviewed in Bluestone and Abbas 2003). These studies have added further support for an important functional role of the recognition of self-antigens by T_R. For example, in a transgenic model of diabetes elicited upon the induction of the pro-inflammatory cytokine TNFα and co-stimulatory molecule CD80 in pancreatic islet β cells, it was shown that as few as 2000 $CD25^+$ T cells isolated from the draining pancreatic lymph nodes were capable of delaying onset of diabetes upon adoptive transfer into a prediabetic host (Green et al. 2002). Thus, these suppressive $CD25^+$ T cells appear to be elicited by the pro-inflammatory environment in the pancreatic islets, although it is unknown whether these cells represent expanded naturally arising T_R or $CD25^-$ T cells converted into T_R. The putative specificity of these T cells for islet cell antigen(s) is underscored by the fact that adoptive transfer of tenfold higher numbers of $CD25^+$ T cells isolated from non-pancreatic lymph nodes was unable to protect recipient mice from diabetes. It must be noted, however, that in addition to TCR specificity, potential differences between the activated "adaptive" regulatory T cells in the draining lymph nodes at the site of inflammation and the naturally arising $CD25^+$ T_R found elsewhere, such as increased suppressor activity or different cytokine and chemokine receptor profiles, could also account for these observations.

Other evidence for the existence of adaptive regulatory T cells specific for self-antigens and their significant biological role comes from studies of tumor immunity. Initial observations suggested that the presence of $CD25^+$ regulatory T cells can diminish anti-tumor responses, but it was not clear whether this effect was antigen-specific (Shimizu et al. 1999). Several recent studies have suggested that adaptive $CD25^+$ T cells may suppress tumor immunity by recognizing self-antigens. For example, $CD25^+$ T cells with suppressor ability can be elicited by gene gun immunization with autoantigens identified in the SEREX screen (Nishikawa et al. 2003). In another example, human T cell clones with a phenotype resembling regulatory T cells were isolated from tumor-infiltrating lymphocytes of melanoma patients (Wang et al. 2004). Some of these clones were identified to be reactive to the self-protein LAGE1. However, it also remains unclear in these experiments whether these cells arose from naturally arising T_R or were elicited from the $CD25^-$ T cell population. Although the lineage relationship between naturally arising and adaptive regulatory T cells has not been definitively addressed, these reports on the self-reactivity of adaptive regulatory T cells are consistent with the self-reactivity of naturally arising T_R described above.

4
The Paradox of Foreign Antigen Recognition by Regulatory T Cells

The above description of self-reactivity within the naturally arising regulatory T cell population fits with the original identification of regulatory T cells as a critical mechanism for the prevention of autoimmunity. However, it has become increasingly evident that T_R play an important role in the regulation of virtually all immune responses. While initial studies focused on defining the progression of a variety of autoimmune responses in the absence or presence of regulatory T cells, more recent studies have examined the role of T_R in the regulation of immune responses to foreign antigens.

For example, it has been reported that infection of mice with *Helicobacter hepaticus* results in the generation of both CD25$^+$ and CD25$^-$ cells capable of producing IL-10 in response to bacterial antigens and suppressing *Helicobacter*-induced inflammatory colitis (Kullberg et al. 2002). As in aforementioned studies, it is not clear whether these IL-10-producing T cells originate from naturally arising CD25$^+$ T_R or differentiate from the CD25$^-$ T cell population. As *Helicobacter* is considered to be a commensal microorganism in immunocompetent hosts, it is intriguing to hypothesize that gut flora may significantly influence the TCR repertoire of "naturally arising" CD25$^+$ T cell populations (as well as CD25$^-$ populations) by facilitating selective expansion of T_R and CD25$^-$ T cell clones bearing TCR reactive to bacterial antigens. Along the same line, studies of oral tolerance to foreign antigens have demonstrated the ability to generate CD25$^+$ T cells with regulatory properties from CD25$^-$ T cells (Thorstenson and Khoruts 2001).

Thus, a portion of the normal naturally arising regulatory CD25$^+$ T cell population in the periphery may actually contain adaptive CD25$^+$ T cells produced upon interactions with foreign antigens. In support of this hypothesis, several groups have reported in vitro generation of CD25$^+$ T cells with regulatory properties from peripheral CD25$^-$ T cells in both human and murine models (Chen et al. 2003; Nagler-Anderson et al. 2004; Walker et al. 2003b). In the latter, TGF-β was shown to play an essential role in the "peripheral conversion" of murine CD25$^-$ T cells into CD25$^+$ T cells with regulatory properties (Chen et al. 2003). Furthermore, von Boehmer's group has also reported on the generation of CD25$^+$ T_R from peripheral CD25$^-$ TCR transgenic x RAG-deficient T cells upon chronic provision of constant levels of the cognate peptide antigen using an osmotic peptide pump as a delivery device (Apostolou and von Boehmer 2004). Thus, these studies serve as a proof of principle that under certain circumstances, such as high levels of TGF-β, CD25$^+$ regulatory T cells can arise from peripheral CD25$^-$ T cells upon encounter with their cognate antigen.

To complicate matters further, recognition of foreign antigen by the naturally arising CD25$^+$ T cell population has also been demonstrated using immunization with hapten 2,4-dinitrofluorobenzene, or infection with *Candida albicans* or *Leishmania major* (Belkaid et al. 2002; Dubois et al. 2003; Montagnoli et al. 2002). For example, adoptive transfer studies revealed that the *Leishmania*-reactive CD25$^+$ T cells accumulating at the sites of infection were derived primarily from the naturally arising CD25$^+$, and not CD25$^-$, donor T cells. In fact, it was observed that persistent immunologic memory to *Leishmania* as well as *Candida* requires the presence of these adaptive T_R

originating from the naturally arising T_R population, arguing for an important biological role for regulatory T cells in the down-modulation of immune responses to pathogens.

These reports describing reactivity to foreign antigens within the naturally arising T_R population appear to be at odds with the prevalent paradigm of T_R development commencing upon recognition of high-affinity self-antigens in the thymus. One scenario that might account for both self- and foreign-antigen reactivity of T_R would be that the TCR specificity requirements for T_R

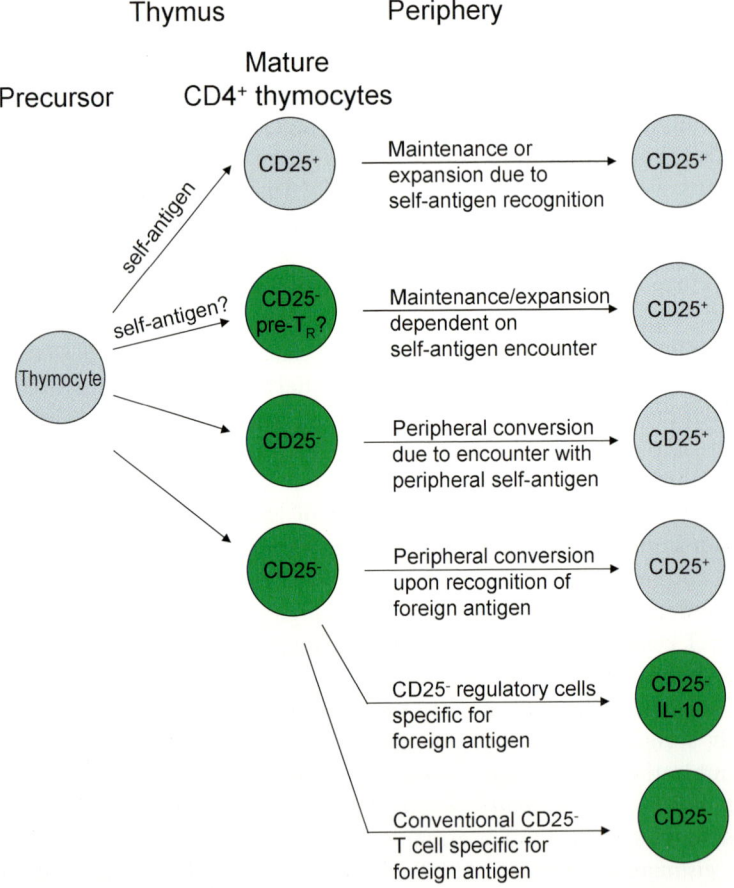

Fig. 2 Development of $CD25^+$ regulatory T cells. Potential TCR-ligand interactions that may result in generation of $CD25^+$ T cells with regulatory properties in the thymus (*left*) and in the periphery (*right*)

development is analogous to conventional CD25⁻ T cell development, except that T_R are simply positively selected based on higher-avidity interactions with self-peptide:MHC class II complexes. A logical extension of this hypothesis is that the T_R TCR repertoire may be functionally as diverse as the CD25⁻ TCR repertoire, allowing for recognition of a wide variety of foreign antigens. The available evidence regarding the diversity of the T_R TCR repertoire does not exclude such a possibility, as it has been shown that Vα and Vβ usage is similar between CD25⁺ and CD25⁻ CD4⁺ T cells (Takahashi et al. 1998). The actual diversity of the T_R TCR repertoire, however, has not been extensively studied until now (see below).

The possibility of a foreign antigen inducing peripheral conversion of CD25⁻ T cells into CD25⁺ regulatory T cells as well as stimulating the expansion of naturally arising CD25⁺ T cells may significantly complicate our view of the development and function of naturally arising T_R (Fig. 2). Thus, it is plausible that there may be several subsets within the peripheral T_R population in regards to specificity of their TCR and their origin. Some peripheral T_R may develop in the thymus as a result of increased avidity recognition of self-antigen, whereas others may have been elicited from CD25⁻ T cells under special conditions, e.g., upon chronic exposure to a foreign or self-antigen in the presence of TGF-β. Finally, thymically derived T_R expanded upon encounter with a high-affinity foreign or self-antigen might also be found within the naturally arising T_R population. The relative size of each of these putative subsets and their functional potential are, however, unknown.

5
T_R Appear to Have a Diverse TCR Repertoire That Is Different from the CD25⁻ TCR Repertoire

To reconcile the findings suggesting that naturally arising regulatory T cells display TCRs having an increased affinity for self-ligands with the observations suggesting that T_R TCRs may also recognize foreign antigens, our group has recently attempted to compare the TCR repertoires displayed by T_R and CD25⁻ CD4⁺ T cells and to test whether the naturally arising T_R population recognizes self-peptide:MHC class II complexes with greater avidity than that of the CD25⁻ T cell population (Hsieh et al. 2004). To directly address these issues, we have analyzed the naturally arising CD25⁺ and CD25⁻ TCR repertoires represented by variable TRAV14 (Vα2) TCRα chains paired with a fixed TCRβ chain in TCRβ transgenic mice. Importantly, T cells were selected in these mice by a highly diverse wild-type array of peptide:MHC class II complexes. Based on the observations regarding CD25⁺ T_R development in TCR transgenic mice with or without RAG expression discussed above, we expected that individual randomly generated TCRα chains will facilitate thymocyte differentiation into either the CD25$^+$ or CD25$^-$ subset.

Direct sequence analyses of the TCR repertoire represented by Vα2 TCRα chains paired with a fixed TCRβ chain suggested that the T$_R$ TCR repertoire is diverse, similar to to the CD25$^-$ T cell subset (Hsieh et al. 2004). In agreement with these results, a remarkable diversity in the T$_R$ TCR repertoire has also been observed using CDR3 spectra-typing analysis of human CD25$^+$ T cells from peripheral blood (Kasow et al. 2004).

This diversity may explain the apparent ability of the naturally arising regulatory T cell population to participate in regulation of immune responses to pathogens such as *Leishmania*. Although T$_R$ were shown to inhibit a sterilizing immune response in the *Leishmania* infection model, thereby allowing for the maintenance of functional "memory" T cells, these and other analogous results provide insufficient support for the idea that the naturally arising T$_R$ population evolved to control infectious immunity. From a general perspective, the potential benefits of preserving a chronic low level infection to maintain functional memory T cells over a sterilizing immune response to pathogens are not immediately obvious. Furthermore, it is possible that T$_R$ involvement in responses to pathogens may be happenstance due to the diversity of the regulatory T cell receptor repertoire and the shared features of inflammation associated with both chronic infection and autoimmunity.

6
A Large Proportion of Peripheral CD25$^+$ TCRs Have Greater Self-Reactivity than CD25$^-$ TCRs

The aforementioned paradigm of regulatory T cell development implies that the CD25$^+$ and CD25$^-$ TCR repertoires are different, as they are selected based on a different avidity for self-antigen. Our sequencing analyses of the TCR repertoire represented by a variable TRAV14 associated with a transgenic TCRβ chain is consistent with this prediction, as we find that there is an overlap estimated at less than 25% between the TCRs isolated between both subsets (Hsieh et al. 2004).

Although increased self-reactivity within the naturally arising regulatory T cell population has been proposed at least a decade ago based on indirect experimental approaches (Taguchi et al. 1994), definitive proof of this hypothesis has been elusive. In vitro studies showed that regulatory T cell recognition of endogenous self-peptide:MHC class II complexes is incapable of inducing suppressor function, and that additional TCR signal is required, e.g., by anti-TCR antibody or mitogen (Takahashi et al. 1998; Thornton and Shevach, 1998). However, there is substantial concern regarding the extent that established methods to assess T_R-mediated suppressor function in vitro represent the physiologic situation in vivo. Thus, this in vitro finding does not exclude the possibility that naturally arising T_R function based on recognition of such self-antigen:MHC class II ligands in vivo. Other in vitro evidence in support of $CD25^+$ T cell self-reactivity obtained by limiting dilution cloning in the presence of syngeneic antigen-presenting cells is hard to interpret because of the difficulty of assessing the cloning efficiency of T_R and the possible contamination of T_R population with activated T cells with up-regulated CD25 expression (Romagnoli et al. 2002). Thus, these in vitro data neither strongly support nor exclude the possibility that T_R recognize self-antigens with greater avidity than $CD25^-$ T cells.

Direct characterization of naturally arising T_R interactions with self-antigens in vivo has also proven difficult, primarily because for some time the only available readout for T_R function in vivo was the prevention of induced or spontaneous pathology. However, it was found independently by several groups that TCR transgenic T_R that develop in the presence of the TCR's cognate peptide ligand encoded by another transgene can proliferate in response to the same neo-self-antigen in vivo (Cozzo et al. 2003; Klein et al. 2003; Walker et al. 2003a; Yamazaki et al. 2003). The proliferative responses of adoptively transferred TCR transgenic T_R in these experimental systems as assessed by dilution of CFSE fluorescence was strictly antigen-specific.

Proliferation within the naturally arising polyclonal T_R populations has also been described in vivo in CSFE dilution or BrDU-labeling experiments (Fisson et al. 2003; Tang et al. 2003). Extrapolating the data described above from TCR transgenic models to these data might suggest then, that naturally arising regulatory T cells are proliferating because of their TCR self-reactivity. However, it is not clear from these data what the precursor frequency of the proliferating cells is. Moreover, the differing proliferative capacity of the $CD25^+$ and $CD25^-$ T cell subsets may be explained by distinct properties unrelated to TCR specificity, such as expression of chemokine receptors or cytokine receptors such as IL-2R. This consideration makes interpretation of these experiments complicated. Although the demonstration of an increased basal level of proliferative turnover within the naturally arising $CD25^+$ T cell population in normal animals is an interesting and important observation, it can be considered only as circumstantial evidence for the self-reactivity of the naturally arising regulatory T cell population.

We have recently addressed these caveats by directly testing whether T_R-derived TCRs exhibit greater self-reactivity than TCRs derived from $CD25^-$

CD4$^+$ T cells (Hsieh et al. 2004). These TCRs were identified in our sequencing studies of TRAV14 TCR-α chain expressing CD25$^+$ and CD25$^-$ CD4 T cells isolated from TCRβ chain transgenic mice. In these experiments, we retrovirally transduced the corresponding TCRα chains into monoclonal CD25$^-$ T cells that express the original transgenic TCRβ chain and are specific for a known foreign peptide antigen. Thus, the transfer of TCRα chains resulted in the recreation of the TCRs from T_R or CD25$^-$ CD4$^+$ T cells and allowed for the meaningful comparison of TCR specificities between the subsets as the intrinsic proliferative capacity and signaling properties of the recipient cells are held constant. The extent and rate of expansion of T_R and CD25$^-$ TCR-transduced T cells adoptively transferred into lymphopenic hosts were used as the most sensitive in vivo readout for the reactivity of TCRs for self-peptide:MHC class II complexes. Using this approach, we found that 40% of the individually expressed T_R TCRs conferred the ability to rapidly expand in vivo while none of the ten CD25$^-$ CD4$^+$ TCRs tested did so. These data therefore suggest that a large proportion of naturally arising T_R TCRs recognize constitutively presented peripheral self-antigens with greater avidity than CD25$^-$ TCRs.

7
What Is the Tissue Distribution of T_R Target Self-Antigens?

We already discussed earlier studies suggesting that regulatory T cells need to specifically recognize tissue-derived self-antigens for their survival and/or functional activity in the periphery (Seddon and Mason 1999; Taguchi et al. 1994) and subsequent work supporting tissue specificity of T_R-mediated protection from autoimmunity (Green et al. 2002; Walker et al. 2003a). However, the recognition of tissue-specific antigens by some T_R does not exclude the recognition of ubiquitously presented self-antigens by others. Such recognition is predicted by TCR transgenic models in which regulatory T cell development is directed by a transgene driving expression of the cognate antigen in a variety of tissues (Cozzo et al. 2003). Furthermore, the development of regulatory T cells in H-2M-deficient mice, which express primarily a single peptide-MHC class II complex, CLIP:I-A^b, or in mice expressing Eα peptide covalently bound to I-A^b molecules, strongly argues for the existence of T_R recognizing ubiquitously presented self-peptides expressed in high copy numbers (Bensinger et al. 2001; Pacholczyk et al. 2002). Our laboratory has obtained analogous results (M. Gavin, J. Fontenot, and A.R., unpublished observations) in studies of previously described single-peptide mice (Barton et al. 2002).

Our aforementioned studies of the regulatory T cell receptor repertoire formed by variable TRAV14 (Vα2) TCRα chains and a fixed TCRβ chain are consistent with the existence of T_R specific for both tissue-specific and ubiquitously expressed MHC class II-bound self-peptides. The latter notion is supported by our observation that complex pools of $CD25^+$- but not $CD25^-$-derived TCRs, conferred the ability of T cells to proliferate in vitro to autologous splenic APCs (Hsieh et al. 2004). When tested individually, however, the proliferative response was observed upon expression of some but not all $CD25^+$ TCRs. TCR recognition of these ligands also appeared to be peptide-specific rather than peptide-promiscuous, as APCs with drastically skewed repertoire of peptides bound to MHC class II molecules failed to induce proliferative in vitro responses (Fig. 3). Thus, these data imply that T_R TCR recognition is peptide-specific and a subset of naturally arising T_R recognizes ubiquitously presented self-peptides with a sufficiently high affinity to be detected in vitro.

On the other hand, T cells transduced with some $CD25^+$, but not $CD25^-$ TCRs, were capable of inducing tissue-specific pathology, e.g., bronchiolitis and lung perivasculitis identified histologically upon adoptive transfer of these T cells into lymphopenic hosts (C.H. and A.R., unpublished observations). In preliminary experiments, we have also observed alveolitis induced by adoptively transferred activated T cells transduced with a single $CD25^+$ TCR. Although it is formally possible that organ-specific pathology, i.e., autoimmunity, in these experiments may result from reactivity of TCR with ubiquitously expressed self-peptides, a more straightforward interpretation of these observations is that some T_R TCR recognize tissue-specific antigens.

How might antigen specificity affect regulatory T cell development? Development of tissue-specific regulatory T cells is likely to require an encounter with the tissue-specific antigen in the thymus, as suggested by an experimental model where TCR transgenic T_R precursors recognize transgene-encoded cognate antigen expressed in the thymus under the rat insulin promoter (Walker et al. 2003a). Presumably, expression of these tissue-specific antigens would be under the control of the AIRE gene. Although the numbers of naturally arising $CD25^+$ $CD4^+$ regulatory T cells are normal in AIRE-deficient mice (Anderson et al. 2002), detailed analysis of the effect of AIRE deficiency on the specificity of regulatory T cells generated in the thymus and their ability to suppress tissue-specific autoimmunity has not been reported. It is expected that the putative tissue-specific T_R would expand and suppress local autoimmune responses upon antigen encounter in the draining lymph nodes and/or peripheral tissues. It can also be hypothesized that the extent of T_R expansion and suppression would correlate with the level of the corresponding self-antigen presented, allowing for more suppression during periods of increased

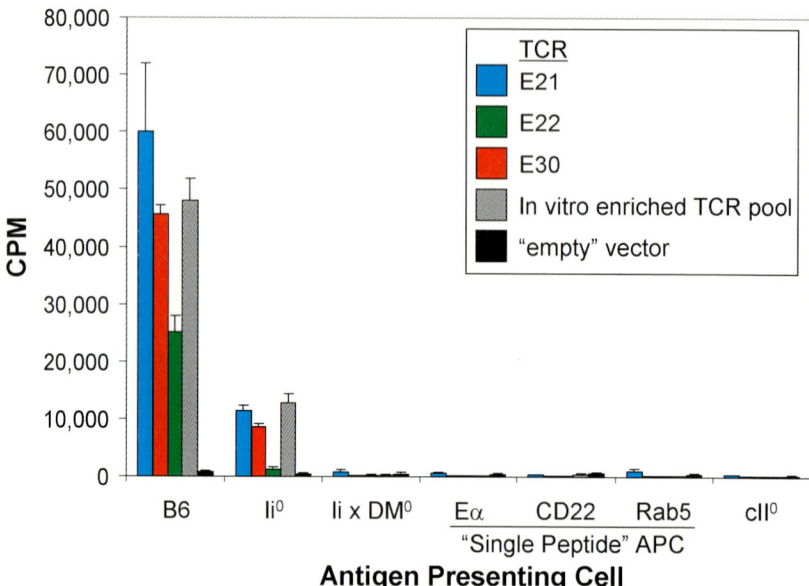

Fig. 3 Recognition of ubiquitous self-peptides displayed by autologous APCs in a peptide-specific manner. Three different individual TRAV14 TCRα chains originally isolated from CD25$^+$ T$_R$ from TCli-β TCRβ transgenic mice were retrovirally transduced into TCli-$\alpha\beta$ TCR transgenic RAG-deficient T cells to reconstitute the original TCRs as described (Hsieh et al. 2004). TCR clones E21, E22, and E30 were isolated from an in vitro-enriched TCR pool obtained by serial passage of T cells transduced with TCRs from a CD25$^+$-derived TCR library in the presence of irradiated autologous splenocytes and IL-2. Retrovirally transduced T cells were rested over 14 days, and then restimulated in the presence of irradiated APCs described below. Incorporation of ^{3}H-thymidine was assessed between 48 and 72 h. T cells transduced with the three individual TCRs or with a pool of TCR (positive control) proliferated, albeit to a differing degree, in response to syngeneic B6 splenic APCs. In contrast, TCli-$\alpha\beta$ TCR transgenic RAG-deficient T cells transduced with the empty vector (negative control) failed to mount a significant proliferative response. The notion that some T$_R$ may recognize ubiquitously expressed self peptides is supported by the observation that two of three individual TCR responded to Ii-deficient APCs. In the absence of Ii, surface expression of MHC class II molecules is decreased five- to tenfold, and they harbor a significantly restricted repertoire of peptides derived primarily from proteins endogenously synthesized by the APCs (Kovats et al. 1998). In contrast, none of the tested TCR was able to recognize Ii x DM double-deficient APCs, which in comparison to Ii-deficient APCs, exhibit a drastic reduction in diversity and expression level of class II-bound self-peptides, but maintain the same overall surface MHC class II expression. Similarly, no response was observed to APCs from previously characterized Eα-dbl^o, Rab-dbl^o, and CD22-dbl^o mice. These single-peptide APCs display wild-type levels of surface MHC class II molecules bound almost exclusively with a single peptide derived from I-Eα, Rab5, or CD22 proteins (Barton et al. 2002)

self-antigen expression or availability, and less suppression during periods of decreased self-antigen expression, permitting tunable suppression of inflammation associated with infection and autoimmunity. Thus, self-recognition would serve as a sensor for a cell-extrinsic negative feedback loop in which regulatory T cells would protect small areas of the body against inadvertent immune responses to excessively presented self-antigens. In a situation of increased efficiency of self-antigen presentation due to infection-associated tissue damage, concurrent innate immune activation via TLR signals induced by microbial ligands during acute infection has been proposed to permit initiation of the adaptive immune response by abrogating or rendering resistance to T_R-mediated suppression (Pasare and Medzhitov 2003). However, we would predict that down-modulation of TLR signals during chronic infection would allow T_R to effectively limit inflammation, as discussed above.

In contrast to tissue-specific regulatory T cells, the potential biological role of T_R recognizing ubiquitously presented antigen appears less obvious. In this regard, we would like to put forward a hypothesis that these T cells make up a significant portion, if not the majority, of the T_R population and provide basal protection against relatively weak low-affinity autoimmune responses of a broad specificity, but cannot efficiently protect from autoimmunity mediated by high-affinity tissue-specific effector T cells. A related intriguing notion is that perhaps these T_R act to preserve tolerance to ubiquitous antigens, such as nuclear antigens potentially involved in systemic lupus erythematosus.

In conclusion, it has become evident that the antigen specificity of naturally arising regulatory T cells is very complex, as their TCR repertoire is arguably as diverse as that of $CD25^-$ T cells. The naturally arising regulatory T cell population found in the periphery is likely largely comprised of the classic, thymus-derived T_R with an increased avidity for self peptide:MHC class II complexes. However, a number of peripheral T_R may also be generated upon repeated or chronic encounters with foreign antigens, such as orally derived or inhaled antigens, as well as commensal non-pathogenic microbes, or self-antigens. These subsets of naturally arising T_R with different antigen specificities for self- or non-self-antigens may then serve to prevent unnecessary tissue damage associated with autoimmunity or chronic infection. Nevertheless, it is clear that there is still much to learn regarding regulatory T cell antigen specificity and its impact on the development, peripheral survival and expansion, and suppressive function mediated by this T cell subset, which is critically important for the maintenance of immune homeostasis. Development of transgenic mice expressing T_R-derived TCR and identification of their foreign and self-peptide ligands will be necessary to further our understanding of the role of TCR-ligand interactions in the development and function of naturally arising regulatory T cells.

Acknowledgements The authors are supported by grants from the National Institutes of Health (C.H. and A.R.), the Howard Hughes Medical Institute (A.R.), and the Arthritis Foundation/American College of Rheumatology (C.H.).

References

Anderson MS, Venanzi ES, Klein L, Chen Z, Berzins SP, Turley SJ, von Boehmer H, Bronson R, Dierich A, Benoist C, Mathis D (2002) Projection of an immunological self shadow within the thymus by the Aire protein. Science 298:1395–1401

Apostolou I, Sarukhan A, Klein L, von Boehmer H (2002) Origin of regulatory T cells with known specificity for antigen. Nat Immunol 3:756–763

Apostolou I, von Boehmer H (2004) In vivo instruction of suppressor commitment in naive T cells. J Exp Med 199:1401–1408

Barton GM, Beers C, deRoos P, Eastman SR, Gomez ME, Forbush KA, Rudensky AY (2002) Positive selection of self-MHC-reactive T cells by individual peptide-MHC class II complexes. Proc Nat Acad Sci U S A 99:6937–6942

Belkaid Y, Piccirillo CA, Mendez S, Shevach EM, Sacks DL (2002) CD4+ CD25+ regulatory T cells control Leishmania major persistence and immunity. Nature 420:502–507

Bensinger SJ, Bandeira A, Jordan MS, Caton AJ, Laufer TM (2001) Major histocompatibility complex class II-positive cortical epithelium mediates the selection of CD4+ CD25+ immunoregulatory T cells. J Exp Med 194:427–438

Bluestone JA, Abbas AK (2003) Natural versus adaptive regulatory T cells. Nat Rev Immunol 3:253–257

Chen W, Jin W, Hardegen N, Lei, K-J, Li L, Marinos N, McGrady G, Wahl SM (2003) Conversion of peripheral CD4+ CD25- naive T cells to CD4+ CD25+ regulatory T cells by TGF-beta induction of transcription factor Foxp3. J Exp Med 198:1875–1886

Cozzo C, Larkin III J, Caton AJ (2003) Cutting edge: self-peptides drive the peripheral expansion of CD4+ CD25+ regulatory T cells. J Immunol 171:5678–5682

Dubois B, Chapat L, Goubier A, Papiernik M, Nicolas J-F, Kaiserlian D (2003) Innate CD4+ CD25+ regulatory T cells are required for oral tolerance and inhibition of CD8+ T cells mediating skin inflammation. Blood 102:3295–3301

Fisson S, Darrasee-Jeze G, Litvinova E, Septier F, Klatzmann D, Liblau R, Salomon BL (2003) Continuous activation of autoreactive CD4+ CD25+ regulatory T cells in the steady state. J Exp Med 198:737–746

Gavin MA, Clarke SR, Negrou E, Gallegos A, Rudensky A (2002) Homeostasis and anergy of CD4+CD25+ suppressor T cells in vivo. Nat Immunol 3:33–41

Green EA, Choi Y, Flavell RA (2002) Pancreatic lymph node-derived CD4+ CD25+ Treg Cells: highly potent regulators of diabetes that require TRANCE-RANK signals. Immunity 16:183–191

Hori S, Haury M, Coutinho A, Demengeot J (2002) Specificity requirements for selection and effector functions of CD25+4+ regulatory T cells in anti-myelin basic protein T cell receptor transgenic mice. Proc Nat Acad Sci U S A 99:8213–8218

Hsieh C-S, Liang Y, Tyznik AJ, Self SG, Liggitt D, Rudensky AY (2004) Recognition of the peripheral self by naturally arising CD25+ CD4+ T cell receptors. Immunity 21:267–277

Itoh M, Takahashi T, Sakaguchi N, Kuniyasu Y, Shimizu J, Otsuka F, Sakaguchi S (1999) Thymus and autoimmunity: production of CD25+ CD4+ naturally anergic and suppressive T cells as a key function of the thymus in maintaining immunologic self-tolerance. J Immunol 162:5317–5326

Jooss K, Gjata B, Danos O, von Boehmer H, Sarukhan A (2001) Regulatory function of in vivo anergized CD4+ T cells. Proc Nat Acad Sci U S A 98:8738–8743

Jordan MS, Boesteanu A, Petrone AL, Holenbeck AE, Lerman MA, Naji A, Caton AJ (2001) Thymic selection of CD4+ CD25+ regulatory T cells induced by an agonist self-peptide. Nat Immunol 2:301–306

Kasow KA, Chen X, Knowles J, Wichlan D, Handgretinger R, Riberdy JM (2004) Human CD4+ CD25+ regulatory T cells share equally complex and comparable repertoires with CD4+ CD25– counterparts. J Immunol 172:6123–6128

Klein L, Khazaie K, von Boehmer H (2003) In vivo dynamics of antigen-specific regulatory T cells not predicted from behavior in vitro. Proc Nat Acad Sci U S A 100:8886–8891

Kovats S, Grubin CE, Eastman SE, deRoos P, Dongre A, Van Kaer L, Rudensky AY (1998) Invariant chain-independent function of H-2M in the formation of endogenous peptide-major histocompatibility complex class II complexes in vivo. J Exp Med 187:245–251

Kullberg MC, Jankovic D, Gorelick PL, Caspar P, Letterio JJ, Cheever AW, Sher A (2002) Bacteria-triggered CD4+ T regulatory cells suppress *Helicobacter hepaticus*-induced colitis. J Exp Med 196:505–515

Maloy KJ, Powrie, F (2001) Regulatory T cells in the control of immune pathology. Nat Immunol 2:816–822

McHugh RS, Whitters MJ, Piccirillo CA, Young DA, Shevach EM, Collins M, Byrne MC (2002) CD4+ CD25+ Immunoregulatory T cells: gene expression analysis reveals a functional role for the glucocorticoid-induced TNF receptor. Immunity 16:311–323

Montagnoli C, Bacci A, Bozza S, Gaziano R, Mosci P, Sharpe AH, Romani, L (2002) B7/CD28-dependent CD4+ CD25+ regulatory T cells are essential components of the memory-protective immunity to *Candida albicans*. J Immunol 169:6298–6308

Nagler-Anderson C, Bhan AK, Podolsky DK, Terhorst C (2004) Control freaks: immune regulatory cells. Nat Immunol 5:119–122

Nishikawa H, Kato T, Tanida K, Hiasa A, Tawara I, Ikeda H, Ikarashi Y, Wakasugi H, Kronenberg M, Nakayama T et al (2003) CD4+ CD25+ T cells responding to serologically defined autoantigens suppress antitumor immune responses. Proc Nat Acad Sci U S A 100:10902–10906

Olivares-Villagomez D, Wang Y, Lafaille JJ (1998) Regulatory CD4$^+$ T cells expressing endogenous T cell receptor chains protect myelin basic protein-specific transgenic mice from spontaneous autoimmune encephalomyelitis. J Exp Med 188:1883–1894

Pacholczyk P, Kraj P, Ignatowicz L (2002) Peptide specificity of thymic selection of CD4+ CD25+ T cells. J Immunol 168:613–620

Pasare C, Medzhitov R (2003) Toll pathway-dependent blockade of CD4+ CD25+ T cell-mediated suppression by dendritic cells. Science 299:1033–1036

Romagnoli P, Hudrisier D, van Meerwijk JPM (2002) Preferential recognition of self antigens despite normal thymic deletion of CD4+ CD25+ regulatory T cells. J Immunol 168:1644–1648

Sakaguchi S, Sakaguchi N, Asano M, Itoh M, Toda M (1995) Immunologic self-tolerance maintained by activated T cells expressing IL-2 receptor alpha-chains (CD25). J Immunol 155:1151–1164

Seddon B, Mason D (1999) Regulatory T cells in the control of autoimmunity: the essential role of transforming growth factor beta and interleukin 4 in the prevention of autoimmune thyroiditis in rats by peripheral CD4+ CD45RC- cells and CD4+ CD8- thymocytes. J Exp Med 189:279–288

Seddon B, Mason D (2000) The third function of the thymus. Immunol Today 21:95–99

Shimizu J, Yamazaki S, Sakaguchi S (1999) Induction of tumor immunity by removing CD25+CD4+ T cells: a common basis between tumor immunity and autoimmunity. J Immunol 163:5211–5218

Taguchi O, Kontani K, Ikeda H, Kezuka T, Takeuchi M, Takahashi T (1994) Tissue-specific suppressor T cells involved in self-tolerance are activated extrathymically by self-antigens. Immunology 82:365–369

Takahashi T, Kuniyasu Y, Toda M, Sakaguchi N, Itoh M, Iwata M, Shimizu J, Sakaguchi S (1998) Immunologic self-tolerance maintained by CD25+ CD4+ naturally anergic and suppressive T cells: induction of autoimmune disease by breaking their anergic/suppressive state. Int Immunol 10:1969–1980

Tang Q, Henriksen KJ, Boden EK, Tooley AJ, Ye J, Subudhi SK, Zheng XX, Strom TB, Bluestone JA (2003) Cutting edge: CD28 controls peripheral homeostasis of CD4+ CD25+ regulatory T cells. J Immunol 171:3348–3352

Thornton AM, Shevach EM (1998) CD4+CD25+ immunoregulatory T cells suppress polyclonal T cell activation in vitro by inhibiting interleukin 2 production. J Exp Med 188:287–296

Thorstenson KM, Khoruts A (2001) Generation of anergic and potentially immunoregulatory CD25+ CD4 T cells in vivo after induction of peripheral tolerance with intravenous or oral antigen. J Immunol 167:188–195

van Santen H-M, Benoist C, Mathis D (2004) Number of T reg cells that differentiate does not increase upon encounter of agonist ligand on thymic epithelial cells. J Exp Med 200:1221–1230

Walker LS, Chodos A, Eggena M, Dooms H, Abbas AK (2003a) Antigen-dependent proliferation of CD4+ CD25+ regulatory T cells in vivo. J Exp Med 198:249–258

Walker MR, Kasprowicz DJ, Gersuk VH, Benard A, Van Landeghen M, Buckner JH, Ziegler SF (2003b) Induction of Foxp3 and acquisition of T regulatory activity by stimulated human CD4+ CD25- T cells. J Clin Invest 112:1437–1443

Wang HY, Lee DA, Peng G, Guo Z, Li Y, Kiniwa Y, Shevach EM, Wang R-F (2004) Tumor-specific human CD4+ regulatory T cells and their ligands: implications for immunotherapy. Immunity 20:107–118

Yamazaki S, Iyoda T, Tarbell K, Olson K, Velinzon K, Inaba K, Steinman RM (2003) Direct expansion of functional CD25+ CD4+ regulatory T cells by antigen-processing dendritic cells. J Exp Med 198:235–247

Thymic Commitment of Regulatory T Cells Is a Pathway of TCR-Dependent Selection That Isolates Repertoires Undergoing Positive or Negative Selection

A. Coutinho · I. Caramalho · E. Seixas · J. Demengeot (✉)

Laboratoire Européen Associé au CNRS, Instituto Gulbenkian de Ciência,
Oeiras, Portugal
jocelyne@igc.gulbenkian.pt

1	Introduction	46
2	Somatically Generated T Cell Receptor Repertoires Are Distributed and Continuous	48
3	The MM96 Solution to the Thymic Sorting of Emergent TCR Repertoires: Differential Roles of TECs and THCs on Treg Selection	50
4	Promiscuous Tissue-Antigen Expression in TECs Selects Treg Repertoires: The Origin and Range of Autoimmune Diseases	52
5	Beyond TCR Repertoires: A Unique Differentiative Lineage, That May Represent Class Regulation Operating Intrathymically	54
6	The Question on the Putative MHC Restriction of Treg: Yet Another Difference Between the Thymic Selection of Treg and Naïve T Cells?	56
7	Selective TLR Expresssion by Treg: Evolutionary Significance and a Possible Handle on Treg Regulation	59
8	Regulatory T Cells Versus Phenomenology on Regulation	61
References		62

Abstract The seminal work of Le Douarin and colleagues (Ohki et al. 1987; Ohki et al. 1988; Salaun et al. 1990; Coutinho et al. 1993) first demonstrated that peripheral tissue-specific tolerance is centrally established in the thymus, by epithelial stromal cells (TEC). Subsequent experiments have shown that TEC-tolerance is dominant and mediated by CD4 regulatory T cells (Treg) that are generated intrathymically by recognition of antigens expressed on TECs (Modigliani et al. 1995; Modigliani et al. 1996a). From these and other observations, in 1996 Modigliani and colleagues derived a general model for the establishment and maintenance of natural tolerance (MM96) (Modigliani et al. 1996b), with two central propositions: (1) T cell receptor (TCR)-dependent sorting of emergent repertoires generates TEC-specific Treg displaying the highest TCR self-affinities below deletion thresholds, thus isolating repertoires undergoing positive and negative selection; (2) Treg are intrathymically committed (and activated) for a unique differentiative pathway with regulatory effector functions. The model explained the embryonic/perinatal time window of natural tolerance acquisition, by developmental programs determining (1) TCR multireactivity, (2) the cellular composition in the thymic stroma (relative abundance of epithelial vs hemopoietic cells), and (3) the dynamics of peripheral lymphocyte pools, built by accumulation of recent thymic emigrants (RTE) that remain recruitable to regulatory functions. We discuss here the MM96 in the light of recent results demonstrating the promiscuous expression of tissue-specific antigens by medullary TECs (Derbinski et al. 2001; Anderson et al. 2002; Gotter et al. 2004) and indicating that Treg represent a unique differentiative pathway (Fontenot et al. 2003; Hori et al. 2003; Khattri et al. 2003), which is adopted by CD4 T cells with high avidity for TEC-antigens (Bensinger et al. 2001; Jordan et al. 2001; Apostolou et al. 2002). In the likelihood that autoimmune diseases (AID) result from Treg deficits, some of which might have a thymic origin, we also speculate on therapeutic strategies aiming at selectively stimulating their de novo production or peripheral function, within recent findings on Treg responses to inflammation (Caramalho et al. 2003; Lopes-Carvalho et al., submitted, Caramalho et al., submitted).

In short, the MM96 argued that natural tolerance is dominant, established and maintained by the activity of Treg, which are selected upon high-affinity recognition of self-ligands on TECs, and committed intrathymically to a unique differentiative pathway geared to anti-inflammatory and antiproliferative effector functions. By postulating the intrathymic deletion of self-reactivities on hemopoietic stromal cells (THC), together with the inability of peripheral resident lymphocytes to engage in the regulatory pathway, the MM96 simultaneously explained the maintenance of responsiveness to non-self in a context of suppression mediating dominant self-tolerance. The major difficulty of the MM96 is related to the apparent tissue specificity of Treg repertoires generated intrathymically. This difficulty has now been principally solved by the work of Hanahan, Kyewski and others (Jolicoeur et al. 1994; Derbinski et al. 2001; Anderson et al. 2002; Gotter et al. 2004), demonstrating the selective expression of a variety of tissue-specific antigens by TECs, in topological patterns that are compatible with the MM96, but difficult to conciliate with recessive tolerance models (Kappler et al. 1987; Kisielow et al. 1988). While the developmentally regulated multireactivity of TCR repertoires (Gavin and Bevan 1995), as well as the peripheral recruitment of Treg among RTE (Modigliani et al. 1996a) might add to this process, it would seem that the establishment of tissue-specific tolerance essentially stems from the "promiscuous expression of tissue antigens" by TEC. The findings of AID resulting from natural mutations (reviewed in Pitkanen and Peterson 2003) or the targeted inactivation (Anderson et al. 2002; Ramsey et al. 2002) of the AIRE transcription factor that regulates promiscuous gene expression on TECs support this conclusion.

The observations on the correlation of natural or forced expression of the Foxp3 transcription factor in CD4 T cells with Treg phenotype and function (Fontenot et al. 2003; Hori et al. 2003; Khattri et al. 2003) provided support for the MM96 contention that Treg represent a unique differentiative pathway that is naturally established inside the thymus. Furthermore, Caton and colleagues (Jordan et al. 2001), as well as several other groups (Bensinger et al. 2001; Apostolou et al. 2002), have provided direct evidence for our postulate that Treg are selected among differentiating CD4 T cells with high affinity for ligands expressed on TECs (Modigliani et al. 1996b).

Finally, the demonstration by Caramalho et al. that Treg express innate immunity receptors (Caramalho et al. 2003) and respond to pro-inflammatory signals and products of inflammation (Caramalho et al., submitted) brought about a new understanding on the peripheral regulation of Treg function. Together with the observation that Treg also respond to ongoing activities of "naïve/effector" T cells—possibly through the IL-2 produced in these conditions—these findings explain the participation of Treg in all immune responses (Onizuka et al. 1999; Shimizu et al. 1999; Annacker et al. 2001; Curotto de Lafaille et al. 2001; Almeida et al. 2002; Shevach 2002; Bach and Francois Bach 2003; Wood and Sakaguchi 2003; Mittrucker and Kaufmann 2004; Sakaguchi 2004), beyond their fundamental role in ensuring self-tolerance (e.g., Modigliani et al. 1996a; Shevach 2000; Hori et al. 2003; Sakaguchi 2004; Thompson and Powrie 2004). Thus, anti-inflammatory and anti-proliferative Treg are amplified by signals that promote or mediate inflammation and proliferation, accounting for the quality control of responses (Coutinho et al. 2001). In turn, such natural regulation of Treg by immune responses to non-self may well explain the alarming epidemiology of allergic and AID in wealthy societies (Wills-Karp et al. 2001; Bach 2002; Yazdanbakhsh et al. 2002), where a variety of childhood infections have become rare or absent. Thus, it is plausible that Treg were evolutionarily set by a given density of infectious agents in the environment. With hindsight, it is not too surprising that natural Treg performance falls once hygiene, vaccination, and antibiotics suddenly (i.e., 100 years) plunged infectious density to below some critical physiological threshold. As the immune system is not adapted to modern clean conditions of postnatal development, clinical immunologists must now deal with frequent Treg deficiencies (allergies and AID) for which they have no curative or rational treatments. It is essential, therefore, that basic immunologists concentrate on strategies to selectively stimulate the production, survival, and activity of this set of lymphocytes that is instrumental in preventing immune pathology. We have argued that the culprit of this inability of basic research to solve major clinical problems has been the self-righteousness of recessive tolerance champions, from Ehrlich to some of our contemporaries. It is ironical, however, that none of us—including the heretic opponents of horror autotoxicus—had understood that self-tolerance, or its robustness at least, is in part determined by the frequency and intensity of the responses to non-self.

In the evolution of ideas on immunological tolerance, the time might be ripe for some kinds of synthesis. First, conventional theory reduced self-tolerance to negative selection and microbial defense to positive selection, while the MM96 solution was the precise opposite: positive selection of autoreactivities for self-tolerance (Treg) and negative selection (of Treg) for ridding responses. In contrast, it would now appear that positive and negative selection of autoreactive T cells are both necessary to establish either self-tolerance or competence to eliminate microbes, two processes that actually reinforce each other in the maintenance of self-integrity. Second, V-region recognition has generally been held responsible for specific discrimination between what should be either tolerated or eliminated from the organism. In contrast again, it would now seem that both processes of self-tolerance and microbial defense (self/non-self discrimination) also operate on the basis of evolutionarily ancient, germ-line-encoded innate, nonspecific receptors (Medzhitov and Janeway 2000) capable of a coarse level of self/non-self discrimination (Coutinho 1975). It could thus be interesting to revisit notions of cooperativity between V-regions and such mitogen receptors, both in single cell functions (Coutinho et al. 1974) and in the system's evolution (Coutinho 1975, 1980) as well. After all, major transitions in evolution were cooperative (Maynard-Smith and Szathmary 1995).

1
Introduction

The last few years have witnessed a radical shift in current notions of self-tolerance and autoimmunity. Recessive tolerance, established by negative selection of self-reactive cells, has had the upper hand ever since Ehrlich declared autoantibodies to be dysteleologic. In the 1980s, the discovery of thymic deletion by antibodies to TCR V-betas (Kappler et al. 1987) launched a large volume of work leading to the conclusion that the establishment of self-tolerance and thymic deletion were one and the same process. This was epitomized by von Boehmer's "the thymus selects the useful, neglects the useless and destroys the harmful," the latter being all autoreactive T cells with productive affinities to self-peptide:MHC complexes (von Boehmer et al. 1989). While this Darwinian tautology could not possibly be wrong, it resulted in little or no progress, and tolerance remained the central question in modern immunology.

For a decade or two, a few groups in the world, working at the margin of prevalent concepts, kept producing evidence and arguments for the alternative notion that tolerance is dominant. For these, the putative solution to natural tolerance was turned up-side down: rather than stemming from the elimination of autoreactive T cells, it would require their positive selection and activation. In a turnaround that seemed sudden to many, dating from the International Congress of Immunology of 2001 in Stockholm, Treg and immune regulation have come forth to the limelight, occupying an increasing place in the literature over the last few years. This was received in widely divergent manners. For some, the topic sounds as if suppressor T cells are back, and this is bad news: after a dozen years of abundant phenomenology, suppressor T cells had been driven out of sight by progress in the molecular biology of lymphocytes, and by the efforts of a few who had never been convinced by often irreproducible, nonquantitative *in vitro* assays. Others were interested in dominant tolerance, for they saw "some reasons why that deletion and anergy cannot satisfactorily explain natural tolerance" (Coutinho et al. 1992), underlining the differences between the old suppressor T cell phenomenology in response to conventional antigens, and the new *in vivo* evidence for Treg operating in self-tolerance. Yet others, who were part of the previous suppressor T cell journey, gladly joined the new trend, again taking up their *in vitro* suppression assays to describe new markers and mechanisms. A large group adapted to fashion by forgetting experiments and models on recessive tolerance to proclaim their novel conviction of dominant regulation. Few, however, gave enough consideration to the fact that models of dominant tolerance must also explain the time window for tolerance acquisition, how Treg develop and have their repertoires selected throughout life, how autoimmune diseases appear and display such a characteristic range of targets, and how conventional immune responses are produced in a context of suppression. In short, if the approaches to natural tolerance seem to be on the right track, fundamental aspects of the organization of the immune system, including the selection of *available* and *actual* T and B cell repertoires in accordance with self-nonself discrimination, remain unsolved. Most importantly, to the dismay of clinicians, the therapeutic approaches to autoimmune patients are today debatable: immunosuppression, as commanded by the classical views, or immunostimulation, as is now suggested by the novel theories.

As stated earlier (Modigliani et al. 1996b), the original observations of Le Douarin on TEC tolerance to peripheral tissues (Ohki et al. 1987, 1988; Salaun et al. 1990; Coutinho et al. 1993), given the postulate for differential roles of TECs and THCs in the presentation of antigens to developing T lymphocytes, had principally solved the core problems of natural tolerance in the framework of dominant mechanisms mediated by thymically committed Treg (Modigliani et al. 1996a). Four types of recent findings strengthen this conviction:

1. Treg represent a unique differentiative lineage of lymphocytes with intrathymic commitment (Fontenot et al. 2003; Hori et al. 2003; Khattri et al. 2003), as proposed.
2. Treg are selected upon high-avidity TCR recognition of antigens expressed on TECs (Bensinger et al. 2001; Jordan et al. 2001; Apostolou et al. 2002), just as postulated.
3. Tissue-specific antigens are selectively expressed by TECs in a promiscuous manner (Derbinski et al. 2001; Anderson et al. 2002; Gotter et al. 2004), providing a simple explanation for the thymic acquisition of tissue-specific tolerance, and supporting our postulate on the differential roles of TECs and THCs in the generation of Treg repertoires; in addition, the respective genetic and cellular mechanisms remind us, as if it were necessary, of the evolutionary relevance of Treg generation, and may explain the acquisition of natural tolerance to self-antigens that are expressed only after the tolerogenic time window.

4. Treg express innate receptors for inflammation-related ligands (Caramalho et al. 2003) and are amplified by ongoing conventional T cell activity (Almeida et al. 2002), opening new leads to their physiology and putative manipulation.

In this conceptual framework, research must now move on. For the benefit of patients, the immunopharmacology of Treg must be explored, while the time may be ripe to address systemic questions of regulation that remain largely unattended: the developmental co-selection of V-region repertoires and functional classes among lymphocyte subsets, the selection, specificity, and population dynamics of natural antibodies and naturally activated T and B cells, including Treg (Pereira et al. 1985), the basis for the life-long memory of the developmental antigenic self.

2
Somatically Generated T Cell Receptor Repertoires Are Distributed and Continuous

The fate of differentiating T cells is ultimately determined by TCR affinity for intrathymic ligands. Conventional selection models (von Boehmer et al. 1989) assume that increasing self-affinities result in neglect, positive and negative selection, in this order. Randomly generated Variable-regions of T cell receptors (TCR) and antibodies, however, are expected to have an interesting property that is necessary in the evolutionary strategy bringing them forth. Populations of V-regions, provided they are sufficiently large, will have a continuous distribution over whatever quantitative parameter we can consider in their interaction with a given antigenic ligand. Immunologists know this well, and have paid a great deal of attention to affinity distributions and degeneracy when considering thresholds for cellular induction or inactivation. It follows that, for a given fixed set of antigenic ligands (such as the thymic environment of an individual[1]), the affinity distribution of an emerging and sufficiently large V-region population (such as the randomly generated TCR diversity of developing T cells) will be continuous.[2] This means that TCRs will distribute continuously below and above a given threshold of cellular

---

[1] For the process of establishing self-tolerance by selecting TCR repertoires, it is essential that the set of selective ligands be fixed, and protected from the ever-changing external antigens that may eventually be brought into the thymus. In this context, it would seem critical that TECs do not present external antigens.

[2] It could be argued that developmentally regulated TCR repertoires, which are essentially germ-line, have been evolutionarily selected for pre-set affinities to a given ensemble of ligands, such that they do not conform to a continuous distribution to

selection and, therefore, that TCRs with very similar affinity to the antigenic environment will fall on either side of that threshold. In the case of thymic negative selection, which aims at purging TCRs that might be activated in the periphery, this property of TCR repertoires poses a central problem. Thus, the antigenic environment in the periphery, where the selected cell will perform, is certainly different from that in the thymus, where cells are selected. First of all, the levels of expression of antigenic ligands and their diversity in peripheral tissues, together with the characteristic degeneracy of TCR-ligand interactions (Mason 1998; Wilson et al. 2004), will bring about critical differences. Moreover, these differences will be functionally amplified by the distinct antigenic contexts in the thymus vs peripheral tissues: the architecture of peripheral lymphoid organs, the expression levels of co-stimulatory molecules, the available cytokine and chemokine milieu, all make it inescapable that TCRs, which were just below the threshold for negative selection in the thymus, will be activated in the periphery. This applies for any postulated level of this affinity threshold. The continuous distribution of TCR affinities would thus allow for the positive selection of naïve T cells with anti-self affinities that are too low to be eliminated in the thymic environment, but high enough to be activated in peripheral contexts of higher antigenic and co-stimulation levels (e.g., inflammation). As these models also assume that positively selected T cells leave the thymus uncommitted as to the class of responses they will produce (e.g., helper vs inflammatory, for CD4 cells), this being determined by activation contexts in the periphery, frequent and indiscriminate development of pathogenic autoreactive responses in the periphery seems unavoidable.

There is, thus, a two-sided difficulty with this particular model of thymic selection that remains widely accepted today: unavoidable wobbling in an all-or-none process (cellular selection) that is controlled by a continuous variable (TCR affinity); no coupling of wobbling TCRs to a particular (nonpathogenic) effector function in the gray range of affinities.

---

such ligands (Cohn and Langman 1990; Langman and Cohn 1992). On the other hand, the major characteristic of these repertoires is their multireactivity (Coutinho et al. 1995) or promiscuity (Gavin and Bevan 1995), indicating an evolutionary strategy that covers all possibilities and would thus conform to continuous distributions, if with high degeneracy. As argued before (Coutinho 2000), this might be particularly relevant in Treg selection at critical developmental times when TCR repertoires are extremely limited in numbers. Hence, the conventional proposal that embryonic/perinatal multireactivity is favored for reasons of anti-infectious defense makes little sense, since this is ensured by mother-derived passive protection that is paramount at precisely these developmental times.

3
The MM96 Solution to the Thymic Sorting of Emergent TCR Repertoires: Differential Roles of TECs and THCs on Treg Selection

The MM96 has solved these two problems, as it proposes that the highest subdeletional TCR self-affinities necessarily result in (activation and) commitment of selected cells to the regulatory pathway. This postulate provides for a double fail-safe mechanism to avoid pathogenic autoreactivity. On the one hand, the process of sorting the emergent TCR diversity includes the affinity-dependent selection of autoreactive Tregs, which conveniently isolates naïve T cell repertoires to well below autoreactivity thresholds, and provides for protecting cells with self-affinities that necessarily supersede those of aggressive cells. In short, a default pathway selects wobbling TCRs to Tregs. On the other hand, the intrathymic commitment of Treg imposes self-protective functions to the most autoreactive TCR repertoires reaching the periphery, thus excluding their association with other effector functions in the Russian roulette of activation contexts.

The MM96, on the other hand, also explains the apparently contradictory findings that high self-affinity may lead to either deletion or Treg generation, by postulating distinct T cell fates following antigen recognition on either epithelial (TECs) or hemopoietic (THCs) stromal cells. For the same TCR, differentiating T cell fate is determined by the type of presenting cell (APCs) on which it recognizes antigen, a postulate that allows for (developmental) regulation of the generation or relative abundance of Treg by varying the differential composition of the thymic stroma. The suggestion that repertoires of high-affinity autoreactive Treg are predominantly directed at self-antigens expressed by deletion-incompetent TECs, but not by THCs, was derived from Le Douarin's experiments (Ohki et al. 1987, 1988; Salaun et al. 1990; Coutinho et al. 1993). Yet, it has now gained new relevance given the observations that a large set of tissue-specific autoantigens is *selectively* expressed by TECs (Derbinski et al. 2001; Anderson et al. 2002; Gotter et al. 2004). Thus, the MM96 predicts that *thymic selection necessarily produces high-affinity, tissue-specific Treg, which cannot be eliminated by deletion-competent THCs that fail to express that set of autoantigens*. Selective expression of tissue-specific antigens by TECs would thus be the key strategy in the construction of autoreactive Treg repertoires. In contrast, *autoreactive TCRs within the same range of affinities but directed to antigens (also) expressed on THCs are deleted, thus purging Treg functions from the peripheral repertoires of positively selected antigen-reactive T cells that respond to foreign peptides presented by professional APCs.* Hence, conventional immune responses would be little, if at all, limited by Treg. Such a division of labor in TCR repertoire selection, together with the genetic mechanisms that allow for promiscuous gene expression (Klein and Kyewski 2000; Derbinski et al. 2001; Anderson et al. 2002; Gotter et al. 2004) and T cell-fate decisions (Fontenot et al. 2003; Hori et al. 2003; Khattri et al. 2003) result in a clear predominance of self-tissue-specific Treg and in their underrepresentation among repertoires directed at non-self antigens and the APCs that handle them. As seen above, this same process contributes to generating the fail-safe mechanism that ensures the absence of potential tissue-specific immune pathology. Thus, productive TCR autoreactivities that are not deleted will necessarily be turned into Treg effector functions, providing for the isolation of autoreactive T cell affinities from those of positively selected T cells.

Within this framework, tolerance to all antigens expressed by THCs has a deletional basis, notwithstanding borderline TCR affinity ranges or cell frequencies, which might always be demonstrated in extreme conditions. This seems to be the case in the experimental system introduced by Medawar and colleagues (Billingham et al. 1953), where tolerance is induced if hemopoietic cells (but not those of other peripheral tissues!) are injected at birth (but not later!) into semi-allogeneic hosts. Thus, if some evidence for dominant, CD4 T cell-dependent mechanisms has been produced (Roser 1989), it seems that Medawar's tolerance essentially results from deletion (Gruchalla and Streilein 1982). Likewise, it would be expected that tolerance to all proteins that are present in circulation at high concentrations, and may be presented by THCs, is recessive as well. This is suggested in classical experiments on physiological tolerance to C5 (Harris et al. 1982; Zal et al. 1994), although Treg may also play a significant role in self-tolerance to this set of antigens (Cairns et al. 1986; Boguniewicz et al. 1989; van den Berg et al. 1991). In contrast, antigens (artificially) introduced in the thymus on cells other than THCs, might be expected to generate Treg and induce dominant tolerance. This has been described for intrathymic grafts of peripheral tissues (Posselt et al. 1990; Gerling et al. 1992; Charlton et al. 1994; Turvey et al. 1999; Salaun et al. 2002), which were shown to overcome and control pathogenic autoimmunity toward the specific tissue.

The model would predict that major deviations from physiology are brought about by alterations in the correct presentation of antigens by TECs or THCs. Treg defects are expected to arise from either deficient promiscuous expression or presentation of tissue antigens by TECs, or else, by their ectopic presentation on THCs (Shih et al. 2004). Likewise, presentation of extrathymic antigens by either cell type may result in pathology, particularly in cases where peripheral self is abnormally expressed by THCs or non-self becomes available on TECs. For example, if peripheral tissue damage releases into circulation tissue-specific proteins that reach the thymus in concentrations that are high enough to be presented by THCs, Treg deletion ensues and tissue-specific autoimmunity may arise. Conversely, non-self (e.g., viral) antigen presentation by TECs, if selective, would be expected to result in specific Treg generation, and in the inability to eliminate the virus. This is probably a very unusual condition, as it can be expected that the same antigens are also presented by THCs and delete virus-specific Treg. On the other hand, in conditions where extensive depletion of THCs takes place, as could be the case in HIV infection, this hypothesis, however strange, should perhaps not be excluded.

4
Promiscuous Tissue-Antigen Expression in TECs Selects Treg Repertoires: The Origin and Range of Autoimmune Diseases

In autoimmune repertoires, a most interesting question relates to the limited number of clinically identified AID. Thus, recessive tolerance models would predict as many distinct diseases as the number of autoreactive clones, or at least, as the number of autoantigens. The limitation in the range of clinical AID led Cohen to suggest that autoreactive repertoires would be focused onto a subset of autoantigens that he designated as "immunological homunculus" (Cohen and Young 1991). Evidence for these notions has been obtained in the analysis of physiological autoreactivities among natural antibodies in healthy individuals, which are restricted to a subset of autoantigens (Nobrega et al. 1993; Mouthon et al. 1995). As Cohen argues for a kind of dominant tolerance, which does not involve sorting of TCR repertoires between Treg and naïve T cells, this bias in both physiological and pathological autoreactivity had to be explained by global properties of T and B cell repertoires, which remain poorly analyzed. In the context of dominant tolerance mediated by a distinct lymphocyte lineage, however, AID can be attributed to failures in the repertoires or functional competence of Treg with unique TCR repertoires, which are selected by the promiscuous subset of thymic autoantigens. It follows that the range of AID would be determined by the original biases in Treg repertoires—ultimately delineated by the antigenic composition of TECs—irrespective of the peripheral availability of potentially pathogenic effector T and B cells to all sorts of autoantigens. This hypothesis is robust. Because it is based on the dominance of a particular repertoire (the Treg repertoire), it accounts for autoreactive repertoire biases in both physiology and disease, and in both T and B cells. Interestingly, recent observations may be used in support of these notions, as they demonstrate that a given genetic defect (e.g., TGFβ, PD-1 KO), possibly associated with Treg function, will vary in its disease manifestations according to the genetic background (Shull et al. 1992; Dang et al. 1995; Yaswen et al. 1996; Nishimura et al. 1998, 1999, 2001). This had already been described in the seminal observations of Kojima who first analyzed the strain dependence of AID manifestations following newborn thymectomy (Kojima and Prehn 1981). Also here, in conditions where disease does result from limitations in Treg (Sakaguchi et al. 1995), AID manifestations vary with the genetic background, while remaining limited in scope and directed to a few typical targets (e.g., thyroid, stomach, ovary, testicles). In other words, *while Treg generation determines health or disease and sets a specific range of tissue targets (following Treg selection on promiscuous TECs), other genes, possibly truly tissue-specific, will determine the precise disease-associated clonal specificities.* In the frame of the MM96, tissue-antigen expression by TECs (Derbinski et al. 2001; Anderson et al. 2002; Gotter et al. 2004) provides a satisfactory explanation for the limitation in AID syndromes, by describing the set of potentially homuncular self-antigens (Cohen and Young 1991), which represent the targets of Treg repertoires. The nature of Treg deficits would determine the range of disease-associated specificities: for localized failures, pathogenic specificities are those found in the physiological autoreactivity of healthy individuals, modified by helper cell-dependent processes of class-switch and affinity maturation. This seems to be the case for autoantibodies in a variety of AID (Shlomchik et al. 1987). In contrast, it could be expected that generalized defects of Treg result in the indiscriminate production of autoantibodies and pathogenic T cells (e.g., TGFβ KO mice) (Shull et al. 1992; Dang et al. 1995; Yaswen et al. 1996).

Finally, this discussion brings forth the notion that AID pathogeny may well begin with deficits in Treg selection on TECs, as it is highly unlikely that Treg defects will ever result from limitations in somatically and randomly generated TCR repertoires. In short, AID may well be TEC diseases, as direct evidence actually indicates (Forsgren et al. 1991; Thomas-Vaslin et al. 1997; Salaun et al. 2002). If some truth exists in these hypotheses, this would suggest a major shift in current research focus, by seeking AID origin elsewhere than in the peripheral antigenic targets. Evidence for the innocent nature of tissue antigen expression in organ-specific AID has been produced by Holmberg et al. in tetraparental mice (Forsgren et al. 1991). Thus, AID development in embryo-fusion chimeras between an autoimmune (NOD) and a normal strain, in which all tissues were variable mosaics of cells from both origins, correlated with the thymic composition, rather than with that of the peripheral target tissues: if most of the thymus (perhaps TECs) happened to be from the NOD donor, AID developed even when pancreatic islands were normal; in contrast, if the thymus was mostly normal, there was no pathogenic autoimmunity toward NOD islands (Forsgren et al. 1991).

5
Beyond TCR Repertoires: A Unique Differentiative Lineage, That May Represent Class Regulation Operating Intrathymically

Results from Hori et al. and others (Fontenot et al. 2003; Hori et al. 2003; Khattri et al. 2003) brought direct support to the MM96 claim that Tregs represent a unique differentiative lineage, committed upon TCR affinity-dependent activation on TECs. This relationship of Treg commitment (expression of FOXP3) with TEC- and TCR-dependent activation, however, has yet to be ascertained, and it may result from the differential expression of Notch-pathway receptors and/or ligands by TECs (Anderson et al. 2001). For the MM96, the key feature is that Treg cell fate is TCR-dependent and established intrathymically, such that a unique self-reactive repertoire is irreversibly associated with a unique effector function (Zelenay et al. 2005). Accordingly, while the results of specific Foxp3 expression in Treg leave room for extrathymic education of naïve T cells into the Treg pathway (Chen et al. 2003; Cobbold et al. 2004; Fantini et al. 2004; Park et al. 2004; Zheng et al. 2004), they also clearly demonstrate commitment of differentiating CD4 T cells inside the thymus, as predicted (Modigliani et al. 1996b). The MM96 also postulated that Treg "positive selection and functional commitment" inside the thymus was accompanied by cellular activation[3], such that the process would be equivalent to the "class regulation" of naïve CD4 T cells in the periphery (Mosmann et al. 1986). Since the fail-safe mechanism to ensure is the sorting of TCRs to a particular functional class before thymic export, however, the postulate of intrathymic activation of Tregs is dispensable if Tregs are committed to a unique functional lineage upon TCR-dependent selection. It should be noted that the MM96 is entirely based on TCR-affinity selection, and it does not require ad hoc postulates on properties of Treg, such as resistance to negative selection. This alternative would require that an independent differentiative lineage of CD4 T cells is committed prior to selection, and it would thus be incompatible with an appropriate sorting of emergent TCR repertoires into naïve vs Treg classes. For the MM96, cell fate determination results from TCR-dependent selection. If Treg lineage determination is equivalent to the process of Th1/Th2 commitment in the periphery, it could be expected that TCR-dependent selection on TECs, within a given affinity range, activates a genetic cascade, which

---

[3] Both the MM96 and its present application to recent findings do not depend on a precise definition of positive selection. It is irrelevant whether Tregs are expanded with or after commitment, or whether such TCRs are simply preserved from deletion at a one-to-one ratio between precursor and mature cells. Thus, either alternative finds abundant room within the wide range of emerging TCR affinities to self-antigens expressed by TECs.

is likely mediated by FOXP3 and involves downstream activation of a set of genes associated with Treg development (CD25, CTLA-4, TLR-4, etc.), as well as inactivation of others (e.g., IL-2). In turn, the suspected involvement of the Notch pathway in the generation of Treg (Anastasi et al. 2003; Vigouroux et al. 2003) possibly owing to differential expression of Notch-ligands by TECs and THCs in thymic stroma, could explain the alternative cell fates (Treg commitment vs cell death), upon productive antigen recognition by developing CD4 T cells on either type of presenting cells.

As discussed in the MM96, other mechanisms must account for the putative generation of Treg with specificities for self-antigens outside the thymus. Based on the observations that recent thymic emigrants (RTE) could be recruited in the periphery for entering the regulatory pathway (Modigliani et al. 1996a), a process that Waldmann and colleagues called "infectious tolerance" (Qin et al. 1993), the peripheral activation-dependent commitment of RTE to regulatory functions was proposed (Modigliani et al. 1996b). This would occur when RTE recognize tissue-antigens in the presence of thymically committed Treg with specificities for other antigens expressed on the same cells, providing for some sort of antigen spreading in self-tolerance. Accordingly, linked suppression mediated by Treg has now been demonstrated in a variety of models (Wise et al. 1998; Honey et al. 2000; Thornton and Shevach 2000; Weiner 2001; Jiang et al. 2003; Graca et al. 2004), and the data of Hori and others (Fontenot et al. 2003; Hori et al. 2003; Khattri et al. 2003) leave room for peripheral commitment of naïve T cells to regulatory functions. At first analysis, promiscuous expression of tissue-specific antigens by TECs would seem to solve the problem of functionally uncommitted (and, thus, potentially pathogenic) naïve tissue-specific cells exiting the thymus. Clearly, however, any model of thymic selection must deal with an emergent TCR diversity toward truly tissue-specific antigens that are not included in the promiscuous subset, at least at high levels of expression. Some of these T cells will necessarily be positively selected and seed the periphery, providing for a range of specific pathogenic potential. The physiological existence of such T cells is readily demonstrated by the experimental induction of AID in healthy individuals (Weigle 1980; Wekerle 1992, 1996; Boon et al. 1994) and by direct determinations on their frequencies (Lohse et al. 1996). Hence, natural tolerance requires either the continuous suppression of naïve autoreactive cells by thymic-derived Treg, or else, the more robust mechanism of their peripheral, antigen-dependent recruitment to Treg functions, as suggested in the MM96. Yet several types of experiments have failed to demonstrate peripheral recruitment of tissue-specific Treg (Hori et al. 2002b) in the absence of manipulations interfering with antigen-recognition by CD4 T cells (Graca et al. 2003; Waldmann 2003). While there is solid evidence for antigen-dependent extrathymic education of naïve T cells to Treg in the latter conditions (Qin et al. 1993; Wise et al. 1998; Honey et al. 2000; Graca et al. 2004), opening great promise in transplantation tolerance, the relevance of infectious dominance for natural tolerance remains unclear.

Interestingly, RTEs, which apparently maintain cell-fate decisions open for some time and are recruitable to the Treg pathway (Modigliani et al. 1996a), may first recognize peripheral antigens on epithelial cells (e.g., at mucosal surfaces). If differentiative rules that apply here are similar to those inside the thymus, this could explain the ease in inducing mucosal tolerance (Wu and Weiner 2003), as well as the findings of dominance in this phenomenon (Weiner 2001; Unger et al. 2003) and of abundant T cells producing TGF-β (a proposed mediator of Treg activity [Fukaura et al. 1996; Weiner 2001]) in the mucosa. Again, particulars of Notch-ligand expression on epithelial cells (Anderson et al. 2001) could apply here as well.

Finally, as discussed below, it is hypothetically plausible that thymically committed Treg are not (all) Class II MHC-restricted. If this were true, and if peripheral recruitment of RTE to the regulatory pathway is a physiologically relevant process, then the Treg population in normal individuals is heterogeneous, containing both thymically committed Treg, as well as cells that have exited the thymus as MHC-restricted, resting naïve T cells. It is perhaps likely that these putative developmental classes of Treg, distinguished by their MHC restriction and, thus, specificity, would also differ in functional competence, patterns of gene expression, markers, population dynamics, and physiological roles. To be confirmed, a period of confusing descriptions and controversies would inevitably occur, which could explain arising disagreements.

6
The Question on the Putative MHC Restriction of Treg: Yet Another Difference Between the Thymic Selection of Treg and Naïve T Cells?

Treg development is far from solved or even principally understood. For example, there is little or no information on the MHC restriction of Treg, if actually these cells are at all MHC-restricted. As MHC restriction results from thymic selection (Bevan 1977; Bevan and Fink 1978; Zinkernagel et al. 1978), there is no a priori reason to exclude that Treg would view antigens as whole proteins, using TCR for an antibody-like recognition of protein surfaces, and remain available for selection in the emergent repertoires, just as occurs for other primitive T cells types (e.g., NK T cells [Bendelac et al. 1997; Taniguchi et al. 2003]) and for conventional T cells exposed to superantigens

(Marrack et al. 1993). Alternatively, Treg may be selected to recognize peptides presented by invariant chaperons, such as HSPs (Gullo and Teoh 2004), in which case their repertoires, while restricted and peptide-specific, would not show MHC-dependent variation. Finally, Treg could be thought to recognize antigenic self-peptides on Class I MHC, as could be indicated by the fact that the promiscuous antigens expressed by TECs are endogenous proteins to the presenting cell and, thus, more likely to engage in this pathway.

On the other hand, if Treg are Class II MHC-restricted, they can only scan tissues under conditions that promote Class II expression (e.g., inflammation), or else, via physiological tissue-antigen transfer to professional APCs, possibly in draining lymph nodes. Either alternative is incompatible with MM96 postulates on thymic selection. Furthermore, the first possibility is also incompatible with the established requirement for peripheral antigen in the physiological survival of Treg (Seddon and Mason 1999; Cozzo et al. 2003; Lerman et al. 2004), while the second poses the central question on how to induce immune responses in a context of dominant suppression, if non-self antigens are presented by the same professional APCs that simultaneously present self-tissue antigens to Treg. In addition, physiological processing and MHC-(cross)presentation of tissue-specific antigens by draining APCs seem to provide conditions that would favor activation of the entire set of tissue peptide-specific autoreactive T cells, which exit the thymus as naïve lymphocytes precisely after selection for MHC-restriction. In short, either Treg and naïve tissue-specific T cells interact on professional APC clusters, in which case responses to self- and non-self-antigens would be equally linked suppressed and self/non-self discrimination jeopardized, or else Treg-dependent suppression relies on other cellular sites or mechanisms. These may be quite diverse, such as Treg-dependent control of tissue immunogenicity or of the expression of tissue-protective genes (Pae et al. 2003). As another nonexclusive scenario, direct interactions of Treg with MHC-restricted naïve T cells may always be possible in species where (activated) CD4 T cells express Class II, and even in mouse if Treg pick up Class II molecules along the course of their thymic development or upon arrival in the periphery. Class II acquisition by activated T cells has been demonstrated (Elliott et al. 1980; Patel et al. 1999; Walker and Mannie 2002; Tsang et al. 2003), and it is expected to preferentially concern Treg as they engage in tissue-specific complexes. These are obviously too many speculations for too few data, but the finding of (some) CD4 T cells in Class II-negative animals, some of which bear Treg markers (Bensinger et al. 2001), could be interpreted by the notion that Treg are also not conventional in regards MHC restriction.

Likewise, little information is available on the age-dependent production of Treg, and on their population dynamics throughout life. These are critical parameters for understanding the time window in natural tolerance acquisition and the physiopathology of Treg, notably that many AID are first manifested around or soon after puberty. The MM96 suggested that Treg are predominantly produced during embryonic and perinatal life, during the time window of natural tolerance acquisition, precisely when the thymus contains self-antigens exclusively and is secluded with certainty from microbial exposure. As seen above, this was explained by the relative predominance of TEC and THC in the composition of the thymic stroma, the former generating (self-specific) Treg, whereas the latter delete them. In contrast, the findings of autoimmune pathology in animals that are thymectomized 3 days after birth has been interpreted to indicate that Treg production and/or export is antedated by the export of tissue-specific naïve, MHC-restricted T cells (Asano et al. 1996). As argued by others, however, alternative interpretations are possible, as the experiments only show that, under those conditions, the physiological balance between Treg and naïve T cells is biased toward the latter in quantitative terms (Suri-Payer et al. 1999; Dujardin et al. 2004). As peripheral T cell pools after thymectomy are built by proliferation of preexisting T cells rather than by accumulation of newly-formed T cells exiting the thymus, as in normal conditions (Modigliani et al. 1994), and given the limitations of Treg to expand (Annacker et al. 2001; Almeida et al. 2002; Gavin et al. 2002), it is expected that such bias will always ensue irrespective of a putative Treg excess at the start. Further arguments in this direction can be invoked from the rather precise time requirements for thymectomy (perhaps representing a unique initial ratio of Treg/Tnaïve that, after expansion, would result in pathogenic imbalance), and from the frequencies and limited range of target-organ specificities of autoimmune manifestations. These are individually variable, and often limited to a particular tissue, indicating that enough Treg toward most self-tissues had been produced at the time of thymectomy. In other words, considering all tissues in all individuals thymectomized, autoimmunity is the exception rather than the rule, the strain specificity of the most frequent manifestations perhaps indicating strain-specific lower rates of Treg production for those particular antigens (possibly due to insufficient TEC expression). The medical relevance of this question is obvious, as AID are typically diseases of young adults, often first manifested at puberty, precisely when thymic production declines. Most unfortunately, other than the fact that thymic involution is autonomously controlled by TEC (Ohki et al. 1988), the molecular and cellular bases of this process are not clear, and we are currently unable to regulate (e.g., stimulate) de novo T cell production by either biological or pharmacological means.

7
Selective TLR Expresssion by Treg: Evolutionary Significance and a Possible Handle on Treg Regulation

Caramalho and colleagues have reported the surprising finding that murine Treg express transcripts for seven of nine Toll-like receptors they have studied, and that four of these are not expressed by conventional CD4 T cells, either before or after activation (Caramalho et al. 2003). Furthermore, they have shown that Treg actually respond to pro-inflammatory agents and inflammatory conditions that are known to involve this set of innate receptors (Caramalho et al., submitted). The expression of TLRs on T cells has been extended to humans (Komai-Koma et al. 2004) and, together with the findings of Treg amplification by conventional T cell responses (Almeida et al. 2002; Caramalho et al., submitted), shed new light on the operation of Treg and the general physiological regulation of this cell subset. In addition, these findings could contain the solution for current controversies on Treg markers, on distinct cellular and molecular mechanisms of regulation, eventually, on the range of Treg specificities. Most importantly, they may provide the explanation for the intimate and twofold relationship of infections with autoimmunity: on the one hand, the surprisingly low frequency of autoimmune manifestations accompanying infections, given the wide range of molecular mimicries (Albert and Inman 1999; Rose and Mackay 2000; Benoist and Mathis 2001), on the other hand, the inverse correlation between certain infections and autoimmune diseases (Oldstone and Dixon 1972; Oldstone et al. 1990; Bras and Aguas 1996; Das et al. 1996; Cooke et al. 1999) or atopy (Matricardi et al. 1997, 2000; Bjorksten et al. 1999; Kalliomaki et al. 2001; Zuany-Amorim et al. 2002; Rodriguez et al. 2003), which has been established epidemiologically (Leibowitz et al. 1966; Greenwood 1968; Kurtzke 1995; Matricardi et al. 1997, 2000; Bjorksten et al. 1999; Group 2000; Kalliomaki et al. 2001) and experimentally demonstrated (Oldstone and Dixon 1972; Oldstone et al. 1990; Bras and Aguas 1996; Das et al. 1996; Cooke et al. 1999; Rodriguez et al. 2003). Thus, in acute infections, stimulation of Treg activity by the infectious inflammatory process itself may explain the natural limitation of the pathological process. Accordingly, absence or deficits of Treg number or function invariably result in marked exacerbation of infection-associated immunopathologies. Thus, depending upon the sites colonized by often opportunistic pathogens, Treg deficiency results in either local inflammatory diseases (e.g., bowel, lung, or skin, [Read et al. 2000; Belkaid et al. 2002; Hori et al. 2002a), or in increased severity of systemic symptoms (E. Seixas, unpublished observations). Conversely, a number of spontaneous autoimmune and allergic manifestations are prevented or ameliorated by infection with a wide variety of pathogens (Bach

2001, 2002; Wills-Karp et al. 2001; Yazdanbakhsh et al. 2002). In all observations that are now available, no specificity of Treg to microbial antigens has been described, suggesting that self-specific Tregs are actually stimulated via TLR recognition of microbial mitogens, as well as by the antigen-dependent activation of microbe-specific naïve T cells.

These considerations are obviously related to the epidemiological evidence for the alarming increases in the frequency of allergic and AID in the Western world, and its explanation by the hygiene hypothesis (Strachan 1989; Wills-Karp et al. 2001; Bach 2002; Yazdanbakhsh et al. 2002). The role of Treg and their physiological stimulation by infectious agents indicate a major evolutionary significance of this cell subset and of their responsiveness to innate signals. In turn, this would suggest that modern medicine, which has eradicated—through hygiene, vaccination, and antibiotics—most common childhood infections, now has to face the clinical consequences of a defective natural stimulation of Treg. The obvious response to the present situation is to discover alternative manners to maintain overall Treg levels above disease thresholds. Given the loss of sustained microbial stimulation of Treg in our societies, increased susceptibility to allergies and AID may reveal partial dysfunctions in any of the developmental processes discussed here, which would otherwise pass unnoticed. Thus, promiscuous autoantigen expression by TECs, repertoire selection/cell-fate decisions in the thymus, maturation of effector functions, and Treg population dynamics are all under genetic controls that are likely to show variability in human populations, and may well be read out as autoimmune susceptibility loci. Likewise, the well-established fact that such complex diseases require environmental interactions with a genetic constitution of variable susceptibility may reflect the frequency of subclinical infections, as well as external influences on Treg generation and performance. Many of these processes relate to thymic function and may represent suitable targets for future therapeutic interventions. Finally, all the genetically controlled physiological mechanisms discussed here must follow quantitative rules that are not even considered in the present discussion. Hence, it is also likely that environmental conditions exist that exceed the physiological levels of Treg operation and will, therefore, result in and/or amplify pathogenicity.

In summary, these recent findings on Treg regulation may offer novel targets for therapeutic intervention and a new understanding of the evolution of mechanisms involved in the establishment of natural tolerance.

8
Regulatory T Cells Versus Phenomenology on Regulation

A final note to clarify a very large set of phenomena pertaining to regulation, which are currently attributed to diverse cellular compartments from the regulatory T cells, warrants discussion here. Thus, with the gain in popularity of notions such as physiological autoreactivity (Coutinho 2000; Coutinho et al. 2001) and dominant tolerance (Shevach 2000; Graca et al. 2003; Sakaguchi 2004; Thompson and Powrie 2004), and with the widespread acceptance of Treg, many types of findings are currently attributed to regulation, and the designation of "regulatory" is given to many a cell or molecule! This is certainly unwarranted and confusing. For example, 7S suppression was the very first phenomenon of regulation ever described (Henry and Jerne 1968), but we do not refer to IgG-secreting plasma cells as regulatory. Thus, plasma cell function is antibody secretion; if the antibodies suppress other antibody responses—or enhance them, as is the case for the IgM class—we do not classify the secreting cells as suppressor and helper plasmacytes, respectively. Seemingly, Th1 cells suppress the generation/activity of Th2 cells and vice-versa. Yet, we do not refer to these differentiated stages of helper T cells as regulatory. It would seem appropriate to reserve the designation of "regulatory T cells" to those lymphocytes that specifically differentiate to the particular function of regulating other cells' activities. Conversely, it may well be that regulatory T cells will end up promoting one or another class of immune responses as a consequence of their regulatory activity. Yet, we will continue to refer to them as regulatory T cells, rather than Th2, Th3, or anything else. This is one of the reasons why we prefer the present designation, as opposed to "suppressor T cells". This argument is strengthened by the notion that Treg represent an independent differentiative lineage of T cell, displaying a specific pattern of gene expression, and following specific rules for selection, population dynamics, and operation. In other words, the criterion for demarcation might be the fundamental difference between Treg and all other varieties of CD4 T cell classes or effector types: Treg are committed intrathymically, while all other T cells exit the thymic womb as naïve, functionally uncommitted cells. Moreover, Treg seem to be selected on nominal antigen (if promiscuously expressed) inside the thymus, while other T cells seem to be merely restricted for the recognition of antigens yet to be encountered in the periphery. Having said this, it would be foolish to ignore many of those regulation processes, which are mediated by lymphocytes or other cells that are not born to regulate. These may well contribute to the overall physiological processes of tolerance and regulation of immune responses.

Acknowledgements This work was supported in part by a project grant on malaria from the Fundação Calouste Gulbenkian, by the Fundação para a Ciência e a Tecnologia (Portugal), and by the Centre National de la Recherche Scientifique (France). The Instituto Gulbenkian de Ciência was founded and is supported by the Fundação Calouste Gulbenkian. We thank our colleagues at the Institutes in Oeiras, Nogent, and Paris for many productive discussions.

References

Albert LJ, Inman RD (1999) Molecular mimicry and autoimmunity. N Engl J Med 341:2068–2074

Almeida AR, Legrand N, Papiernik M, Freitas AA (2002) Homeostasis of peripheral CD4+ T cells: IL-2R alpha and IL-2 shape a population of regulatory cells that controls CD4+ T cell numbers. J Immunol 169:4850–4860

Anastasi E, Campese AF, Bellavia D, Bulotta A, Balestri A, Pascucci M, Checquolo S, Gradini R, Lendahl U, Frati L, Gulino A, Di Mario U, Screpanti I (2003) Expression of activated Notch3 in transgenic mice enhances generation of T regulatory cells and protects against experimental autoimmune diabetes. J Immunol 171:4504–4511

Anderson G, Pongracz J, Parnell S, Jenkinson EJ (2001) Notch ligand-bearing thymic epithelial cells initiate and sustain Notch signaling in thymocytes independently of T cell receptor signaling. Eur J Immunol 31:3349–3354

Anderson MS, Venanzi ES, Klein L, Chen Z, Berzins SP, Turley SJ, von Boehmer H, Bronson R, Dierich A, Benoist C, Mathis D (2002) Projection of an immunological self shadow within the thymus by the aire protein. Science 298:1395–1401

Annacker O, Pimenta-Araujo R, Burlen-Defranoux O, Barbosa TC, Cumano A, Bandeira A (2001) CD25+ CD4+ T cells regulate the expansion of peripheral CD4 T cells through the production of IL-10. J Immunol 166:3008–3018

Apostolou I, Sarukhan A, Klein L, von Boehmer H (2002) Origin of regulatory T cells with known specificity for antigen. Nat Immunol 3:756–763

Asano M, Toda M, Sakaguchi N, Sakaguchi S (1996) Autoimmune disease as a consequence of developmental abnormality of a T cell subpopulation. J Exp Med 184:387–396

Bach JF (2001) Protective role of infections and vaccinations on autoimmune diseases. J Autoimmun 16:347–353

Bach JF (2002) The effect of infections on susceptibility to autoimmune and allergic diseases. N Engl J Med 347:911–920

Bach JF, Francois Bach J (2003) Regulatory T cells under scrutiny. Nat Rev Immunol 3:189–198

Belkaid Y, Piccirillo CA, Mendez S, Shevach EM, Sacks DL (2002) CD4+CD25+ regulatory T cells control Leishmania major persistence and immunity. Nature 420:502–507

Bendelac A, Rivera MN, Park SH, Roark JH (1997) Mouse CD1-specific NK1 T cells: development, specificity, and function. Annu Rev Immunol 15:535–562

Benoist C, Mathis D (2001) Autoimmunity provoked by infection: how good is the case for T cell epitope mimicry? Nat Immunol 2:797–801

Bensinger SJ, Bandeira A, Jordan MS, Caton AJ, Laufer TM (2001) Major histocompatibility complex class II-positive cortical epithelium mediates the selection of CD4(+)25(+) immunoregulatory T cells. J Exp Med 194:427–438

Bevan MJ (1977) In a radiation chimaera, host H-2 antigens determine immune responsiveness of donor cytotoxic cells. Nature 269:417–418

Bevan MJ, Fink PJ (1978) The influence of thymus H-2 antigens on the specificity of maturing killer and helper cells. Immunol Rev 42:3–19

Billingham RE, Brent L, Medawar PB (1953) Activity acquired tolerance of foreign cells. Nature 172:603–606

Bjorksten B, Naaber P, Sepp E, Mikelsaar M (1999) The intestinal microflora in allergic Estonian and Swedish 2-year-old children. Clin Exp Allergy 29:342–346

Boguniewicz M, Sunshine GH, Borel Y (1989) Role of the thymus in natural tolerance to an autologous protein antigen. J Exp Med 169:285–290

Boon T, Cerottini JC, Van den Eynde B, van der Bruggen P, Van Pel A (1994) Tumor antigens recognized by T lymphocytes. Annu Rev Immunol 12:337–365

Bras A, Aguas AP (1996) Diabetes-prone NOD mice are resistant to Mycobacterium avium and the infection prevents autoimmune disease. Immunology 89:20–25

Cairns L, Rosen FS, Borel Y (1986) Mice naturally tolerant to C5 have T cells that suppress the response to this antigen. Eur J Immunol 16:1277–1282

Caramalho I, Lopes-Carvalho T, Ostler D, Zelenay S, Haury M, Demengeot J (2003) Regulatory T cells selectively express toll-like receptors and are activated by lipopolysaccharide. J Exp Med 197:403–411

Charlton B, Taylor-Edwards C, Tisch R, Fathman CG (1994) Prevention of diabetes and insulitis by neonatal intrathymic islet administration in NOD mice. J Autoimmun 7:549–560

Chen W, Jin W, Hardegen N, Lei KJ, Li L, Marinos N, McGrady G, Wahl SM (2003) Conversion of peripheral CD4+CD25– naive T cells to CD4+CD25+ regulatory T cells by TGF-beta induction of transcription factor Foxp3. J Exp Med 198:1875–1886

Cobbold SP, Castejon R, Adams E, Zelenika D, Graca L, Humm S, Waldmann H (2004) Induction of foxP3+ regulatory T cells in the periphery of T cell receptor transgenic mice tolerized to transplants. J Immunol 172:6003–6010

Cohen IR, Young DB (1991) Autoimmunity, microbial immunity and the immunological homunculus. Immunol Today 12:105–110

Cohn M, Langman RE (1990) The protection: the unit of humoral immunity selected by evolution. Immunol Rev 115:11–147

Cooke A, Tonks P, Jones FM, O'Shea H, Hutchings P, Fulford AJ, Dunne DW (1999) Infection with Schistosoma mansoni prevents insulin dependent diabetes mellitus in non-obese diabetic mice. Parasite Immunol 21:169–176

Coutinho A (1975) The theory of the 'one nonspecific signal' model for B cell activation. Transplant Rev 23:49–65

Coutinho A (1980) The self-nonself discrimination and the nature and acquisition of the antibody repertoire. Ann Immunol (Paris). 131D:235–253

Coutinho A (2000) Germ-line selection ensures embryonic autoreactivity and a positive discrimination of self mediated by supraclonal mechanisms. Semin Immunol 12:205–213; discussion 257–344

Coutinho A, Gronowicz E, Bullock WW, Moller G (1974) Mechanism of thymus-independent immunocyte triggering. Mitogenic activation of B cells results in specific immune responses. J Exp Med 139:74–92

Coutinho A, Coutinho G, Grandien A, Marcos MA, Bandeira A (1992) Some reasons why deletion and anergy do not satisfactorily account for natural tolerance. Res Immunol 143:345–354

Coutinho A, Salaun J, Corbel C, Bandeira A, Le Douarin N (1993) The role of thymic epithelium in the establishment of transplantation tolerance. Immunol Rev 133:225–240

Coutinho A, Kazatchkine MD, Avrameas S (1995) Natural autoantibodies. Curr Opin Immunol 7:812–818

Coutinho A, Hori S, Carvalho T, Caramalho I, Demengeot J (2001) Regulatory T cells: the physiology of autoreactivity in dominant tolerance and "quality control" of immune responses. Immunol Rev 182:89–98

Cozzo C, Larkin J 3rd, Caton AJ (2003) Cutting edge: self-peptides drive the peripheral expansion of CD4+CD25+ regulatory T cells. J Immunol 171:5678–5682

Curotto de Lafaille MA, Muriglan S, Sunshine MJ, Lei Y, Kutchukhidze N, Furtado GC, Wensky AK, Olivares-Villagomez D, Lafaille JJ (2001) Hyper immunoglobulin E response in mice with monoclonal populations of B, T lymphocytes. J Exp Med 194:1349–1359

Dang H, Geiser AG, Letterio JJ, Nakabayashi T, Kong L, Fernandes G, Talal N (1995) SLE-like autoantibodies and Sjogren's syndrome-like lymphoproliferation in TGF-beta knockout mice. J Immunol 155:3205–3212

Das MR, Cohen A, Zamvil SS, Offner H, Kuchroo VK (1996) Prior exposure to superantigen can inhibit or exacerbate autoimmune encephalomyelitis: T-cell repertoire engaged by the autoantigen determines clinical outcome. J Neuroimmunol 71:3–10

Derbinski J, Schulte A, Kyewski B, Klein L (2001) Promiscuous gene expression in medullary thymic epithelial cells mirrors the peripheral self. Nat Immunol 2:1032–1039

Dujardin HC, Burlen-Defranoux O, Boucontet L, Vieira P, Cumano A, Bandeira A (2004) Regulatory potential and control of Foxp3 expression in newborn $CD4^+$ T cells. Proc Natl Acad Sci U S A. 101:14473–14478

Elliott BE, Nagy ZA, Takacs BJ, Ben-Neriah Y, Givol D (1980) Antigen-binding receptors on T cells from long-term MLR. evidence of binding sites for allogeneic and self-MHC products. Immunogenetics 11:177–190

Fantini MC, Becker C, Monteleone G, Pallone F, Galle PR, Neurath MF (2004) Cutting edge: TGF-beta induces a regulatory phenotype in CD4+CD25− T cells through Foxp3 induction and down-regulation of Smad7. J Immunol 172:5149–5153

Fontenot JD, Gavin MA, Rudensky AY (2003) Foxp3 programs the development and function of CD4+CD25+ regulatory T cells. Nat Immunol 4:330–336

Forsgren S, Dahl U, Soderstrom A, Holmberg D, Matsunaga T (1991) The phenotype of lymphoid cells and thymic epithelium correlates with development of autoimmune insulitis in NOD in equilibrium with C57BL/6 allophenic chimeras. Proc Natl Acad Sci U S A 88:9335–9339

Fukaura H, Kent SC, Pietrusewicz MJ, Khoury SJ, Weiner HL, Hafler DA (1996) Induction of circulating myelin basic protein and proteolipid protein-specific transforming growth factor-beta1-secreting Th3 T cells by oral administration of myelin in multiple sclerosis patients. J Clin Invest 98:70–77

Gavin MA, Bevan MJ (1995) Increased peptide promiscuity provides a rationale for the lack of N regions in the neonatal T cell repertoire. Immunity 3:793–800

Gavin MA, Clarke SR, Negrou E, Gallegos A, Rudensky A (2002) Homeostasis and anergy of CD4(+)CD25(+) suppressor T cells in vivo. Nat Immunol 3:33–41

Gerling IC, Serreze DV, Christianson SW, Leiter EH (1992) Intrathymic islet cell transplantation reduces beta-cell autoimmunity and prevents diabetes in NOD/Lt mice. Diabetes 41:1672–1676

Gotter J, Brors B, Hergenhahn M, Kyewski B (2004) Medullary epithelial cells of the human thymus express a highly diverse selection of tissue-specific genes colocalized in chromosomal clusters. J Exp Med 199:155–166

Graca L, Le Moine A, Cobbold SP, Waldmann H (2003) Dominant transplantation tolerance. Opinion. Curr Opin Immunol 15:499–506

Graca L, Le Moine A, Lin CY, Fairchild PJ, Cobbold SP, Waldmann H (2004) Donor-specific transplantation tolerance: the paradoxical behavior of CD4+CD25+ T cells. Proc Natl Acad Sci U S A 101:10122–10126

Greenwood BM (1968) Autoimmune disease and parasitic infections in Nigerians. Lancet 2:380–382

Group EAS (2000) Variation and trends in incidence of childhood diabetes in Europe. EURODIAB ACE Study Group. Lancet 355:873–876

Gruchalla RS, Streilein JW (1982) Analysis of neonatally induced tolerance of H-2 alloantigens. II. Failure to detect alloantigen-specific T-lymphocyte precursors and suppressors. Immunogenetics 15:111–127

Gullo CA, Teoh G (2004) Heat shock proteins: to present or not, that is the question. Immunol Lett 94:1–10

Harris DE, Cairns L, Rosen FS, Borel Y (1982) A natural model of immunologic tolerance. Tolerance to murine C5 is mediated by T cells, and antigen is required to maintain unresponsiveness. J Exp Med 156:567–584

Henry C, Jerne NK (1968) Competition of 19S and 7S antigen receptors in the regulation of the primary immune response. J Exp Med 128:133–152

Honey K, Cobbold SP, Waldmann H (2000) Dominant tolerance and linked suppression induced by therapeutic antibodies do not depend on Fas-FasL interactions. Transplantation 69:1683–1689

Hori S, Carvalho TL, Demengeot J (2002a) CD25+CD4+ regulatory T cells suppress CD4+ T cell-mediated pulmonary hyperinflammation driven by Pneumocystis carinii in immunodeficient mice. Eur J Immunol 32:1282–1291

Hori S, Haury M, Lafaille JJ, Demengeot J, Coutinho A (2002b) Peripheral expansion of thymus-derived regulatory cells in anti-myelin basic protein T cell receptor transgenic mice. Eur J Immunol 32:3729–3735

Hori S, Nomura T, Sakaguchi S (2003) Control of regulatory T cell development by the transcription factor Foxp3. Science 299:1057–1061

Jiang S, Camara N, Lombardi G, Lechler RI (2003) Induction of allopeptide-specific human CD4+CD25+ regulatory T cells ex vivo. Blood 102:2180–2186

Jolicoeur C, Hanahan D, Smith KM (1994) T-cell tolerance toward a transgenic beta-cell antigen and transcription of endogenous pancreatic genes in thymus. Proc Natl Acad Sci U S A 91:6707–6711

Jordan MS, Boesteanu A, Reed AJ, Petrone AL, Holenbeck AE, Lerman MA, Naji A, Caton AJ (2001) Thymic selection of CD4+CD25+ regulatory T cells induced by an agonist self-peptide. Nat Immunol 2:301–306

Kalliomaki M, Salminen S, Arvilommi H, Kero P, Koskinen P, Isolauri E (2001) Probiotics in primary prevention of atopic disease: a randomised placebo-controlled trial. Lancet 357:1076–1079

Kappler JW, Roehm N, Marrack P (1987) T cell tolerance by clonal elimination in the thymus. Cell 49:273–280

Khattri R, Cox T, Yasayko SA, Ramsdell F (2003) An essential role for Scurfin in CD4+CD25+ T regulatory cells. Nat Immunol 4:337–342

Kisielow P, Bluthmann H, Staerz UD, Steinmetz M, von Boehmer H (1988) Tolerance in T-cell-receptor transgenic mice involves deletion of nonmature CD4+8+ thymocytes. Nature 333:742–746

Klein L, Kyewski B (2000) Self-antigen presentation by thymic stromal cells: a subtle division of labor. Curr Opin Immunol 12:179–186

Kojima A, Prehn RT (1981) Genetic susceptibility to post-thymectomy autoimmune diseases in mice. Immunogenetics 14:15–27

Komai-Koma M, Jones L, Ogg GS, Xu D, Liew FY (2004) TLR2 is expressed on activated T cells as a costimulatory receptor. Proc Natl Acad Sci U S A 101:3029–3034

Kurtzke JF (1995) MS epidemiology world wide. One view of current status. Acta Neurol Scand Suppl 161:23–33

Langman RE, Cohn M (1992) What is the selective pressure that maintains the gene loci encoding the antigen receptors of T, B cells? A hypothesis. Immunol Cell Biol 70: 397–404

Leibowitz U, Antonovsky A, Medalie JM, Smith HA, Halpern L, Alter M (1966) Epidemiological study of multiple sclerosis in Israel. II. Multiple sclerosis and level of sanitation. J Neurol Neurosurg Psychiatry 29:60–68

Lerman MA, Larkin J 3rd, Cozzo C, Jordan MS, Caton AJ (2004) CD4+ CD25+ regulatory T cell repertoire formation in response to varying expression of a neo-self-antigen. J Immunol 173:236–244

Lohse AW, Dinkelmann M, Kimmig M, Herkel J, Meyer zum Buschenfelde KH (1996) Estimation of the frequency of self-reactive T cells in health and inflammatory diseases by limiting dilution analysis and single cell cloning. J Autoimmun 9:667–675

Marrack P, Winslow GM, Choi Y, Scherer M, Pullen A, White J, Kappler JW (1993) The bacterial and mouse mammary tumor virus superantigens; two different families of proteins with the same functions. Immunol Rev 131:79–92

Mason D (1998) A very high level of crossreactivity is an essential feature of the T-cell receptor. Immunol Today 19:395–404

Matricardi PM, Rosmini F, Ferrigno L, Nisini R, Rapicetta M, Chionne P, Stroffolini T, Pasquini P, D'Amelio R (1997) Cross-sectional retrospective study of prevalence of atopy among Italian military students with antibodies against hepatitis A virus. BMJ 314:999–1003

Matricardi PM, Rosmini F, Riondino S, Fortini M, Ferrigno L, Rapicetta M, Bonini S (2000) Exposure to foodborne and orofecal microbes versus airborne viruses in relation to atopy and allergic asthma: epidemiological study. BMJ 320:412–417

Maynard-Smith J, Szathmary E (1995) The major transitions in evolution. Oxford. Freeman & Co.

Medzhitov R, Janeway CA Jr (2000) How does the immune system distinguish self from nonself? Semin Immunol 12:185–188; discussion 257–344

Mittrucker HW, Kaufmann SH (2004) Mini-review: regulatory T cells and infection: suppression revisited. Eur J Immunol 34:306–312

Modigliani Y, Coutinho G, Burlen-Defranoux O, Coutinho A, Bandeira A (1994) Differential contribution of thymic outputs and peripheral expansion in the development of peripheral T cell pools. Eur J Immunol 24:1223–1227

Modigliani Y, Thomas-Vaslin V, Bandeira A, Coltey M, Le Douarin NM, Coutinho A, Salaun J (1995) Lymphocytes selected in allogeneic thymic epithelium mediate dominant tolerance toward tissue grafts of the thymic epithelium haplotype. Proc Natl Acad Sci U S A 92:7555–7559

Modigliani Y, Coutinho A, Pereira P, Le Douarin N, Thomas-Vaslin V, Burlen-Defranoux O, Salaun J, Bandeira A (1996a) Establishment of tissue-specific tolerance is driven by regulatory T cells selected by thymic epithelium. Eur J Immunol 26:1807–1815

Modigliani Y, Bandeira A, Coutinho A (1996b) A model for developmentally acquired thymus-dependent tolerance to central and peripheral antigens. Immunol Rev 149:155–120

Mosmann TR, Cherwinski H, Bond MW, Giedlin MA, Coffman RL (1986) Two types of murine helper T cell clone. I. Definition according to profiles of lymphokine activities and secreted proteins. J Immunol 136:2348–2357

Mouthon L, Nobrega A, Nicolas N, Kaveri SV, Barreau C, Coutinho A, Kazatchkine MD (1995) Invariance and restriction toward a limited set of self-antigens characterize neonatal IgM antibody repertoires and prevail in autoreactive repertoires of healthy adults. Proc Natl Acad Sci U S A 92:3839–3843

Nishimura H, Minato N, Nakano T, Honjo T (1998) Immunological studies on PD-1 deficient mice: implication of PD-1 as a negative regulator for B cell responses. Int Immunol 10:1563–1572

Nishimura H, Nose M, Hiai H, Minato N, Honjo T (1999) Development of lupus-like autoimmune diseases by disruption of the PD-1 gene encoding an ITIM motif-carrying immunoreceptor. Immunity 11:141–151

Nishimura H, Okazaki T, Tanaka Y, Nakatani K, Hara M, Matsumori A, Sasayama S, Mizoguchi A, Hiai H, Minato N, Honjo T (2001) Autoimmune dilated cardiomyopathy in PD-1 receptor-deficient mice. Science 291:319–322

Nobrega A, Haury M, Grandien A, Malanchere E, Sundblad A, Coutinho A (1993) Global analysis of antibody repertoires. II. Evidence for specificity, self-selection and the immunological "homunculus" of antibodies in normal serum. Eur J Immunol 23:2851–2859

Ohki H, Martin C, Corbel C, Coltey M, Le Douarin NM (1987) Tolerance induced by thymic epithelial grafts in birds. Science 237:1032–1035

Ohki H, Martin C, Coltey M, Le Douarin NM (1988) Implants of quail thymic epithelium generate permanent tolerance in embryonically constructed quail/chick chimeras. Development 104:619–630

Oldstone MB, Dixon FJ (1972) Inhibition of antibodies to nuclear antigen and to DNA in New Zealand mice infected with lactate dehydrogenase virus. Science 175:784–786

Oldstone MB, Ahmed R, Salvato M (1990) Viruses as therapeutic agents. II. Viral reassortants map prevention of insulin-dependent diabetes mellitus to the small RNA of lymphocytic choriomeningitis virus. J Exp Med 171:2091–2100

Onizuka S, Tawara I, Shimizu J, Sakaguchi S, Fujita T, Nakayama E (1999) Tumor rejection by in vivo administration of anti-CD25 (interleukin-2 receptor alpha) monoclonal antibody. Cancer Res 59:3128–3133

Pae HO, Oh GS, Choi BM, Chae SC, Chung HT (2003) Differential expressions of heme oxygenase-1 gene in CD25– and CD25+ subsets of human CD4+ T cells. Biochem Biophys Res Commun 306:701–705

Park HB, Paik DJ, Jang E, Hong S, Youn J (2004) Acquisition of anergic and suppressive activities in transforming growth factor-beta-costimulated CD4+CD25– T cells. Int Immunol 16:1203–1213

Patel DM, Arnold PY, White GA, Nardella JP, Mannie MD (1999) Class II MHC/peptide complexes are released from APC and are acquired by T cell responders during specific antigen recognition. J Immunol 163:5201–5210

Pereira P, Larsson EL, Forni L, Bandeira A, Coutinho A (1985) Natural effector T lymphocytes in normal mice. Proc Natl Acad Sci U S A 82:7691–7695

Pitkanen J, Peterson P (2003) Autoimmune regulator: from loss of function to autoimmunity. Genes Immun 4:12–21

Posselt AM, Barker CF, Tomaszewski JE, Markmann JF, Choti MA, Naji A (1990) Induction of donor-specific unresponsiveness by intrathymic islet transplantation. Science 249:1293–1295

Qin S, Cobbold SP, Pope H, Elliott J, Kioussis D, Davies J, Waldmann H (1993) "Infectious" transplantation tolerance. Science 259:974–977

Ramsey C, Winqvist O, Puhakka L, Halonen M, Moro A, Kampe O, Eskelin P, Pelto-Huikko M, Peltonen L (2002) Aire deficient mice develop multiple features of APECED phenotype and show altered immune response. Hum Mol Genet 11:397–409

Read S, Malmstrom V, Powrie F (2000) Cytotoxic T lymphocyte-associated antigen 4 plays an essential role in the function of CD25(+)CD4(+) regulatory cells that control intestinal inflammation. J Exp Med 192:295–302

Rodriguez D, Keller AC, Faquim-Mauro EL, de Macedo MS, Cunha FQ, Lefort J, Vargaftig BB, Russo M (2003) Bacterial lipopolysaccharide signaling through Toll-like receptor 4 suppresses asthma-like responses via nitric oxide synthase 2 activity. J Immunol 171:1001–1008

Rose NR, Mackay IR (2000) Molecular mimicry: a critical look at exemplary instances in human diseases. Cell Mol Life Sci 57:542–551

Roser BJ (1989) Cellular mechanisms in neonatal and adult tolerance. Immunol Rev 107:179–202

Sakaguchi S (2004) Naturally arising CD4+ regulatory T cells for immunologic self-tolerance and negative control of immune responses. Annu Rev Immunol 22:531–562
Sakaguchi S, Sakaguchi N, Asano M, Itoh M, Toda M (1995) Immunologic self-tolerance maintained by activated T cells expressing IL-2 receptor alpha-chains (CD25). Breakdown of a single mechanism of self-tolerance causes various autoimmune diseases. J Immunol 155:1151–1164
Salaun J, Bandeira A, Khazaal I, Calman F, Coltey M, Coutinho A, Le Douarin NM (1990) Thymic epithelium tolerizes for histocompatibility antigens. Science 247:1471–1474
Salaun J, Simmenauer N, Belo P, Coutinho A, Le Douarin NM (2002) Grafts of supplementary thymuses injected with allogeneic pancreatic islets protect nonobese diabetic mice against diabetes. Proc Natl Acad Sci U S A 99:874–877
Seddon B, Mason D (1999) Peripheral autoantigen induces regulatory T cells that prevent autoimmunity. J Exp Med 189:877–882
Shevach EM (2000) Regulatory T cells in autoimmmunity. Annu Rev Immunol 18:423–449
Shevach EM (2002) CD4+ CD25+ suppressor T cells: more questions than answers. Nat Rev Immunol 2:389–400
Shih FF, Mandik-Nayak L, Wipke BT, Allen PM (2004) Massive Thymic deletion results in systemic autoimmunity through elimination of CD4+ CD25+ T regulatory cells. J Exp Med 199:323–335
Shimizu J, Yamazaki S, Sakaguchi S (1999) Induction of tumor immunity by removing CD25+CD4+ T cells: a common basis between tumor immunity and autoimmunity. J Immunol 163:5211–5218
Shlomchik MJ, Marshak-Rothstein A, Wolfowicz CB, Rothstein TL, Weigert MG (1987) The role of clonal selection and somatic mutation in autoimmunity. Nature 328:805–811
Shull MM, Ormsby I, Kier AB, Pawlowski S, Diebold RJ, Yin M, Allen R, Sidman C, Proetzel G, Calvin D et al (1992) Targeted disruption of the mouse transforming growth factor-beta 1 gene results in multifocal inflammatory disease. Nature 359:693–699
Strachan DP (1989) Hay fever, hygiene, and household size. BMJ 299:1259–1260
Suri-Payer E, Amar AZ, McHugh R, Natarajan K, Margulies DH, Shevach EM (1999) Post-thymectomy autoimmune gastritis: fine specificity and pathogenicity of anti-H/K ATPase-reactive T cells. Eur J Immunol 29:669–677
Taniguchi M, Harada M, Kojo S, Nakayama T, Wakao H (2003) The regulatory role of Valpha14 NKT cells in innate and acquired immune response. Annu Rev Immunol 21:483–513
Thomas-Vaslin V, Damotte D, Coltey M, Le Douarin NM, Coutinho A, Salaun J (1997) Abnormal T cell selection on nod thymic epithelium is sufficient to induce autoimmune manifestations in C57BL/6 athymic nude mice. Proc Natl Acad Sci U S A 94:4598–4603
Thompson C, Powrie F (2004) Regulatory T cells. Curr Opin Pharmacol 4:408–414
Thornton AM, Shevach EM (2000) Suppressor effector function of CD4+CD25+ immunoregulatory T cells is antigen nonspecific. J Immunol 164:183–190

Tsang JY, Chai JG, Lechler R (2003) Antigen presentation by mouse CD4+ T cells involving acquired MHC class II:peptide complexes: another mechanism to limit clonal expansion? Blood 101:2704–2710

Turvey SE, Hara M, Morris PJ, Wood KJ (1999) Mechanisms of tolerance induction after intrathymic islet injection: determination of the fate of alloreactive thymocytes. Transplantation 68:30–39

Unger WW, Jansen W, Wolvers DA, van Halteren AG, Kraal G, Samsom JN (2003) Nasal tolerance induces antigen-specific CD4+CD25– regulatory T cells that can transfer their regulatory capacity to naive CD4+ T cells. Int Immunol 15:731–739

Van den Berg CW, Hofhuis FM, Rademaker PM, van Dijk H (1991) Induction of active immunological hypo/non-responsiveness to C5 in adult C5-deficient DBA/2 mice. Immunology 74:380–385

Vigouroux S, Yvon E, Wagner HJ, Biagi E, Dotti G, Sili U, Lira C, Rooney CM, Brenner MK (2003) Induction of antigen-specific regulatory T cells following overexpression of a Notch ligand by human B lymphocytes. J Virol 77:10872–10880

Von Boehmer H, Teh HS, Kisielow P (1989) The thymus selects the useful, neglects the useless and destroys the harmful. Immunol Today 10:57–61

Waldmann H (2003) The new immunosuppression. Curr Opin Chem Biol 7:476–480

Walker MR, Mannie MD (2002) Acquisition of functional MHC class II/peptide complexes by T cells during thymic development and CNS-directed pathogenesis. Cell Immunol 218:13–25

Weigle WO (1980) Analysis of autoimmunity through experimental models of thyroiditis and allergic encephalomyelitis. Adv Immunol 30:159–273

Weiner HL (2001) Oral tolerance: immune mechanisms and the generation of Th3-type TGF-beta-secreting regulatory cells. Microbes Infect 3:947–954

Wekerle H (1992) Myelin specific, autoaggressive T cell clones in the normal immune repertoire: their nature and their regulation. Int Rev Immunol 9:231–241

Wekerle H, Bradl M, Linington C, Kaab G, Kojima K (1996) The shaping of the brain-specific T lymphocyte repertoire in the thymus. Immunol Rev 149:231–243

Wills-Karp M, Santeliz J, Karp CL (2001) The germless theory of allergic disease: revisiting the hygiene hypothesis. Nat Rev Immunol 1:69–75

Wilson DB, Wilson DH, Schroder K, Pinilla C, Blondelle S, Houghten RA, Garcia KC (2004) Specificity and degeneracy of T cells. Mol Immunol 40:1047–1055

Wise MP, Bemelman F, Cobbold SP, Waldmann H (1998) Linked suppression of skin graft rejection can operate through indirect recognition. J Immunol 161:5813–5816

Wood KJ, Sakaguchi S (2003) Regulatory T cells in transplantation tolerance. Nat Rev Immunol 3:199–210

Wu HY, Weiner HL (2003) Oral tolerance. Immunol Res 28:265–284

Yaswen L, Kulkarni AB, Fredrickson T, Mittleman B, Schiffman R, Payne S, Longenecker G, Mozes E, Karlsson S (1996) Autoimmune manifestations in the transforming growth factor-beta 1 knockout mouse. Blood 87:1439–1445

Yazdanbakhsh M, Kremsner PG, van Ree R (2002) Allergy, parasites, and the hygiene hypothesis. Science 296:490–494

Zal T, Volkmann A, Stockinger B (1994) Mechanisms of tolerance induction in major histocompatibility complex class II-restricted T cells specific for a blood-borne self-antigen. J Exp Med 180:2089–2099

Zheng SG, Wang JH, Gray JD, Soucier H, Horwitz DA (2004) Natural and induced CD4+CD25+ cells educate CD4+CD25− cells to develop suppressive activity: the role of IL-2, TGF-beta, and IL-10. J Immunol 172:5213–5221

Zelenay S, Lopes-Carvalho T, Caramalho I, Moraes-Fontes MF, Rebelo M, Demengeot J (2005) Foxp3$^+$CD25$^-$CD4 T cells constitute a reservoir of committed regulatory cells that regain CD25 expression upon homeostatic expansion. Proc Natl Acad Sci U S A 102:4091–4096

Zinkernagel RM, Callahan GN, Althage A, Cooper S, Klein PA, Klein J (1978) On the thymus in the differentiation of "H-2 self-recognition" by T cells: evidence for dual recognition? J Exp Med 147:882–896

Zuany-Amorim C, Sawicka E, Manlius C, Le Moine A, Brunet LR, Kemeny DM, Bowen G, Rook G, Walker C (2002) Suppression of airway eosinophilia by killed Mycobacterium vaccae-induced allergen-specific regulatory T-cells. Nat Med 8:625–629

Selection and Behavior of CD4⁺ CD25⁺ T Cells In Vivo: Lessons from T Cell Receptor Transgenic Models

L. Klein[1] (✉) · J. Emmerich[1] · L. d'Cruz[1] · K. Aschenbrenner[1] · K. Khazaie[2]

[1]Research Institute of Molecular Pathology, Dr. Bohr-Gasse 7, 1030 Vienna, Austria
klein@imp.univie.ac.at
[2]Harvard Medical School, Dana-Farber Cancer Institute, 44 Binney Street, Boston, MA 02115, USA

1	Selection of Suppressor T Cells in the Thymus	74
2	Thymic Epithelium and Suppressor T Cells	76
3	Extrathymic Differentiation of Suppressor T Cells	78
4	Factors That Shape the Repertoire of CD25⁺ Suppressor T Cells in the Periphery	79
5	Toward an Understanding of the Behavior of Suppressor T Cells In Vivo	81
6	Anergy of CD25⁺ Suppressor T Cells: An In Vitro Artifact?	82
7	Concluding Remarks	84
References		85

Abstract Despite great interest in CD4⁺ CD25⁺ suppressor T cells, many of the fundamental properties of these cells remain enigmatic. This is in part due to experimental limitations inherent to the study of polyclonal suppressor T cells, and the extensive use of in vitro assays. This review article intends to outline recent advances in our understanding of the biology of suppressor T cells that have emerged from the analysis of T cell receptor (TCR) transgenic models. Several laboratories have taken advantage of model systems in which suppressor T cells of defined antigen-specificity are naturally selected in order to characterize the selection and behavior of these cells in vivo. In addition to providing valuable insights into the mechanism of differentiation of suppressor T cells, these systems now offer new possibilities for understanding the mode of action of suppressor T cells. For example, adoptive transfer of small numbers of ex vivo isolated TCR transgenic suppressor T cells allows for the visualization of the fate of such cells when confronted with cognate antigen in a quasi-normal, nonlymphopenic environment. Characteristic features of the currently available TCR transgenic models of suppressor T cells will be highlighted, and particular issues pertaining to the differentiation, function, and homeostasis of this T cell subset that have emerged from these models will be discussed.

1
Selection of Suppressor T Cells in the Thymus

Soon after the first description of $CD4^+$ $CD25^+$ suppressor T cells, it became evident that intrathymic selection/differentiation processes play a major role in their generation. Thus, $CD25^+$ CD4 single-positive cells with full suppressive capacity in vitro can be found in the thymus in a frequency similar to that observed in the peripheral repertoire. Furthermore, these cells do not appear to have re-immigrated into the thymus from the periphery [1, 2]. Based on these observations, it was suggested that the $CD25^+$ "lineage" of CD4 T cells branches off from the CD4 single-positive lineage upon encounter of self-antigen in the thymic medulla, as a result of "altered negative selection." However, although conceptionally certainly attractive, it remained hard to prove that the encounter of self-antigen was indeed involved in the shaping of the $CD25^+$ suppressor T cell pool, and conclusive evidence in polyclonal systems remained elusive.

New insight into this issue was provided by recent observations in two T cell receptor transgenic model systems, that populations of T cells with known specificity for antigen adopt a suppressive phenotype in an antigen-dependent fashion. Thus, definitive evidence for the role of intrathymically expressed self-antigen was obtained by Jordan et al., who showed that expression of an agonist ligand under control of the ubiquitous SV40 promoter (HA28) drives the intrathymic selection of specific CD4 T cells into the $CD25^+$ lineage in a T cell receptor transgenic system [3]. The T cell receptor transgenic model used in this report and recently in several other studies on the biology of suppressor T cells is the TCR-HA system. Here, a TCR specific for influenza hemagglutinin (HA) is expressed on CD4 T cells, and specific T cells can be followed by staining with the anti-clonotypic antibody 6.5 [4]. In the TCR-HA x HA28 system used by Jordan et al., antigen expression by radioresistant cell types, most probably thymic epithelial cells, was necessary and sufficient for the selection of HA-specific $CD25^+$ suppressor T cells. Thus, reconstitution of HA28 single transgenic animals with TCR-HA transgenic bone marrow recapitulated the phenotype of TCR-HA x HA28 double-transgenic animals, i.e., efficient intrathymic generation of HA-specific $CD25^+$ suppressor T cells. In contrast, reconstitution of wild-type animals with TCR-HA x HA28 double-transgenic bone marrow did not induce suppressor T cells.

The TCR-HA transgenic system had already been used earlier by von Boehmer and colleagues in an attempt to define conditions that tolerize CD4 T cells. TCR-HA mice were crossed with mice expressing HA under control of the B cell-specific Igκ promoter in order to address the consequences of widespread expression of self-antigen in hematopoietic cells of the B lineage.

These mice exhibited almost complete intrathymic deletion of TCR-HA CD4 T cells; however, a distinct population of clonotype-positive CD4 T cells in the periphery were observed. Upon isolation and stimulation, these CD4 T cells turned out to be anergic in vitro [5]. In follow-up studies using a gene transfer system where HA-antigen was expressed in skeletal muscle using adenoviral vectors, it was shown that concomitant adoptive transfer of TCR-HA CD4 T cells from TCR-HA x Igκ-HA mice could prevent the immune response that normally accompanies adenoviral gene delivery [6]. Thus, these in vitro anergic T cells possess suppressive properties in vivo. When the expression of CD25 was assessed on the anergic cells from TCR-HA x Igκ-HA mice, it was found that only a minor fraction was positive for this marker.

Apostolou et al. went on to address whether the suppressive properties would eventually segregate with expression of CD25 in the TCR-HA x Igκ-HA system [7]. When purified and tested in vitro, both the minor (<15%) subpopulation of CD25$^+$ and the major (>85%) subpopulation of CD25$^-$ TCR-HA CD4 T cells were anergic and displayed suppressive properties in the standard in vitro assay. This is in marked contrast to the observations in the TCR-HA x HA28 system established by Jordan et al., where a co-existence of anergic and suppressive CD25$^+$ T cells and apparently naïve (nonanergic and nonsuppressive) CD25$^-$ T cells, both expressing the TCR-HA, was observed. Apostolou and colleagues hypothesized that the somewhat puzzling split phenotype of suppressive T cells in the TCR-HA x Igκ-HA system may reflect tolerogenic antigen encounter on different compartments. Therefore, a careful re-analysis of the intrathymic expression pattern of HA under control of the presumably B cell-specific Igκ promoter was performed. This indeed revealed a more widespread expression pattern than anticipated, in that the transgenic antigen was expressed not only in thymic B cells, but also in epithelial cells (cortical and medullary) as well as very weakly in dendritic cells and macrophages. In order to elucidate how far antigen expression by different thymic stromal cell compartments (hematopoietic vs nonhematopoietic) could, in fact, account for the induction of suppressor T cells with different phenotypes, thymus and bone marrow chimeras of Igκ-HA mice were generated. It turned out that expression of HA exclusively by thymic epithelium predominantly mediated the intrathymic differentiation of HA-specific CD4 T cells into CD25$^+$ suppressors, while expression in hematopoietic cells mostly led to the intrathymic generation of CD25$^-$ suppressors. Taken together, the findings in the TCR-HA x Igκ-HA model support the notion that thymic epithelium is critical for the differentiation of CD25$^+$ suppressor T cells, while antigen recognition on hematopoietic elements may rather induce CD25$^-$ suppressor T cells. The exact conditions that favor the latter phenotype remain to be addressed, as well as the question of how far these cells are similar to so-called T_R1 CD4

T cells, which are induced upon antigen recognition on immature dendritic cells [8].

In a third model using the TCR-HA T cell receptor transgenic system, we have recently found that expression of HA under control of the ubiquitous pgk-promoter induces intrathymic selection of $CD25^+$ TCR-HA CD4 T cells [9]. Transplantation of the pgk-HA transgenic thymus into TCR-HA single transgenic animals faithfully reproduced the thymic phenotype of pgk-HA x TCR-HA double-transgenic animals, again underscoring the essential role of antigen expression by thymic epithelium for the induction of $CD25^+$ suppressor T cells. By and large, the phenotype of this double transgenic system resembles that of the above-mentioned TCR-HA x HA28 system, although the fraction of HA-specific T cells that express CD25 is somewhat higher in the thymus of pgk-HA x TCR-HA animals. In addition, the peripheral CD4 T cells expressing the transgenic TCR at a high level essentially all fall into the $CD25^+$ category, while $CD25^-$ TCR-HA^{hi} cells are virtually absent.

A second TCR transgenic system in which, under particular circumstances of transgenic antigen expression, the selection of CD4 T cells into the $CD25^+$ lineage has been observed is the ovalbumin-specific DO11.10 system. Kawahata et al. and Walker et al. have reported that in mice expressing transgenic Ovalbumin under the control of the MHC class I promoter (Ld-nOva) [10] or of the rat insulin promoter (RIP-mOva) [11], respectively, Ova-specific TCR transgenic CD4 T cells (DO11.10) were selected into the $CD25^+$ lineage. In both models, induction of the $CD25^+$ phenotype appeared to occur in the thymus, in line with the important role of thymic epithelium, although this remains to be formally demonstrated.

2
Thymic Epithelium and Suppressor T Cells

Only a few years ago, one would have interpreted the expression of model antigens under control of a B-cell-specific (Igκ) or pancreas-specific (RIP-mOva) promoter in the thymus as an experimental artifact of transgenesis. However, the phenomenon of "promiscuous" expression of peripheral antigens in thymic epithelium is now well documented and widely accepted [12–14]. Thus, rather than being of accidental nature, "ectopic" intrathymic expression of transgenes under the control of tissue-specific promoters in many cases actually reflects the normal physiology of the thymus. In view of the accumulating evidence from TCR transgenic models, for the essential role of thymic epithelium in the generation of $CD25^+$ suppressor T cells, it is tempting to postulate a link between the promiscuous expression of organ-specific self-antigens in the thymus and the intrathymic shaping of suppressor T cell pools with specificities for peripheral organs. Along these lines, the findings in TCR transgenic models explain many of the classical observations concerning induction of dominant tolerance upon xenogeneic or allogeneic transplantation of the thymic *anlage* (i.e., pure thymic epithelium) [15–17]. In these elegant experiments, the nature of the cells mediating dominant tolerance initially remained elusive. Yet later these cells were shown to reside within the pool of CD4 T cells [18]. Now, as the link between thymic epithelium and the induction of $CD4^+$ $CD25^+$ suppressor T cells has been documented in a number of TCR transgenic systems, we are facing the challenge of exactly delineating the T cell–stromal cell interactions that underlie the differentiation of a developing T cell into a $CD25^+$ suppressor T cell. In analogy to the— not undisputed—compartmentalization of positive and negative selection to cortex and medulla of the thymus, respectively, it may be hypothesized that differentiation of suppressor T cells is either a consequence of altered positive selection (cortex) or altered negative selection (medulla) within the respective thymic compartments. Such a compartmentalization would in turn determine the scope of self-antigens to which suppressor T cells are induced, as promiscuous expression of organ-specific antigens appears to be predominantly a feature of medullary epithelial cells, while the cortex is unlikely to display as broad a representation of self as the medulla [19].

Attempts have been made to address this issue in TCR transgenic models, but the studies remain as yet inconclusive. Thus, in the Igκ-HA and pgk-HA mice the neo-antigen was found to be expressed in cortical as well as medullary epithelial cells ([7] and our unpublished observation). The HA28 as well as the Ld-nOva system use strong ubiquitous promoters, and although detailed expression analyses with respect to intrathymic compartmentalization have not been performed in these systems, a strict confinement of antigen expression to only one epithelial cell type appears highly unlikely. The RIP-mOva system, in which the intrathymic expression pattern likewise has yet to be elucidated, may represent a particularly interesting case, as the insulin gene itself has been shown to be expressed in medullary epithelial cells (mTEC), but not in cortical epithelial cells (cTEC) [12]. If the RIP-mOva transgene indeed recapitulates the expression pattern of the endogenous insulin gene, this would provide a link between mTEC as the major cell type expressing peripheral antigens in the thymus and induction of CD4 $CD25^+$ suppressor T cells. However, at present such a connection remains tentative, and it should be noted that some experimental evidence argues against a role of mTEC in suppressor T cell induction. Thus, it was shown that in mice expressing MHC class-II exclusively on cortical epithelial cells (K14-A_β^b), induction of an apparently normal population of polyclonal $CD25^+$ CD4 T cells occurred [20].

Here, the term "normal" refers to the fact that these CD25$^+$ T cells are functional suppressors when tested either in vitro in the co-culture assay or in vivo in the lymphopenia-induced colitis model. However, the question of whether the repertoire of these mice indeed is equivalent to that of normal mice in terms of the TCR specificities represented among the suppressor population remains open. Another and more important caveat is that the strict confinement of class-II expression to cTEC in this model was essentially based on histological evidence; however, the definitive absence of class-II on mTEC was not rigorously tested in functional assays of isolated cells.

An alternative view of the intrathymic differentiation of CD25$^+$ suppressor T cells is that it is not the stromal interaction partner per se that determines the outcome of self-antigen recognition in the thymus, but rather the strength of the interaction may be a crucial factor. This topic bears some obvious resemblance to the controversial issue of positive selection of T cells [21]. Thus, the affinity/avidity model of T cell selection postulates that the choice between positive and negative selection is occurring within a continuum of TCR signal strength, largely independent of the nature of the peptide ligand and the stromal interaction partner [22]. In analogy, it may now be postulated that a signal of intermediate strength could induce the differentiation into the CD25$^+$ lineage. Again, experimental evidence in favor of this scenario is mostly based on correlations [3].

Taken together, there has not yet been a verdict on to what extent intrathymic selection of CD25$^+$ suppressor T cells is the result of a unique type of T cell–stromal cell interaction or whether it occurs within a particular window of avidity–affinity, irrespective of the stromal interaction partner. Notably, antigen-specific induction of TCR transgenic CD25$^+$ suppressor T cells was often accompanied by a drastic reduction in the frequency of TCR transgenic CD4 T cells in the thymus. Thus, the possibility of a stochastic component contributing to the choice between deletion and suppressor T cell differentiation should not be ignored.

3
Extrathymic Differentiation of Suppressor T Cells

Is antigen recognition on thymic epithelium the only natural way of induction of CD25$^+$ suppressor T cells? This question is intimately related to the issue of whether the choice to become a CD25$^+$ suppressor T cell can only be made at an immature stage of development, or whether a mature, naïve T cell can, under particular circumstances, differentiate into a suppressor T cell. The emerging picture is that post-thymic mechanisms of suppressor

T cell development do indeed exist, with obvious implications for potential therapeutic applications of suppressor T cells. Therefore, one would ultimately want to define conditions under which a T cell of particular specificity would predictably and reliably turn into a suppressor T cell.

Using adoptive transfer of naïve DO11.10 TCR transgenic CD4 CD25$^-$ T cells, Mahnke and colleagues showed that targeting of Ovalbumin (Ova) to immature DCs using anti-DEC205-coupled antigen led to a brief phase of expansion followed by induction of anergy in the residual Ova-specific TCR transgenic CD4 T cells. These cells displayed a CD25$^+$/CTLA4$^+$ phenotype as well as the typical functional properties of suppressor T cells in vitro [23]. Similar observations were reported using transfer of TCR-HA cells into recipients that expressed HA under the control of the Igκ-promoter [7]. Transferred cells went through a phase of contraction and expansion and, after 2 weeks, segregated into CD25$^+$ and CD25$^-$ subpopuations. Both populations were anergic to antigenic stimulation in vitro and inhibited the proliferation of co-cultured naïve cells. An identical outcome was observed when the experiment was repeated using T cell deficient (rag$^{-/-}$) Igκ-HA recipients, showing that under these circumstances the extrathymic induction of suppressor T cells was not dependent on any kind of tutoring by a thymus-derived preformed population of endogenous suppressor T cells, as has been inferred from certain polyclonal systems [18]. Thorstensen and Khoruts transferred CD25$^-$ DO11.10 obtained from DO11.10 rag$^{-/-}$ mice into normal recipients and treated these animals with low doses of antigen. They found a reduction in the number of transferred cells, and some of the residual cells had adopted a CD25$^+$ phenotype [24]. Finally, Zhang and colleagues showed that oral administration of Ovalbumin induced an increase in the proportion of DO11.10 CD4 CD25$^+$ cells [25]. However, as the latter experiments did not involve adoptive transfer of naïve, CD25$^-$ cells, they did not distinguish between de novo induction of suppressor T cells and expansion of pre-existing CD25$^+$ T cells.

Taken together, it is clear that there are extrathymic pathways of suppressor T cell development, and it is reasonable to assume that under physiological conditions, a certain fraction of the polyclonal CD25$^+$ CD4 T cell repertoire may be generated through such mechanisms. Bluestone and Abbas have recently proposed classifying regulatory T cells into natural and adaptive subsets according to their intra- or extrathymic origin, respectively [26]. However, such discrimination may perhaps be misleading, as it implies that extrathymic generation of suppressor T cells occurs predominantly under the influence of experimental manipulation rather than in a steady-state immune system.

4
Factors That Shape the Repertoire of CD25+ Suppressor T Cells in the Periphery

For several reasons, it is unlikely that the composition of the suppressor T cell pool as it exists in a normal immune system is a linear projection of the intrathymically generated pool. First, extrathymic conversion of conventional, naïve CD4 T cells into suppressor T cells may modulate the composition of the peripheral suppressor T cell pool. Although this has at present only been demonstrated in certain experimental systems (see preceding section), it appears reasonable to assume that the normal immune system in the steady state exploits similar pathways. Furthermore, there is accumulating evidence that the repertoire of suppressor T cells undergoes dynamic changes that are dictated by competition for survival factors such as access to cognate antigen or "niches" in the immune system. Among polyconal (non-TCR-transgenic) model systems, the most straightforward evidence in favor of interplay between an intra- and extrathymic encounter of self-antigen in the shaping of the repertoire of suppressor T cells has been obtained in a model of autoimmune thyroiditis in neonatally thymectomized rats [27]. In this model, transfer of peripheral or thymic CD4 T cells from normal, euthymic rats prevented the development of the disease. Strikingly, when the thyroid of the donor animals had been ablated with ^{131}I, only thymic, but not peripheral CD4 T cells prevented disease. The most reasonable interpretation is that thyroid-specific suppressor T cells are generated in the thymus, and that after exit into the periphery these cells require continuous access to the respective self-antigen(s) in order to maintain functional suppressive activity toward a particular organ [27]. Unless the antigen-specific suppressor T cells can be directly visualized, it remains unclear whether this loss of suppressive potential indicates a physical loss of the respective suppressor T cells or persisting cells have lost their suppressive activity. Again, TCR transgenic models of antigen-specific suppressor T cells can be expected to be instrumental in clarifying this issue.

When Walker et al. compared the frequency of Ova-specific CD25+ suppressor T cells within several peripheral lymphoid organs in the RIP-mOva x DO11.10 model, they found that these cells were enriched in the pancreatic lymph node [11]. This clearly documents that suppressor T cells are "aware" of their cognate antigen in the steady state in vivo, and it is tempting to speculate that organ-specific suppressor T cells, after their generation in the thymus, preferentially occupy antigen-exposed microenvironments, i.e., those lymph nodes that drain the respective organ. Thus, each draining lymph node may harbor a particular ensemble of suppressive specificities that reflects the local representation of self-antigen. Since at present this experimental system is quite unique, more experimental evidence is needed to verify this hypothesis, and to what extent this observation can be generalized remains open. Two, mutually nonexclusive, hypotheses may be put forward to explain the enrichment of specific suppressor T cells in antigen-exposed microenvironments. First, after their generation in the thymus, suppressor T cells may circulate through the body very much like conventional T cells. Upon specific antigen recognition it may be that they change their migration behavior, resulting in their specific retention and accumulation at antigen-exposed sites. Alternatively, peripheral antigen recognition may induce proliferation and expansion of specific suppressor T cells in situ, wherever cognate antigen is presented, likewise leading to an enrichment of particular antigen specificities in a permissive microenvironment. The latter scenario is in obvious contradiction to the concept of anergy of $CD25^+$ suppressor T cells, yet, as will be discussed later, there is accumulating experimental evidence challenging the view that $CD25^+$ suppressor T cells are truly anergic. As a consequence, specificities for antigens presented by APC in the thymus, but not in the periphery, may have a selective disadvantage and may be gradually lost from the pool of suppressor T cells.

Taken together, it appears that post- or extrathymic encounter of self-antigen plays a critical and dynamic role in shaping the repertoire of suppressor T cells.

5
Toward an Understanding of the Behavior of Suppressor T Cells In Vivo

With the availability of the appropriate T cell receptor transgenic models, adoptive transfer of TCR transgenic suppressor T cells into wild-type (antigen negative) recipients now permits access to a number of questions that so far could not at all or at best only indirectly be addressed in polyclonal systems. The basic strategy of the adoptive transfer approach was pioneered by the lab of Mark Jenkins a decade ago. By transferring a small number of conventional naïve TCR transgenic cells the normal repertoire of mice was spiked with a traceable cohort of cells of known specificity to visualize the consequences of tolerogenic or immunogenic regimens of antigen administration in vivo [28]. The rationale was to circumvent the potential artifacts that can arise when studying largely monoclonal immune systems, as is the case with TCR transgenic animals. Ever since this approach was first applied in the early 1990s, there has been a continuous wealth of knowledge emerging from adoptive transfer experiments using conventional naïve T cells with respect to various aspects of T cell physiology, such as the dynamics of antigen-driven expansion, induction of peripheral tolerance, T cell trafficking, as well as the induction and maintenance of memory T cells [29]. Similarly, adoptive transfer of antigen-specific suppressor T cells can now be expected to extend our understanding of the in vivo behavior of these cells. Perhaps one of the least complex questions to be addressed is whether suppressor T cells persist in a similar fashion to their naïve counterparts when transferred into an antigen-negative host. This question is of more than just academic interest if one considers adoptive transfer of autoantigen-specific suppressor T cells—generated or isolated by as yet to be established protocols—into autoimmune patients as a potential therapeutic approach. In such a setting, it is instrumental to make sure that these cells first of all persist at all, and second, that they display a stable phenotype, because an eventual reversal to a conventional effector T cell phenotype may have obvious adverse effects. Fisson et al. found that upon adoptive transfer of polyclonal $CD25^+$ CD4 T cells, these cells remain phenotypically stable for more than 2 months [30]. Although these data show that under steady-state conditions there is no conversion of $CD25^+$ into $CD25^-$ cells, the interpretation is complicated by the fact that this approach does not allow for discriminating whether the $CD25^+$ phenotype is stable per se or continuous encounter of self-antigen is essential. These limitations can be overcome using adoptive transfer of antigen-specific suppressor T cells. Using adoptive transfer of HA-specific $CD25^+$ suppressor T cells isolated from pgk-HA x TCR-HA mice, we found that the $CD25^+$ phenotype is indeed stable upon adoptive transfer, at least within a time frame of up to 2 weeks after transfer [9]. Not only did these cells maintain expression of CD25, but more importantly, their functional characteristics, such as anergy and suppressive function in vitro, were retained upon re-isolation after having been "parked" in an antigen-free host for several days. Nevertheless, at present these data should be regarded as somewhat preliminary, as the long-term survival and phenotypic stability were not rigorously addressed and definitely warrant further examination.

6
Anergy of $CD25^+$ Suppressor T Cells: An In Vitro Artifact?

Based on the characterization of $CD25^+$ CD4 T cells in vitro, anergy was regarded as a hallmark of this class of T cells [31]. The general perception has been that conditions that break the anergy, i.e., co-stimulation or addition of high levels of exogenous IL-2 in the standard in vitro assay, would abolish suppression. Whether these in vitro characteristics actually represent the behavior of CD25$^+$ T cells upon antigen encounter in vivo remained elusive because of experimental limitations inherent to the study of polyclonal CD25$^+$ CD4 T cells, where the antigen specificity is unknown. The observation that CD25$^+$ CD4 T cells enter a phase of MHC class-II dependent homeostatic proliferation upon transfer into a lymphopenic environment could be cited as evidence that these cells are not absolutely locked in a nonproliferative state [32, 33]. However, it may be argued that such a rather artificial situation may not represent the normal antigen-driven behavior of a T cell. Gavin et al. were the first to use adoptive transfer of TCR transgenic CD25$^+$ T cells to address the behavior of these cells when confronted with a strong immunogenic stimulus in vivo [33]. CD25$^+$ or CD25$^-$ CD4 T cells from a TCR transgenic mouse expressing a TCR recognizing the human invariant chain peptide hCLIP in the context of I-A^b were labeled with CFSE and transferred into normal BL/6 mice prior to immunization of the recipient mice with hCLIP in complete Freund's adjuvants (CFA). It was observed that in contrast to CD25$^-$ cells, the CD25$^+$ cells were indeed hyporesponsive, i.e., only few of these cells proliferated in the draining lymph node. While this report argues in favor of anergy of CD25$^+$ CD4 T cells in vivo, two more recent reports used a very similar approach and came to the opposite conclusion. Walker at al. and Klein et al. adoptively transferred CFSE-labeled TCR transgenic CD25$^+$ T cells from the RIP-mOva x DO11.10 or the pgk-HA x TCR-HA model, respectively, and immunized with peptide antigen in incomplete Freund's adjuvant (IFA) [9, 11]. In both studies, a pattern of cell division of CD25$^+$ cells was observed that was almost identical to that observed with CD25$^-$ cells under identical conditions. How can these discrepancies be reconciled? It appears unlikely that the mode of antigen administration (complete vs incomplete adjuvants) can account for the different outcomes, in particular since the presumably stronger stimulus failed to induce proliferation in the hCLIP model. Steinman and colleagues recently showed that the anergy of CD25$^+$ CD4 T cells can be broken in vitro through stimulation with mature dendritic cells [34]. It is likely that the antigen-presenting cell in the draining lymph node upon immunization in IFA or CFA is functionally equivalent to the bone marrow-derived dendritic cells used in these experiments. As a consequence, the expected outcome of antigen encounter on mature DCs, be it in vitro or in vivo, should be proliferation of specific CD25$^+$ suppressor T cells. However, as it is at present unclear whether the polyclonal repertoire of CD25$^+$ CD4 T cells eventually comprises distinct subsets of suppressor T cells with varying degrees of unresponsiveness to antigen, it is possible that the behavior of the hCLIP-specific CD25$^+$ T cells may be representative for a subclass of CD25 suppressor T cells that are locked in "deeper" state of anergy. In this context, the recent finding that polyclonal CD25$^+$ CD4 T cells can apparently be subdivided into two subsets, one that appears quiescent and has a long life span and a second that appears to extensively cycle under steady-state conditions deserves mentioning [30]. Further characterization of the respective systems will be needed to clarify whether suppressor T cells from the different TCR transgenic models eventually represent one or the other subset.

So far, the in vivo response of $CD25^+$ suppressor T cells to bona-fide immunogenic stimuli has been discussed. In addition, it is becoming more and more evident that the postulated anergy of $CD25^+$ suppressor T cells is broken in vivo not only upon deliberate experimental immunization, but that even steady-state conditions of self-antigen presentation may favor expansion of suppressor T cells. Walker and colleagues used the DO11.10 / RIP-Ova system to compare the behavior of Ova-specific $CD25^+$ CD4 T cells when adoptively transferred into either RIP-mOva mice or transgene negative litter mates. Strikingly, the recovery of $CD25^+$ T cells from RIP-mOva mice was higher than that from antigen-negative litter mates. CFSE-labeling experiments indicated that this was indeed due to proliferation and expansion in response to antigen. When naïve DO11.10 CD4 T cells were analyzed in a similar fashion, not unexpectedly these cells were to a large extend depleted from the immune system of antigen-expressing animals, consistent with the well-studied phenomenon of tolerance through peripheral deletion of mature T cells [5, 35]. The crucial point here is the reciprocal regulation of the clone size of either autoreactive $CD25^+$ or autoreactive naïve CD4 T cells in response to self-antigen, whereby identical signals, i.e., antigen encounter in a tolerogenic steady-state fashion, lead to opposing outcomes. Along the same lines, it was reported that intravenous injection of soluble antigen promotes proliferation of antigen-specific suppressors in vivo [34]. Collectively, the data obtained using TCR transgenic models have revealed a surprisingly dynamic lifestyle of antigen-specific $CD25^+$ suppressor T cells when confronted with cognate antigen in vivo. From a teleological point of view, one may argue that such behavior would be beneficial for the maintenance of self-tolerance, as it favorably tips the balance between suppressor T cells and potentially dangerous naïve T cells.

7
Concluding Remarks

TCR transgenic systems in which suppressor T cells with known specificity for antigen are naturally generated have significantly contributed to our understanding of several aspects of the physiology and homeostasis of these cells.

The role of antigen-expression by thymic epithelium for the intrathymic differentiation of $CD25^+$ suppressor T cells has become a well-accepted concept. Nevertheless, the fundamental question remains under which circumstances intrathymic encounter of self-antigen leads to suppressor T cell differentiation as opposed to negative selection. Since alternative, extrathymic pathways for suppressor T cell differentiation exist, great effort is now being invested in the establishment of experimental manipulations by which naïve T cells can be converted into suppressor T cells. Adoptive transfer of antigen-specific suppressor T cells from TCR-transgenic animals and subsequent challenge of recipient animals with antigen has led to the notion that some of the basic features of suppressor T cells deduced from their characterization in vitro have to be revised. For instance, the dynamic behavior of suppressor T cells that was observed when antigen-specific suppressors were confronted with cognate antigen in vivo, either in a tolerogenic or immunogenic context, was not predicted from their apparent anergy in vitro. As $CD25^+$ suppressor T cells readily expand in vivo in response to self-antigen, they obviously compete with potentially harmful autoreactive $CD25^-$ T cells for access to antigen, growth-factors and space wherever self-antigens are exposed. Thus, it may turn out that competition is an essential component of suppressor T cell function. In the near future, experiments using co-transfer of suppressor T cells and conventional T cells can be expected to clarify the prerequisites for efficient immune regulation in vivo.

Acknowledgements This work was supported by the Austrian Science Fund FWF, Boehringer Ingelheim and the European Union ("EUROTHYMAIDE"). KK is supported by NIH grant DAMD 17–02-1-0361.

References

1. Papiernik M et al (1998) Regulatory CD4 T cells: expression of IL-2R alpha chain, resistance to clonal deletion and IL-2 dependency. Int Immunol 10:371–378
2. Itoh M et al (1999) Thymus and autoimmunity: production of CD25+CD4+ naturally anergic and suppressive T cells as a key function of the thymus in maintaining immunologic self-tolerance. J Immunol 162:5317–5326
3. Jordan MS et al (2001) Thymic selection of CD4+CD25+ regulatory T cells induced by an agonist self-peptide. Nat Immunol 2:301–306
4. Kirberg J et al (1994) Thymic selection of CD8+ single positive cells with a class II major histocompatibility complex-restricted receptor. J Exp Med 180:25–34
5. Lanoue A et al (1997) Conditions that induce tolerance in mature CD4+ T cells. J Exp Med 185:405–414
6. Jooss K et al (2001) Regulatory function of in vivo anergized CD4(+) T cells. Proc Natl Acad Sci U S A 98:8738–8743

7. Apostolou I et al (2002) Origin of regulatory T cells with known specificity for antigen. Nat Immunol 3:756–763
8. Wakkach A et al (2003) Characterization of dendritic cells that induce tolerance and T regulatory 1 cell differentiation in vivo. Immunity 18:605–617
9. Klein L, Khazaie K, von Boehmer H(2003) In vivo dynamics of antigen-specific regulatory T cells not predicted from behavior in vitro. Proc Natl Acad Sci U S A 100:8886–8891
10. Kawahata K et al (2002) Generation of CD4(+)CD25(+) regulatory T cells from autoreactive T cells simultaneously with their negative selection in the thymus and from nonautoreactive T cells by endogenous TCR expression. J Immunol 168:4399–4405
11. Walker LS et al (2003) Antigen-dependent proliferation of CD4+ CD25+ regulatory T cells in vivo. J Exp Med 198:249–258
12. Derbinski J et al (2001) Promiscuous gene expression in medullary thymic epithelial cells mirrors the peripheral self. Nat Immunol 2:1032–1039
13. Kyewski B et al (2002) Promiscuous gene expression and central T-cell tolerance: more than meets the eye. Trends Immunol 23:364–371
14. Anderson MS. et al (2002) Projection of an immunological self shadow within the thymus by the aire protein. Science 298:1395–1401
15. Ohki H et al (1987) Tolerance induced by thymic epithelial grafts in birds. Science 237:1032–1035
16. Salaun J et al (1990) Thymic epithelium tolerizes for histocompatibility antigens. Science 247:1471–1474
17. Le Douarin N et al (1996) Evidence for a thymus-dependent form of tolerance that is not based on elimination or anergy of reactive T cells. Immunol Rev 149:35–53
18. Modigliani Y et al (1996) Establishment of tissue-specific tolerance is driven by regulatory T cells selected by thymic epithelium. Eur J Immunol 26:1807–1815
19. Klein L, Kyewski B (2000) Self-antigen presentation by thymic stromal cells: a subtle division of labor. Curr Opin Immunol 12:179–186
20. Bensinger SJ et al (2001) Major histocompatibility complex class II-positive cortical epithelium mediates the selection of CD4(+)25(+) immunoregulatory T cells. J Exp Med 194:427–438
21. Starr TK, Jameson SC, Hogquist KA (2003) Positive and negative selection of T cells. Annu Rev Immunol 21:139–176
22. Sebzda E et al (1994) Positive and negative thymocyte selection induced by different concentrations of a single peptide. Science 263:1615–1618
23. Mahnke K et al (2003) Induction of CD4+/CD25+ regulatory T cells by targeting of antigens to immature dendritic cells. Blood 101:4862–4869
24. Thorstenson KM, Khoruts A (2001) Generation of anergic and potentially immunoregulatory CD25+CD4 T cells in vivo after induction of peripheral tolerance with intravenous or oral antigen. J Immunol 167:188–195
25. Zhang X et al (2001) Activation of CD25(+)CD4(+) regulatory T cells by oral antigen administration. J Immunol 167:4245–4253
26. Bluestone JA, Abbas AK (2003) Natural versus adaptive regulatory T cells. Nat Rev Immunol 3:253–257
27. Seddon B, Mason D (1999) Peripheral autoantigen induces regulatory T cells that prevent autoimmunity. J Exp Med 189:877–882

28. Kearney ER et al (1994) Visualization of peptide-specific T cell immunity and peripheral tolerance induction in vivo. Immunity 1:327–339
29. Pape KA et al (1997) Use of adoptive transfer of T-cell-antigen-receptor-transgenic T cell for the study of T-cell activation in vivo. Immunol Rev 156:67–78
30. Fisson S et al (2003) Continuous activation of autoreactive CD4+ CD25+ regulatory T cells in the steady state. J Exp Med 198:737–746
31. Shevach EM (2002) CD4+ CD25+ suppressor T cells: more questions than answers. Nat Rev Immunol 2:389–400
32. Annacker O et al (2001) CD25+ CD4+ T cells regulate the expansion of peripheral CD4 T cells through the production of IL-10. J Immunol 166:3008–3018
33. Gavin MA et al (2002) Homeostasis and anergy of CD4(+)CD25(+) suppressor T cells in vivo. Nat Immunol 3:33–41
34. Yamazaki S et al (2003) Direct expansion of functional CD25+ CD4+ regulatory T cells by antigen-processing dendritic cells. J Exp Med 198:235–247
35. Rocha B, von Boehmer H (1991) Peripheral selection of the T cell repertoire. Science 251:1225–1228

Migration Rules: Functional Properties of Naive and Effector/Memory-Like Regulatory T Cell Subsets

J. Huehn (✉) · K. Siegmund · A. Hamann

Exp. Rheumatology, Charité Universitaetsmedizin Berlin, Campus Mitte,
Berlin, Germany
huehn@drfz.de

1	Introduction	90
2	Characterization of Tregs	90
2.1	CD25$^+$CD4$^+$ Tregs Can Suppress a Variety of Immune Reactions	90
2.2	Suppressor Mechanisms	91
2.3	Identification of Activation-Independent Treg Markers	92
2.4	Further Subsets with Suppressive Capacity	93
2.5	In Vivo Behavior of Tregs	94
3	Origin of Tregs: Thymus and Peripheral Induction	95
4	The Integrin $\alpha_E\beta_7$ Is a Marker for Peculiar Treg Subsets	97
5	Are α_E-Expressing Tregs Prototypes of Peripherally Induced or Expanded Adaptive Tregs?	99
6	Distinct Migratory Behavior of Treg Subsets Correlates with Their Suppressive Capacity in Certain Models	101
7	Division of Labor Between Distinct Treg Subsets?	106
	References	107

Abstract Suppressor T cells were first described in the early 1970s, but since the hypothetical soluble suppressor factor could not be identified on a molecular level and since appropriate cellular markers were lacking, the suppressor T cell concept vanished for a long time. The discovery by Sakaguchi and co-workers, that the adoptive transfer of CD25$^+$CD4$^+$-depleted T cells induced several organ-specific autoimmune diseases in immunodeficient recipients, put the suppressor T cell model back into the focus of many immunologists. CD25$^+$CD4$^+$ T cells were named regulatory T cells (Treg) and since then have been intensively characterized by many groups. It has now been well documented in a variety of models that CD25$^+$CD4$^+$ Tregs, in addition to cell-intrinsic peripheral tolerance mechanisms such as anergy induction and peripheral deletion, play indispensable roles in the maintenance of natural self-tolerance, in averting autoimmune responses as well as in controlling inflammatory reactions. However, a number of fundamental questions concerning their origin, mechanism of action, and the sites of suppression remain elusive and are currently a matter of debate. Notably, the potential heterogeneity of Tregs with respect to phenotype and function deserves attention and is a major issue discussed in this review.

1
Introduction

Suppressor T cells have first been described in the early 1970s (Gershon and Kondo 1970; Gershon 1975), but since the hypothetical soluble suppressor factor could not be identified on a molecular level and since appropriate cellular markers were lacking, the suppressor T cell concept vanished for a considerable time. The discovery made by Sakaguchi and coworkers, that the adoptive transfer of $CD25^+CD4^+$-depleted T cells induced several organ-specific autoimmune diseases in immunodeficient recipients, put the suppressor T cell model back into the focus of many immunologists (Sakaguchi et al. 1995).

$CD25^+CD4^+$ T cells were named regulatory T cells (Treg) and since then have been intensively characterized by many groups (reviewed by Maloy and Powrie 2001; Shevach 2002; Sakaguchi 2004). It has now been well documented in a variety of models that $CD25^+CD4^+$ Tregs, in addition to cell-intrinsic peripheral tolerance mechanisms such as anergy induction and peripheral deletion, play indispensable roles in the maintenance of natural self-tolerance, in averting autoimmune responses, as well as in controlling inflammatory reactions.

However, a number of fundamental questions concerning their origin, mechanism of action, and the sites of suppression remain elusive and are currently a matter of debate. Notably, the potential heterogeneity of Tregs with respect to phenotype and function deserves attention and is a major issue discussed in this review.

2
Characterization of Tregs

2.1
$CD25^+CD4^+$ Tregs Can Suppress a Variety of Immune Reactions

$CD25^+CD4^+$ Tregs are pluripotent suppressors modulating many different immune reactions. They efficiently inhibit naive $CD4^+$ T cell proliferation and differentiation (Thornton and Shevach 1998; Oldenhove et al. 2003), prevent cytotoxic activity of $CD8^+$ T cells both in vitro and in vivo (Piccirillo and Shevach 2001; Murakami et al. 2002; Suvas et al. 2003; Dittmer et al. 2004), suppress the activation and antibody production of B cells (Sakaguchi et al. 1995; Bystry et al. 2001) and limit the activity of cells from the innate immune system such as NK cells, neutrophils, and monocytes (Maloy et al. 2003). Moreover, $CD25^+CD4^+$ Tregs can efficiently limit the stimulatory capacity of antigen-presenting cells (APCs) by downregulating cell surface expression of costimulatory molecules such as CD80 and CD86 (Cederbom et al. 2000).

2.2
Suppressor Mechanisms

The precise molecular mechanisms by which $CD25^+CD4^+$ Tregs suppress the different target cells are currently controversial and under intense investigation. In vitro studies have shown that Tregs have to be activated via their T cell receptor (TCR) to exert their suppressive activity, but once they have been activated they can suppress antigen nonspecifically. Under these in vitro conditions, $CD25^+CD4^+$ Tregs suppress their target cells in a cell–cell contact-dependent and cytokine–soluble factor-independent manner (Takahashi et al. 1998; Thornton and Shevach 1998). This in vitro suppressive cell contact was not due to killing of the responder T cell population via the Fas/FasL- or TNF/TNF receptor-dependent pathway (Takahashi et al. 1998). However, killing of antigen-presenting B cells by $CD25^+CD4^+$ Tregs in vitro in a Fas/FasL-dependent manner has recently been reported (Janssens et al. 2003).

In contrast to the in vitro situation, the mechanisms via which Tregs regulate immune responses in vivo seem to be far more complicated, and several immunosuppressive cytokines such as IL-10 and TGFβ have been implicated in Treg suppressor function. A critical contribution of IL-10 to $CD25^+CD4^+$ Treg-mediated suppression was initially shown in the adoptive transfer colitis model (Asseman et al. 1999; Annacker et al. 2001) as well as in models of transplantation tolerance, graft-versus-host disease, chronic parasite infection and other autoimmune models (reviewed in Hori et al. 2003b). However, Tregs from IL-10-deficient mice, although not capable of suppressing colitis induction, are fully capable of suppressing autoimmune gastritis in the same mouse, indicating a tissue-specific role for this cytokine (Suri-Payer and Cantor 2001).

The contribution of TGFβ to $CD25^+CD4^+$ Treg-mediated suppression remains controversial as its cellular sources are numerous and may include effector T cells, nonlymphoid tissues such as epithelium, which are targets of autoimmune attack or in the process of healing, or even Tregs themselves (Asano et al. 1996; Prud'homme and Piccirillo 2000). TGFβ blockade has been shown to abrogate suppression in the induced SCID colitis model (Powrie et al. 1996; Read et al. 2000), and Nakamura and colleagues reported that activated $CD25^+CD4^+$ Tregs, but not $CD25^-CD4^+$ T cells, expressed functional $TGF\beta$ in a cell surface-bound manner (Nakamura et al. 2001). However, in a different study a functional role of $TGF\beta$ for the suppressive capacity of $CD25^+CD4^+$ Tregs could not be observed (Piccirillo et al. 2002).

Another molecule that has been implicated in the function of $CD25^+CD4^+$ Tregs is CTLA-4. In contrast to conventional naive $CD25^-CD4^+$ T cells, Tregs in normal mice constitutively express CTLA-4 and several studies using neutralizing antibodies indicate a critical role for this molecule in Treg-mediated suppression (Read et al. 2000; Salomon et al. 2000; Takahashi et al. 2000). These results collectively indicated that signals through CTLA-4 may activate $CD25^+CD4^+$ Tregs to exert suppression and that blockade of the signal lead to a failure in their activation and thereby to attenuation of the Treg-mediated suppression. However, another suppressor mechanism involving CTLA-4 has been suggested involving a direct T–T interaction and reverse signaling through the costimulatory molecules CD80/CD86 being expressed on activated target T cells leading to their inhibition (Gavin and Rudensky 2003). So far, it is unknown whether $CD25^+CD4^+$ Tregs can use all these different suppressor mechanisms concomitantly or whether specialized subsets exist that exert suppression just via one mechanism.

2.3
Identification of Activation-Independent Treg Markers

In addition to CD25 and CTLA-4, another molecule named GITR has been shown to be constitutively expressed on $CD25^+CD4^+$ Tregs (Shimizu et al. 2002; McHugh et al. 2002). However, the usage of these molecules to identify Tregs is problematic, because their expression is strongly dependent on the activation status of the cell (Table 1). CD25 expression, for example, is transiently upregulated on activated cells and therefore is not sufficient to discriminate between recently activated T cells and Tregs constitutively expressing CD25.

The best marker currently known for $CD4^+$ Tregs seems to be the recently identified transcription factor Foxp3, a forkhead family transcriptional regulator, which has been shown to be expressed almost exclusively in $CD25^+CD4^+$ Tregs and to be essential for both the generation and function of $CD25^+CD4^+$ Tregs (Hori et al. 2003a; Khattri et al. 2003; Fontenot et al. 2003). Most importantly, activation of $CD25^-CD4^+$ T cells or differentiated Th1/Th2 cells failed to induce Foxp3 expression (Hori et al. 2003a; Fontenot et al. 2003). Strikingly, retroviral transfection of $CD25^-CD4^+$ T cells with Foxp3 induces Treg-like cells both phenotypically and functionally, indicating that the tran-

Table 1 CD4$^+$ Treg markers[a]

	Induced upon activation on naive conventional CD4$^+$ T cells	Proposed functional involvement in the suppressor mechanism
CD25	Yes	IL-2 competition
CTLA-4	Yes	Costimulatory signals and *trans*-signaling
GITR	Yes	Ligation abrogates suppressive activity
$\alpha_E\beta_7$	No	Retention of Tregs at inflamed sites
Foxp3	No	Required for generation and effector function
Neuropilin-1	No	Immunological synapse formation

[a] This table summarizes molecular markers currently used to identify CD4$^+$ T cells with suppressive capacity and states whether these markers are capable of discriminating between Tregs and recently activated T cells. Moreover, putative functions of these molecules in the action of Tregs are listed. For details and references see text.

scription factor itself is sufficient to induce Tregs (Hori et al. 2003a; Khattri et al. 2003; Fontenot et al. 2003). In humans, mutations in the Foxp3 gene have been shown to be associated with the development of several autoimmune diseases (Gambineri et al. 2003).

Although Foxp3 so far is widely accepted as the best marker to identify Tregs, its intracellular expression does not allow isolating Foxp3-expressing Tregs, as it is possible for the cell surface markers CD25, CTLA-4, or GITR. A comprehensive attempt to find better Treg cell surface markers recently screened CD25$^+$CD4$^+$ Tregs for molecules, which are specifically and stably expressed on CD25$^+$CD4$^+$ Tregs and which are not induced on CD25$^-$CD4$^+$ T cells upon activation. Neuropilin-1 was identified as a novel activation-independent cell surface Treg marker, which might even be involved in the suppressive function (Bruder et al. 2004).

2.4
Further Subsets with Suppressive Capacity

In addition to CD25$^+$CD4$^+$ Tregs, other T cell subsets bearing suppressive capacity have been described (reviewed by Jonuleit and Schmitt 2003). Among those the most prominent were Tr1 and Th3 cells, which have been shown to be peripherally induced as a consequence of antigen exposure under certain tolerogenic conditions and which are characterized by the production of the immunosuppressive cytokines IL-10 and TGFβ, respectively (Roncarolo et al. 2001; Weiner 2001).

Tr1 cells were first described by Groux and colleagues and, in contrast to $CD25^+CD4^+$ Tregs, were shown to solely depend on the expression of IL-10 to exert their suppressive capacity (Groux et al. 1997). Th3 cells were originally identified in mice after oral tolerance induction to an autoantigen, preferentially produced TGFβ and established a state of systemic tolerance that prevented the development of autoimmunity and that was reversible by neutralizing antibodies against TGFβ (Chen et al. 1994). Although the contribution of TGFβ to $CD25^+CD4^+$ Treg-mediated suppression is still discussed controversially, it cannot be excluded that cells described as Th3 cells in fact might belong to the population of $CD25^+CD4^+$ Tregs.

Moreover, there is a substantial amount of data that $CD45RB^{low}$ T cells in the $CD25^-CD4^+$ T cell population in normal naive rodents bear similar suppressive activity in vivo and in vitro as their $CD25^+$ counterparts (Stephens and Mason 2000; Read et al. 2000; Annacker et al. 2001; Kullberg et al. 2002; Hori et al. 2002b). Recent efforts to further characterize these Tregs in the $CD25^-CD45RB^{low}CD4^+$ T cell population in terms of Foxp3 expression and in vitro suppressive activity have revealed that they are $CTLA-4^+$ and $GITR^{high}$, similar to $CD25^+CD4^+$ Tregs (Sakaguchi 2004). This indicates that expression of CD25 on $CD4^+$ T cells is not sufficient to identify a cell as Treg, and that a significant heterogeneity among cells with suppressive function might exist.

2.5
In Vivo Behavior of Tregs

Numerous in vitro studies suggested that $CD25^+CD4^+$ Tregs own an anergic phenotype with poor proliferation upon TCR triggering as well as growth dependence on exogenous IL-2 (Asano et al. 1996; Thornton and Shevach 1998; Papiernik et al. 1998). However, recent publications demonstrated that $CD25^+CD4^+$ Tregs display a completely different behavior in vivo, showing a high homeostatic as well as antigen-induced proliferation in different systems (Hori et al. 2002c; Klein et al. 2003; Oldenhove et al. 2003; Walker et al. 2003; Yamazaki et al. 2003; Fisson et al. 2003; Cozzo et al. 2003). These findings suggest that, in normal naive mice, a fraction of $CD25^+CD4^+$ Tregs is slowly proliferating without exogenous antigenic stimulation, presumably by recognizing self-antigens in the periphery (Fisson et al. 2003; Cozzo et al. 2003; Sakaguchi et al. 2003). Thus, $CD25^+CD4^+$ Tregs show antigen-specific expansion and consequently augment antigen-specific suppression with each successive exposure to a particular antigen.

Another important aspect regarding the in vivo suppressive capacity of $CD25^+CD4^+$ Tregs has only very recently been addressed and concerns the localization and migratory behavior of Tregs. Whereas in vitro data can only give limited information about the suppressive capacity of Treg subsets per se, the in vivo situation might be completely different, as the Tregs need the ability to migrate to the sites where suppression is required. The impact of the migratory behavior for the in vivo suppressive capacity of $CD25^+CD4^+$ Tregs will be discussed in more detail below.

3
Origin of Tregs: Thymus and Peripheral Induction

A number of findings provide ample evidence that the majority of $CD25^+CD4^+$ Tregs are produced within the thymus in the process of thymic selection as a functionally distinct and mature subpopulation of T cells. It is currently not known whether Tregs develop from a unique lineage precursor, or whether any $CD4^+CD8^-$ thymocyte can differentiate into a Treg under particular conditions.

In a normal thymus, 2%–5% of $CD4^+CD8^-$ thymocytes express CD25, and these cells are functionally competent, as illustrated by their ability to suppress naive T cell activation in vitro and to protect mice from developing autoimmunity upon adoptive transfer (Itoh et al. 1999). Similar to their peripheral counterparts, $CD25^+CD4^+CD8^-$ thymocytes express Foxp3, and in Foxp3-deficient mice both populations are lacking (Hori et al. 2003a; Fontenot et al. 2003). Furthermore, an earlier study reported that neonatal day 3 thymectomy results in the development of organ-specific autoimmunity due to the diminished number of $CD25^+CD4^+$ Tregs in the periphery (Sakaguchi et al. 1995). These studies indicate that the normal thymus is continuously producing potentially pathogenic self-reactive $CD25^-CD4^+$ T cells as well as functionally mature $CD25^+CD4^+$ Tregs. Thus, the thymus contributes to the maintenance of self-tolerance not only by deleting or inactivating the majority of self-reactive T cells during the process of negative selection but also by producing $CD25^+CD4^+$ Tregs.

The repertoire of antigen specificities of $CD25^+CD4^+$ Tregs is thought to be as broad as that of naive T cells, and they conceivably are capable of recognizing a wide array of both self- and non-self-antigens, thus enabling them to control various immune responses (Sakaguchi et al. 2003; Takahashi et al. 1998; Romagnoli et al. 2002; Pacholczyk et al. 2002; Hori et al. 2002b). There are accumulated findings indicating that the thymic development of $CD25^+CD4^+$ Tregs requires unique interactions of their TCRs, with self-peptides being presented on MHC molecules expressed on thymic stromal cells. In a double-transgenic model in which mice expressing a transgenic TCR of known specificity are crossed with mice that express the corresponding antigen in the thymus, antigen-specific Treg cells appear to require high-affinity antigen recognition in the thymus to develop (Jordan et al. 2001). Under these circumstances, if high-affinity antigen-specific thymocytes recognize their antigen being expressed on thymic epithelial cells, the vast majority of these thymocytes developed into $CD25^+CD4^+$ Tregs (Apostolou et al. 2002; Kawahata et al. 2002; Jordan et al. 2001).

In addition to the thymic generation of $CD25^+CD4^+$ Tregs, a number of reports have shown that $CD4^+$ T cells bearing suppressive capacity can be induced in the periphery from conventional $CD25^-CD4^+$ precursors upon antigen exposure under tolerogenic conditions. Two major types of these induced Tregs have already been mentioned and were described as Tr1 (Roncarolo et al. 2001) and Th3 cells (Weiner 2001). However, even $CD25^+CD4^+$ Tregs showing the same characteristics as thymus-derived $CD25^+CD4^+$ Tregs could be peripherally induced from antigen-specific $CD25^-CD4^+$ T cells by either intravenous or oral administration of low-dose peptide antigen or by adoptive transfer of naive transgenic T cells to antigen-expressing transgenic mice (Thorstenson and Khoruts 2001; Apostolou et al. 2002). This induction process neither requires an intact thymus nor the presence of thymus-derived $CD25^+CD4^+$ Tregs as observed in a skin allograft model (Karim et al. 2004).

Recent data from von Boehmer's group support these findings, showing that continuous systemic low-dose antigen delivery by osmotic pumps induced long-lived highly potent $CD25^+CD4^+$ Tregs from TCR-transgenic $CD25^-CD4^+$ T cells or even from the endogenous T cell pool (Apostolou 2004). However, it remains to be determined whether these peripherally generated Tregs are de novo induced from naive T cells or derived from Treg-precursors ($Foxp3^+CTLA-4^+GITR^{high}$) present in the $CD25^-CD4^+$ T cell population. Further comprehensive studies are required to compare the phenotypic and functional properties of such apparently de novo induced Tregs with thymic-derived $CD25^+CD4^+$ Tregs.

In order to classify the diverse subtypes of suppressive T cells, Bluestone and Abbas recently suggested the nomenclature of "natural" and "adaptive" Tregs (Bluestone and Abbas 2003). In their terminology, natural Tregs comprise those Tregs that develop as $CD25^+CD4^+$ Tregs within the thymus and that are specialized to regulate immune homeostasis and to maintain self-tolerance. In contrast, those suppressive T cells that develop in the periphery either from naive T cells or from natural Tregs upon antigen-induced differentiation/expansion under certain tolerogenic conditions were named adaptive Tregs, and this type of Tregs also includes Tr1 and Th3 cells.

4
The Integrin $\alpha_E\beta_7$ Is a Marker for Peculiar Treg Subsets

Recently, several groups have identified the integrin $\alpha_E\beta_7$ as a marker for murine CD4$^+$ Tregs isolated from secondary lymphoid organs (Lehmann et al. 2002; Zelenika et al. 2002; Gavin et al. 2002; McHugh et al. 2002; Banz et al. 2003). So far, the integrin $\alpha_E\beta_7$ has been well known as a marker for intraepithelial lymphocytes (IEL) residing in the gut wall and other epithelial compartments such as skin or lung, and its expression was shown to be largely controlled by TGFβ (Cerf-Bensussan et al. 1987; Kilshaw and Murant 1991). However, only very limited knowledge exists on the function of the integrin $\alpha_E\beta_7$ on CD4$^+$ T cells.

In contrast to the related integrin $\alpha_4\beta_7$, which acts as a homing receptor for mucosa-seeking lymphocytes by recognizing the mucosal addressin cell adhesion molecule-1 (MAdCAM-1) (Hamann et al. 1994), $\alpha_E\beta_7$ seems not to play a role in the migration of lymphocytes into mucosal or epithelial sites (Austrup et al. 1995). Instead, it has been suggested that the interaction between $\alpha_E\beta_7$ and its ligand E-cadherin, which is expressed on epithelial cells but not on endothelium (Cepek et al. 1994), might be involved in the retention of lymphocytes within epithelial compartments. This assumption is supported by the phenotype of α_E-deficient mice, which showed a reduction in the number of mucosal T lymphocytes (Schon et al. 1999). Furthermore, these mice developed mild cutaneous inflammatory disorders (Schon et al. 2000), which led to the suggestion that the integrin might be important for the control of autoimmunity in the skin.

In addition to intraepithelial lymphocytes, the integrin $\alpha_E\beta_7$ is expressed on a small subpopulation of about 5–6% CD4$^+$ T cells from secondary lymphoid organs. Initial characterization of this subset in our laboratory revealed that the majority of this subpopulation co-expresses CD25 and is localized within the CD45RB^{low} compartment (Lehmann et al. 2002). The integrin not only subdivides the CD25$^+$ compartment into CD25 single positive (α_E^-CD25$^+$) and α_E^+CD25$^+$ cells, but also identifies CD25-negative α_E single positive cells (α_E^+CD25$^-$). Since CD25 and CD45RB^{low} have been described as Treg markers, we analyzed whether the α_E-expressing subsets exhibit suppressive capacity (Fig. 1).

Functional studies both in vitro (suppression of naive T cell proliferation) and in vivo (inhibition of induced SCID colitis) revealed that α_E^+ T cell subsets irrespective of their CD25 expression showed regulatory activity (Lehmann et al. 2002; Banz et al. 2003). Throughout all settings, α_E^+CD25$^+$ cells turned out to be the most potent suppressors. In vitro, the α_E^+CD25$^-$ subpopulation displayed only moderate suppressive activity comparable to total CD45RB^{low}

$\alpha_E^-CD25^+$
- intermediate suppressive capacity in vitro and in vivo
- CTLA-4$^+$ / ICOS$^-$
- cytokine^{low}
- Foxp3$^+$

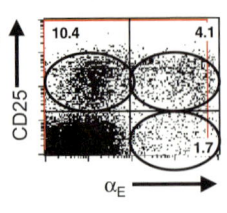

$\alpha_E^+CD25^+$
- high suppressive capacity
- CTLA-4^{+++} / ICOS^{+++}
- cytokine^{neg}
- Foxp3$^+$

$\alpha_E^+CD25^-$
- high suppressive capacity only in vivo
- CTLA-4^{+++} / ICOS^{+++}
- cytokine^{high} (Th1/Th2)
- Foxp3$^+$

Fig. 1 Phenotype of a_E^- and a_E^+ Treg subsets. For details see text

CD4$^+$ cells, but strikingly α_E single positive cells were potent regulators in vivo, being as effective as CD25 single positive cells in inhibiting the development of SCID colitis (Lehmann et al. 2002). Furthermore, Foxp3 mRNA was present in all three Treg subsets with a similar expression level in α_E single positive cells compared to both CD25 expressing subsets (Huehn et al. 2004). This latter finding underlines the regulatory function of $\alpha_E^-CD25^+$, $\alpha_E^+CD25^+$ as well as $\alpha_E^+CD25^-$ CD4$^+$ T cells in the murine system.

However, the integrin $\alpha_E\beta_7$ does not account as a marker for Tregs from the human peripheral blood as $\alpha_E^+CD25^+$ cells are absent in the peripheral blood CD4$^+$ T cell compartment and the small subset of $\alpha_E^+CD25^-$ CD4$^+$ T cells does not contain any suppressive capacity (unpublished observations; Iellem et al. 2003; Stassen 2004).

Further characterization of α_E-expressing as well as $\alpha_E^-CD25^+$ Tregs revealed striking differences between these subsets, supporting the concept that a high degree of heterogeneity exists within the suppressor T cell pool (Fig. 1). Whereas $\alpha_E^-CD25^+$ and especially $\alpha_E^+CD25^+$ cells fulfilled the hallmark of Tregs by expressing only low frequencies of both proinflammatory and Th2-type cytokines upon restimulation, the $\alpha_E^+CD25^-$ subset showed a rather peculiar cytokine expression pattern, producing high levels of both Th1- and Th2-type cytokines (Lehmann et al. 2002). Additionally, the $\alpha_E^-CD25^+$ subset showed only minor frequencies of CTLA-4$^+$ cells, whereas both α_E-expressing subsets expressed this immunomodulatory molecule at high frequencies (Lehmann et al. 2002). However, we did not observe any differences with regard to GITR expression, as all three subsets showed a comparable high expression of this molecule (unpublished observation). Nevertheless, the considerable heterogeneity in the Treg pool with respect to suppressive capacity, cytokine secretion, and expression of CTLA-4 suggests distinct functional profiles of these subsets.

5
Are α_E-Expressing Tregs Prototypes of Peripherally Induced or Expanded Adaptive Tregs?

To get a more comprehensive picture of molecular differences between α_E^+ and α_E^- Treg subsets, we performed global gene expression analyses. The results suggested a fundamental dichotomy with regard to phenotype and developmental stage, allowing the differentiation into naive- and effector/memory-like Tregs (Table 2; Huehn et al. 2004).

CD25 single positive cells, although expressing CD45RB at low levels, displayed a rather naive-like phenotype with high expression levels of CD62L as well as expression of functional CCR7. Their CD62L expression was comparable to α_E^-CD25$^-$ control cells, which largely are composed of conventional naive T cells bearing a CD45RB^{high} phenotype.

In contrast, both α_E-expressing subsets and especially the α_E^+CD25$^-$ cells showed an activated effector/memory-like phenotype with low expression levels of CD45RB and CD62L combined with high levels of certain effector/memory markers (CD44, ICOS, CD29, LFA-1). Additionally, other markers known to characterize antigen-experienced or recently activated CD4$^+$

Table 2 Phenotypic characteristics and functional properties of α_E^+ and α_E^- Treg subsets (for details see text)

	α_E^-CD25$^+$	α_E^+CD25$^+$	α_E^+CD25$^-$
Effector/memory-like phenotype	–	++	+++
Naive-like phenotype	+++	+	–
TREC content	+++	++	+
CD62L expression	+++	++	+
E/P-selectin ligand expression	–	++	+++
Chemokine responsiveness			
CCR7 ligand	+++	++	+
CXCR3 ligand	+	++	+++
CCR4 ligand	+	++	+++
CCR6 ligand	+	+++	++
In vivo suppression			
Induced SCID colitis	++	+++	+++
Antigen-induced arthritis	–	+++	++
Skin inflammation	+	+++*	+++*

* in this model only total α_E^+ Tregs were analyzed in comparison to α_E^-CD25$^+$ Tregs

T cells including CD69, Ki67 (Brown and Gatter 2002), granzyme B (Jacob and Baltimore 1999) and CD8 (Nascimbeni et al. 2004) were also upregulated within the α_E-expressing Treg subsets.

The highly differentiated effector/memory-like phenotype of α_E-expressing Tregs suggested that these cells have been activated in the periphery upon contact with their cognate antigen, leading to their differentiation and expansion. Indeed, when we were analyzing the TREC (T cell receptor excision circles) content of the Treg subsets, which is an indicator of their expansion after recombination of the TCR, we observed a relatively high TREC numbers in CD25 single positive cells, similar to the predominantly naive $\alpha_E^- CD25^-$ control cells. This reflects a limited proliferative activity of CD25 single positive cells during development. In contrast, both α_E-expressing subsets and especially $\alpha_E^+ CD25^-$ cells showed a strongly reduced TREC content indicating that these cells have undergone repetitive cell divisions after maturation within the thymus (Huehn et al. 2004). Our data on the proliferative history of α_E-expressing Treg subsets support recently published observations from different groups showing a strong in vivo proliferative capacity of $CD25^+ CD4^+$ Tregs (reviewed in von Boehmer 2003).

Interestingly, Fisson and colleagues have postulated that the $CD25^+ CD4^+$ Treg compartment is composed of two Treg subsets showing distinct phenotypes and homeostasis under steady-state conditions (Fisson et al. 2003). Upon adoptive transfer of natural $CD62L^{high} CD25^+ CD4^+$ Tregs, which largely corresponds to the $\alpha_E^- CD25^+$ Treg subset, a substantial fraction of these cells underwent repetitive cell divisions upon contact with tissue self-antigen. Strikingly, those cells that were dividing extensively acquired an effector/memory-like phenotype ($CD44^{high}$ $CD69^+$ $CD134^+$ $CD62L^{low}$). Whether these cells also express the integrin $\alpha_E \beta_7$ was not addressed in that study, but our own data would suggest that these cells become α_E^+ Tregs, indicating that adaptive effector/memory-like Tregs can develop from natural $CD25^+ CD4^+$ precursors.

However, as already mentioned above, von Boehmer and colleagues have shown in an antigen-specific adoptive transfer model that continuous peripheral low-dose delivery of specific peptide antigen by osmotic pumps generates $CD25^+ CD4^+$ Tregs from conventional naive $CD25^- CD4^+$ T cells. Interestingly, when analyzing the phenotype of these de novo induced Tregs through gene array technology, not only the key Treg marker Foxp3, but also the integrin α_E was found to be strongly upregulated in the antigen-specific T cells (H. von Boehmer and J. Buer, personal communication).

Together these data suggest that α_E-expressing effector/memory Tregs can be derived either from conventional naive $CD25^- CD4^+$ T cells or from

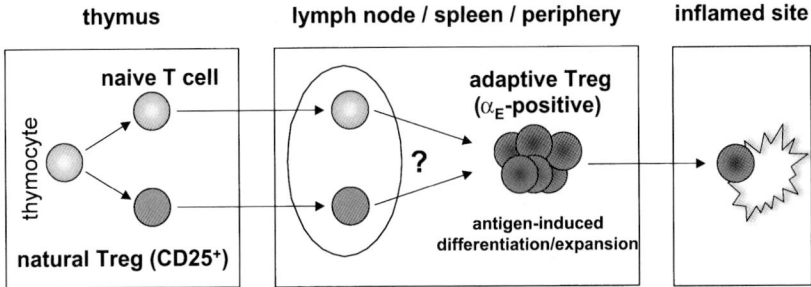

Fig. 2 CD25 single positive cells represent natural Tregs, whereas a_E-expressing subsets are prototypes of adaptive Tregs

natural naive-like CD25$^+$CD4$^+$ Tregs, strengthening our current view that the expression of the integrin $\alpha_E\beta_7$ on CD4$^+$ Treg subsets is indicative of their antigen-specific differentiation and expansion in the periphery (Fig. 2). Where in the organism the conversion into adaptive Tregs takes place has not been addressed sufficiently yet. However, it is very likely that this scenario involves secondary lymphoid organs as the precursors, either naive conventional CD25$^-$CD4$^+$ T cells or naive-like natural CD25$^+$CD4$^+$ Tregs, both express high levels of CD62L and CCR7 and therefore display remarkable tropism for these sites (Mackay et al. 1990; Moser and Loetscher 2001).

Despite these numerous findings supporting the hypothesis of the peripheral generation of α_E-expressing Treg subsets, the inter-relationship between α_E^+CD25$^+$ and α_E single positive cells remains largely unknown and needs further investigation. It is unlikely that α_E^+CD25$^-$ Tregs merely represent a nonactivated and thereby CD25-negative precursor state of α_E^+CD25$^+$ cells, as the α_E single positive cells display the most differentiated phenotype with respect to the expression of cytokines, effector/memory markers, and reduced TREC numbers (Lehmann et al. 2002; Huehn et al. 2004). On the other hand, α_E single positive cells express relatively high levels of CD25 mRNA and rapidly acquire CD25 expression upon activation, suggesting some flexibility in the phenotypes with regard to this marker (Lehmann et al. 2002).

6
Distinct Migratory Behavior of Treg Subsets Correlates with Their Suppressive Capacity in Certain Models

The gene array based analysis of α_E^+ and α_E^- Treg subsets not only revealed differences in the expression of effector/memory markers, unraveling a dichotomy within the Treg compartment with respect to antigen experience and developmental stage. Striking differences were also observed with respect to the expression of certain adhesion molecules and chemokine receptors, suggesting that in vivo α_E^+ and α_E^- Treg subsets are not equally distributed throughout the body and that specialized Treg subsets exist that can patrol through distinct sites of the body (Table 2; Huehn et al. 2004).

These observations fit to our current concept that α_E-expressing Tregs have acquired their effector/memory-like phenotype in the periphery, as it is known that antigen recognition in secondary lymphoid tissues not only results in clonal expansion and differentiation into effector/memory cells with distinct functional properties, but also induces a change in the expression of adhesion molecules and chemokine receptors that allows the exit from the lymph nodes and the migration into distinct effector sites (Mackay et al. 1990; Austrup et al. 1997; Tietz et al. 1998; Masopust et al. 2001; Campbell and Butcher 2002).

Indeed, migration studies of α_E^+ and α_E^- Treg subsets revealed that the observed phenotypic differences between the Treg subsets precisely correspond to their behavior in vivo (Huehn et al. 2004). Naive-like CD25 single positive cells efficiently migrated into lymph nodes fitting to their combinatorial high CD62L expression and high responsiveness toward CCR7 ligands. Both molecules have been shown to be a prerequisite for the entry into lymph nodes (Gallatin et al. 1983; Forster et al. 1999; Luther et al. 2000). In contrast, both α_E-expressing Treg subsets and especially α_E single positive cells showed increased frequencies of E/P selectin ligand expression combined with a substantial downregulation of CD62L, high expression levels for LFA-1, β_1-integrin, and ICAM-1, as well as a high responsiveness toward a number of inflammatory chemokines. Corresponding to these phenotypes, effector/memory-like Treg subsets displayed only a rather poor capacity to migrate into lymph nodes, but, in contrast, efficiently entered inflamed sites.

Overall, the in vivo migration data identified naive-like α_E^-CD25$^+$ as a recirculating subset, whereas the effector/memory-like α_E-expressing Tregs proved to be rather inflammation-seeking (Huehn et al. 2004). The observed migration behavior of α_E^+ and α_E^- Treg subsets largely corresponds to findings in a number of recent publications studying adhesion molecule expression or chemokine responsiveness of Treg subsets (Iellem et al. 2001; Iellem et al. 2003; Goulvestre et al. 2002; Colantonio et al. 2002; Sebastiani et al. 2001; Gavin et al. 2002; Fu et al. 2004). Most strikingly, Szanya et al., by separating the CD25$^+$CD4$^+$ compartment into CD62L^{high} and CD62L^{low} cells, which largely correspond to CD25 single positive and α_E^+CD25$^+$ cells, respectively, were able to show enhanced expression of CCR7 on the CD62L^{high} subset, whereas levels of CCR2, CCR4, and CXCR3 were much higher on CD62L^{low} cells (Szanya et al. 2002).

The migratory phenotype of Treg subsets is discussed more controversially in the human system. Iellem et al. have observed an enrichment in E-selectin-binding and CCR4$^+$ cells among CD25$^+$CD4$^+$ Tregs accompanied by a paucity of gut-homing ($\alpha_4\beta_7{}^+$, CCR9$^+$) cells, suggesting that these cells most likely would home into the skin as well as inflamed sites (Iellem et al. 2003). This report contrasts with a recent finding from Jonuleit and colleagues who have shown that 15%–30% of human CD25$^+$CD4$^+$ Tregs expressed the integrin $\alpha_4\beta_7$, suggesting that these cells would preferentially migrate into the mucosa (Stassen 2004). However, in the murine system we did not observe a preferential migration of any of the analyzed Treg subsets into both noninflamed and inflamed mucosal tissues, although all subsets expressed the integrin $\alpha_4\beta_7$ at reasonable frequencies (30%) (Huehn et al. 2004 and unpublished observations). These findings indicate that Tregs similar to conventional effector/memory T cells display a heterogenous migration pattern, which is not biased toward a single tissue.

Despite accumulating knowledge on the chemokine responsiveness of certain Treg subsets, only limited data exist on where distinct Treg subsets localize in vivo. Whereas it has been shown that the CD62L^{high} subset of CD25$^+$CD4$^+$ Tregs preferentially migrates into peripheral lymph nodes (Fisson et al. 2003), the phenotype of those Tregs that have been isolated from effector sites such as synovial fluid of rheumatoid arthritis patients (Cao et al. 2003), lung tumors (Woo et al. 2002), transplants (Graca et al. 2002), skin lesion of *Leishmania major*-infected mice (Belkaid et al. 2002), lungs of *Pneumocystis carinii*-infected mice (Hori et al. 2002a), islets of Langerhans in a diabetes model (Lepault and Gagnerault 2000; Green et al. 2002), or the inflamed intestine in the induced colitis model (Mottet et al. 2003) remains largely unknown. However, it is tempting to speculate that those Tregs largely correspond to adaptive effector/memory-like Tregs displaying an activated phenotype.

Interestingly, Tregs from the inflamed intestine showed strong signs of proliferation (Mottet et al. 2003) and those Tregs that were recovered from the inflamed islets in the diabetes model were mainly CD62L^{low} (Lepault and Gagnerault 2000), indicating some similarities with α_E-expressing Tregs. This latter finding was recently supported by observations of Mathis and colleagues who analyzed the phenotype of Tregs isolated directly from the inflamed pancreatic islets in BDC2.5/NOD mice using gene array technology. Interestingly, these inflammation-derived Tregs showed an enhanced expression of the integrin $\alpha_E\beta_7$ and also displayed increased mRNA for the inflammatory chemokine receptors CCR2, CCR5, and CXCR3 (A. Herman, C. Benoist and D. Mathis, personal communication), fitting to our own observations that only α_E-expressing Tregs, which show an enhanced migratory response toward inflammatory chemokines, can enter such inflamed sites (Huehn et al. 2004).

Moreover, α_E-expressing Tregs have also been observed in the aforementioned *Leishmania major* infection model. In this model, antigen-specific Tregs could be isolated from skin lesions of infected mice and have been shown to play a crucial role in the immune response against the parasite (Belkaid et al. 2002). Belkaid and colleagues now have observed in a follow-up study that up to 80% of Tregs from the skin lesions stained positive for the integrin $\alpha_E\beta_7$. Strikingly, using a monoclonal antibody that blocked the interaction of the integrin $\alpha_E\beta_7$ with its ligand E-cadherin, they could show that the number of Tregs in the chronic site of infection were significantly reduced, leading to the hypothesis that the expression of the integrin $\alpha_E\beta_7$ on the skin-resident Tregs has a functional role mediating the retention of the Tregs within the skin lesions of infected mice (Y. Belkaid, personal communication).

However, a general functional role for the integrin $\alpha_E\beta_7$ in the retention of effector/memory-like Tregs at any site of acute inflammation could not be supported by Annacker et al., who did not observe a significant difference in the suppressive capacity of $CD25^+CD4^+$ Tregs derived from wild-type or α_E-deficient mice in the induced SCID colitis model (Annacker 2003). This latter finding corresponds to data obtained with $CD4^+$ or $CD8^+$ effector T cells, for which a role of $\alpha_E\beta_7$ in homing into or retention within epithelial sites could not be demonstrated (Austrup et al. 1995; Lefrancois et al. 1999).

The conspicuous different migration phenotypes of α_E^+ and α_E^- Treg subsets also turned out to be of functional significance when the suppressive capacities of these subsets were compared in an inflammation model, the antigen-induced arthritis. Strikingly, only the α_E-positive cells, which efficiently migrated into the inflamed site, could significantly reduce acute knee joint swelling as well as signs of chronic inflammation. In contrast, CD25 single positive cells, which showed no preferential migration to the inflamed knee joint, lacked suppressive activity under these acute inflammatory conditions (Huehn et al. 2004).

In order to generalize the concept that the suppressive capacity of Treg subsets is correlated with their in vivo migration behavior, we have established another inflammation model affecting the skin. This model is based on the adoptive transfer of in vitro generated, fully differentiated TCR-transgenic Th1 cells, and the inflammation is elicited by the subsequent injection of the cognate antigen into the footpad. Similar to the antigen-induced arthritis model, CD25 single positive cells, which showed no migration into the inflamed site, were not effective in suppressing the acute inflammatory response, whereas α_E^+ Tregs, which efficiently entered the inflamed skin, significantly suppressed the Th1-mediated footpad swelling (unpublished observations).

Recently, another group published data supporting our view of the functional relevance of the appropriate localization of Tregs for their in vivo suppressive capacity using a contact hypersensitivity model. In this model, hapten-specific Tregs induced by ultraviolet radiation were capable of inhibiting the induction phase of the skin inflammation, but showed no suppressive capacity during the effector phase (Schwarz et al. 2004). These hapten-specific Tregs expressed high levels of CD62L, but not the ligands for the skin-homing receptors E- and P-selectin. This phenotype most likely allows the migration into lymph nodes, the site of the induction phase, but not into the skin, where the effector response takes place. However, if these hapten-specific Tregs were injected directly into the effector site they could even suppress the challenge reaction. This finding indicates that hapten-specific Tregs, although in principle able to inhibit T effector cells, do not suppress the effector phase, because they obviously do not migrate into the skin (Schwarz et al. 2004).

The observation that effector/memory-like Tregs express certain adhesion molecules and chemokine receptors that allow their efficient migration into inflamed sites has important implications for the use of such molecules as targets for anti-inflammatory therapies. Inhibition of migratory functions might not only prevent the infiltration of effector cells but also that of highly effective adaptive Tregs.

This issue was addressed in a recent publication demonstrating a crucial role of CCR2-expressing Tregs in a model of collagen-induced arthritis (Bruhl et al. 2004). Whereas blockade of CCR2 using monoclonal antibodies during the disease initiation phase markedly improved the signs of arthritis, blockade during the later phase of arthritis progression significantly aggravated clinical and histological signs of arthritis (Bruhl et al. 2004). The authors postulate that this latter effect was most likely due to the interference with the proper in vivo localization of CCR2$^+$CD25$^+$CD4$^+$ Tregs, which seemed to be essential for the control of the inflammatory response. Interestingly, CCR2 expression on CD25$^+$CD4$^+$ Tregs strongly correlated with the expression of the integrin $\alpha_E\beta_7$ (Bruhl et al. 2004), supporting our view that α_E-expressing effector/memory-like Tregs are important for the control of already ongoing inflammatory reactions (Fig. 2).

In contrast to the inflammation models, in which naive-like α_E^-CD25$^+$ Tregs showed almost no suppressive activity, recent reports demonstrated potent suppressive capacity of CD62L-expressing CD25$^+$CD4$^+$ Tregs in other models. Strikingly, CD62L^{high} but not CD62L^{low} CD25$^+$CD4$^+$ Tregs were capable of preventing the development of autoimmunity in the NOD diabetes model, indicating that the homeostatic regulation by naive-like Tregs is of major importance under conditions where the initiation of the immune response has to be controlled (Herbelin et al. 1998; Lepault and Gagnerault 2000; Szanya et al. 2002). Similar results were observed in the murine model of allogeneic bone marrow transplantation, in which only adoptive transfer of donor $CD62L^{high}CD25^+CD4^+$ Tregs protects recipient mice from lethal acute graft-versus-host disease (aGVHD) induced by donor $CD25^-CD4^+$ T cells (J. Ermann, personal communication).

Most studies report a similar in vitro suppressive capacity of $CD62L^{high}$ and $CD62L^{low}$ Treg subsets (Kuniyasu et al. 2000; Thornton and Shevach 2000; Szanya et al. 2002). Only one recent report showed increased in vitro suppressive activity within the $CD62L^{high}$ subset (Fu et al. 2004). Thus, the differential regulatory capacities of the $CD62L^{high}$ and $CD62L^{low}$ subsets in the diabetes model most likely reflect differences in homing properties rather than suppressor potential per se. As adoptive Treg transfer in the NOD model was performed before the onset of diabetes, the control of the induction of autoimmunity apparently takes place in the lymph node, where antigen-specific T cells get activated and become effector cells. Since only $CD62L^{high}CD25^+CD4^+$ Tregs efficiently can enter lymph nodes (Fisson et al. 2003; Huehn et al. 2004), the development of these effector cells and thereby the induction of autoimmunity could only be prevented by $CD62L^{high}$ Tregs.

Results supporting this hypothesis were again obtained from the aGVHD model, in which early after transplantation a higher number of donor-type Treg cells could be recovered from host spleen and mesenteric lymph nodes when $CD62L^{high}CD25^+CD4^+$ Tregs were transferred as compared to the $CD62L^{low}$ subset, suggesting that the ability of Treg cells to efficiently enter secondary lymphoid organs is a prerequisite for their protective function in this model (J. Ermann, personal communication). Finally, these data were supported by Oldenhove and colleagues, showing that $CD25^+CD4^+$ Tregs limit the development of Th1 cells directly within the lymph node draining the site of antigen injection, suggesting that $CD62L^{high}$ Tregs were involved in this part of immune regulation (Oldenhove et al. 2003).

7
Division of Labor Between Distinct Treg Subsets?

Phenotype and localization properties let suggest a subdivision of the Treg compartment into distinct lineages or differentiation stages according to the aforementioned model of Bluestone and Abbas proposing the existence of so-called natural and adaptive Tregs (Bluestone and Abbas 2003). CD25 single positive cells might be good candidates for these natural Tregs, as they preferentially migrate into lymph nodes where they control the priming phase of immune responses. In contrast, α_E-expressing Tregs subsets bearing an effector/memory-like, inflammation-seeking phenotype seem to be good candidates for the adaptive Tregs specialized for the suppression of already ongoing immune reactions. These α_E-expressing Treg subsets are thought to be tasked when the lymph node-residing natural Tregs have failed or when immune reactions are going out of control.

However, as these types of immune reactions take place at peripheral effector sites this "fail-safe" system of peripheral tolerance absolutely requires specialized Tregs, which harbor the capacity to enter inflamed effector sites. Therefore, to allow the suppression of such established immune reactions, Tregs do not merely require extraordinarily potent inhibitory mechanisms but also need to efficiently enter the hot spots of the inflammatory reaction. We assume that the localization of Treg subsets is of equal importance as their direct suppressive capacity as exemplified by α_E single positive cells having only poor in vitro, but high in vivo suppressive potential (Lehmann et al. 2002, Huehn et al. 2004). Therefore, considerations on the migratory capacities of Treg populations have to be taken into account when future therapeutic strategies based on the adoptive transfer of Treg subsets become attractive.

References

Annacker O, Pimenta-Araujo R, Burlen-Defranoux O, Barbosa TC, Cumano A, Bandeira A (2001) CD25+ CD4+ T cells regulate the expansion of peripheral CD4 T cells through the production of IL-10. J Immunol 166:3008–3018

Annacker O, Malmstroem V, Bournbe T, Parker CM, Powrie F (2003) Essential role for CD103 in the T cell-mediated regulation of experimental colitis (abstract). Immunology 110:117

Apostolou I, Sarukhan A, Klein L, von Boehmer H (2002) Origin of regulatory T cells with known specificity for antigen. Nat Immunol 3:756–763

Apostolou I, von Boehmer H (2004) In vivo induction of suppressor commitment in naive T cells. J Exp Med 199:1401–1408

Asano M, Toda M, Sakaguchi N, Sakaguchi S (1996) Autoimmune disease as a consequence of developmental abnormality of a T cell subpopulation. J Exp Med 184:387–396

Asseman C, Mauze S, Leach MW, Coffman RL, Powrie F (1999) An essential role for interleukin 10 in the function of regulatory T cells that inhibit intestinal inflammation. J Exp Med 190:995–1004

Austrup F, Rebstock S, Kilshaw PJ, Hamann A (1995) TGF beta1-induced expression of the mucosa-related integrin alpha E on lymphocytes is not associated with mucosa-specific homing. Eur J Immunol 25:1487–1491

Austrup F, Vestweber D, Borges E, Löhning M, Bräuer R, Herz U, Renz H, Hallmann R, Scheffold A, Radbruch A, Hamann A (1997) P-and E-selectin mediate recruitment of T helper 1 but not T helper 2 cells into inflamed tissues. Nature 385:81–83

Banz A, Peixoto A, Pontoux C, Cordier C, Rocha B, Papiernik M (2003) A unique subpopulation of CD4+ cells regulatory T cells controls wasting disease IL-10 secretion and T cell homeostasis. Eur J Imm 33:2419–2428

Belkaid Y, Piccirillo CA, Mendez S, Shevach EM, Sacks D L (2002) CD4+CD25+ regulatory T cells control Leishmania major persistence and immunity. Nature 420:502–507

Bluestone JA, Abbas AK (2003) Natural versus adaptive regulatory T cells. Nat Rev Immunol 3:253–257

Brown DC, Gatter K C (2002) Ki67 protein: the immaculate deception? Histopathology 40:2–11

Bruder D, Probst-Kepper M, Westendorf AM, Geffers R, Beissert S, Loser K, von Boehmer H, Buer J, Hansen W (2004) Neuropilin-1: a surface marker of regulatory T cells. Eur J Immunol 34:623–630

Bruhl H, Cihak J, Schneider MA, Plachy J, Rupp T, Wenzel I, Shakarami M, Milz S, Ellwart JW, Stangassinger M et al (2004) Dual role of CCR2 during initiation and progression of collagen-induced arthritis: evidence for regulatory activity of CCR2+ T cells. J Immunol 172:890–898

Bystry RS, Aluvihare V, Welch KA, Kallikourdis M, Betz AG (2001) B cells and professional APCs recruit regulatory T cells via CCL4. Nat Immunol 2:1126–1132

Campbell DJ, Butcher EC (2002) Rapid acquisition of tissue-specific homing phenotypes by CD4+ T cells activated in cutaneous or mucosal lymphoid tissues. J Exp Med 195:135–141

Cao D, Malmstrom V, Baecher-Allan C, Hafler D, Klareskog L, Trollmo C (2003) Isolation and functional characterization of regulatory CD25brightCD4+ T cells from the target organ of patients with rheumatoid arthritis. Eur J Immunol 33:215–223

Cederbom L, Hall H, Ivars F (2000) CD4+CD25+ regulatory T cells down-regulate co-stimulatory molecules on antigen-presenting cells. Eur J Immunol 30:1538–1543

Cepek KL, Shaw SK, Parker CM, Russell GJ, Morrow JS, Rimm DL, Brenner MB (1994) Adhesion between epithelial cells and T lymphocytes mediated by E-cadherin and the alpha E beta 7 integrin. Nature 372:190–193

Cerf-Bensussan N, Jarry A, Brousse N, Lisowska-Grospierre B, Guy-Grand D, Griscelli C (1987) A monoclonal antibody (HML-1) defining a novel membrane molecule present on human intestinal lymphocytes. Eur J Immunol 17:1279–1285

Chen Y, Kuchroo VK, Inobe J, Hafler DA, Weiner HL (1994) Regulatory T cell clones induced by oral tolerance: suppression of autoimmune encephalomyelitis. Science 265:1237–1240

Colantonio L, Iellem A, Sinigaglia F, D'Ambrosio D (2002) Skin-homing CLA+ T cells and regulatory CD25+ T cells represent major subsets of human peripheral blood memory T cells migrating in response to CCL1/I-309. Eur J Immunol 32:3506–3514

Cozzo C, Larkin J 3rd, Caton AJ (2003) Cutting edge: self-peptides drive the peripheral expansion of CD4+CD25+ regulatory T cells. J Immunol 171:5678–5682

Dittmer U, He H, Messer RJ, Schimmer S, Olbrich AR, Ohlen C, Greenberg PD, Stromnes IM, Iwashiro M, Sakaguchi S et al (2004) Functional impairment of CD8(+) T cells by regulatory T cells during persistent retroviral infection. Immunity 20:293–303

Fisson S, Darrasse-Jeze G, Litvinova E, Septier F, Klatzmann D, Liblau R, Salomon BL (2003) Continuous activation of autoreactive CD4+ CD25+ regulatory T cells in the steady state. J Exp Med 198:737–746

Fontenot JD, Gavin MA, Rudensky AY (2003) Foxp3 programs the development and function of CD4+CD25+ regulatory T cells. Nat Immunol 4:330–336

Forster R, Schubel A, Breitfeld D, Kremmer E, Renner Muller I, Wolf E, Lipp M (1999) CCR7 coordinates the primary immune response by establishing functional microenvironments in secondary lymphoid organs. Cell 99:23–33

Fu S, Yopp AC, Mao X, Chen D, Zhang N, Mao M, Ding Y, Bromberg JS (2004) CD4+ CD25+ CD62+ T-regulatory cell subset has optimal suppressive and proliferative potential. Am J Transplant 4:65–78

Gallatin WM, Weissman IL, Butcher EC (1983) A cell-surface molecule involved in organ-specific homing of lymphocytes. Nature 304:30–34

Gambineri E, Torgerson TR, Ochs HD (2003) Immune dysregulation, polyendocrinopathy, enteropathy X-linked inheritance (IPEX), a syndrome of systemic autoimmunity caused by mutations of FOXP3, a critical regulator of T-cell homeostasis. Curr Opin Rheumatol 15:430–435

Gavin M, Rudensky A (2003) Control of immune homeostasis by naturally arising regulatory CD4+ T cells. Curr Opin Immunol 15:690–696

Gavin MA, Clarke SR, Negrou E, Gallegos A, Rudensky A (2002) Homeostasis and anergy of CD4+CD25+ suppressor T cells in vivo. Nat Immunol 3:33–41

Gershon RK (1975) A disquisition on suppressor T cells. Transplant Rev 26:170–185

Gershon RK, Kondo K (1970) Cell interactions in the induction of tolerance: the role of thymic lymphocytes. Immunology 18:723–737

Goulvestre C, Batteux F, Charreire J (2002) Chemokines modulate experimental autoimmune thyroiditis through attraction of autoreactive or regulatory T cells. Eur J Immunol 32:3435–3442

Graca L, Cobbold SP, Waldmann H (2002) Identification of regulatory T cells in tolerated allografts. J Exp Med 195:1641–1646

Green EA, Choi Y, Flavell RA (2002) Pancreatic lymph node-derived CD4(+)CD25(+) Treg cells: highly potent regulators of diabetes that require TRANCE-RANK signals. Immunity 16:183–191

Groux H, O'Garra A, Bigler M, Rouleau M, Antonenko S, de Vries JE, Roncarolo MG (1997) A CD4+ T-cell subset inhibits antigen-specific T-cell responses and prevents colitis. Nature 389:737–742

Hamann Andrew DP, Jablonski-Westrich D, Holzmann B, Butcher EC (1994) Role of a4-integrins in lymphocyte homing to mucosal tissues in vivo. J Immunol 152:3282–3293

Herbelin A, Gombert JM, Lepault F, Bach JF, Chatenoud L (1998) Mature mainstream TCR alpha beta+CD4+ thymocytes expressing L-selectin mediate "active tolerance" in the nonobese diabetic mouse. J Immunol 161:2620–2628

Hori S, Carvalho TL, Demengeot J (2002a) CD25+CD4+ regulatory T cells suppress CD4+ T cell-mediated pulmonary hyperinflammation driven by Pneumocystis carinii in immunodeficient mice. Eur J Immunol 32:1282–1291

Hori S, Haury M, Coutinho A, Demengeot J (2002b) Specificity requirements for selection and effector functions of CD25+4+ regulatory T cells in anti-myelin basic protein T cell receptor transgenic mice. Proc Natl Acad Sci U S A 99:8213–8218

Hori S, Haury M, Lafaille JJ, Demengeot J, Coutinho A (2002c) Peripheral expansion of thymus-derived regulatory cells in anti-myelin basic protein T cell receptor transgenic mice. Eur J Immunol 32:3729–3735

Hori S, Nomura T, Sakaguchi S (2003a) Control of regulatory T cell development by the transcription factor Foxp3. Science 299:1057–1061

Hori S, Takahashi T, Sakaguchi S (2003b) Control of autoimmunity by naturally arising regulatory CD4+ T cells. Adv Immunol 81:331–371

Huehn J, Siegmund K, Lehmann J, Siewert C, Haubold U, Feuerer M, Debes GF, Lauber J, Frey O, Przybylski GK et al (2004) Developmental stage, phenotype and migration distinguish naive- and effector/memory-like CD4+ regulatory T cells. J Exp Med 199:303–313

Iellem A, Mariani M, Lang R, Recalde H, Panina-Bordignon P, Sinigaglia F, D'Ambrosio D (2001) Unique chemotactic response profile and specific expression of chemokine receptors CCR4 and CCR8 by CD4(+)CD25(+) regulatory T cells. J Exp Med 194:847–853

Iellem A, Colantonio L, D'Ambrosio D (2003) Skin-versus gut-skewed homing receptor expression and intrinsic CCR4 expression on human peripheral blood CD4+CD25+ suppressor T cells. Eur J Immunol 33:1488–1496

Itoh M, Takahashi T, Sakaguchi N, Kuniyasu Y, Shimizu J, Otsuka F, Sakaguchi S (1999) Thymus and autoimmunity: production of CD25+CD4+ naturally anergic and suppressive T cells as a key function of the thymus in maintaining immunologic self-tolerance. J Immunol 162:5317–5326

Jacob J, Baltimore D (1999) Modelling T-cell memory by genetic marking of memory T cells in vivo [see comments]. Nature 399:593–597

Janssens W, Carlier V, Wu B, VanderElst L, Jacquemin MG, Saint-Remy JM (2003) CD4+CD25+ T cells lyse antigen-presenting B cells by Fas-Fas ligand interaction in an epitope-specific manner. J Immunol 171:4604–4612

Jonuleit H, Schmitt E (2003) The regulatory T cell family: distinct subsets and their interrelations. J Immunol 171:6323–6327

Jordan MS, Boesteanu A, Reed AJ, Petrone AL, Holenbeck AE, Lerman MA, Naji A, Caton AJ (2001) Thymic selection of CD4+CD25+ regulatory T cells induced by an agonist self-peptide. Nat Immunol 2:301–306

Karim M, Kingsley CI, Bushell AR, Sawitzki BS, Wood KJ (2004) Alloantigen-induced CD25+CD4+ regulatory T cells can develop in vivo from CD25-CD4+ precursors in a thymus-independent process. J Immunol 172:923–928

Kawahata K, Misaki Y, Yamauchi M, Tsunekawa S, Setoguchi K, Miyazaki J, Yamamoto K (2002) Generation of CD4(+)CD25(+) regulatory T cells from autoreactive T cells simultaneously with their negative selection in the thymus and from nonautoreactive T cells by endogenous TCR expression. J Immunol 168:4399–4405

Khattri R, Cox T, Yasayko SA, Ramsdell F (2003) An essential role for Scurfin in CD4+CD25+ T regulatory cells. Nat Immunol 4:337–342

Kilshaw PJ, Murant SJ (1991) Expression and regulation of beta 7(beta p) integrins on mouse lymphocytes: relevance to the mucosal immune system. Eur J Immunol 21:2591–2597

Klein L, Khazaie K, von Boehmer H (2003) In vivo dynamics of antigen-specific regulatory T cells not predicted from behavior in vitro. Proc Natl Acad Sci U S A 100:8886–8891

Kullberg MC, Jankovic D, Gorelick PL, Caspar P, Letterio JJ, Cheever AW, Sher A (2002) Bacteria-triggered CD4(+) T regulatory cells suppress Helicobacter hepaticus-induced colitis. J Exp Med 196:505–515

Kuniyasu Y, Takahashi T, Itoh M, Shimizu J, Toda G, Sakaguchi S (2000) Naturally anergic and suppressive CD25(+)CD4(+) T cells as a functionally and phenotypically distinct immunoregulatory T cell subpopulation. Int Immunol 12:1145–1155

Lefrancois L, Parker CM, Olson S, Muller W, Wagner N, Puddington L (1999) The role of beta7 integrins in CD8 T cell trafficking during an antiviral immune response. J Exp Med 189:1631–1638

Lehmann J, Huehn J, Rosa MDl, Maszyna F, Kretschmer U, Brunner M, Scheffold A, Krenn V, Hamann A (2002) Expression of the integrin alphaEbeta7 identifies unique subsets of CD25+ as well as CD25-regulatory T cells. Proceed Natl Acad Sci U S A 99:13031–13036

Lepault F, Gagnerault MC (2000) Characterization of peripheral regulatory CD4+ T cells that prevent diabetes onset in nonobese diabetic mice. J Immunol 164:240–247

Luther SA, Tang HL, Hyman PL, Farr AG, Cyster JG (2000) Coexpression of the chemokines ELC and SLC by T zone stromal cells and deletion of the ELC gene in the plt/plt mouse. Proc Natl Acad Sci U S A 97:12694–12699

Mackay CR, Marston WL, Dudler L (1990) Naive and memory T cells show distinct pathways of lymphocyte recirculation. J Exp Med 171:801–817

Maloy KJ, Powrie F (2001) Regulatory T cells in the control of immune pathology. Nat Immunol 2:816–822

Maloy KJ, Salaun L, Cahill R, Dougan G, Saunders NJ, Powrie F (2003) CD4+CD25+ T(R) cells suppress innate immune pathology through cytokine-dependent mechanisms. J Exp Med 197:111–119

Masopust D, Vezys V, Marzo AL, Lefrancois L (2001) Preferential localization of effector memory cells in nonlymphoid tissue. Science 291:2413–2417

McHugh R, Whitters MJ, Piccorillo CA, Young DA, Shevach EM, Collins M, Byrne MC (2002) CD4+CD25+ immunoregulatory T cells: gene expression analysis reveals a functional role for the glucocorticoid-induced TNF receptor. Immunity 16:311–323

Moser B, Loetscher P (2001) Lymphocyte traffic control by chemokines. Nat Immunol 2:123–128

Mottet C, Uhlig HH, Powrie F (2003) Cutting edge: cure of colitis by CD4(+)CD25(+) regulatory T cells. J Immunol 170:3939–3943

Murakami M, Sakamoto A, Bender J, Kappler J, Marrack P (2002) CD25+CD4+ T cells contribute to the control of memory CD8+ T cells. Proc Natl Acad Sci U S A 99:8832–8837

Nakamura K, Kitani A, Strober W (2001) Cell contact-dependent immunosuppression by CD4(+)CD25(+) regulatory T cells is mediated by cell surface-bound transforming growth factor beta. J Exp Med 194:629–644

Nascimbeni M, Shin EC, Chiriboga L, Kleiner DE, Rehermann B (2004) Peripheral CD4/CD8 double-positive T cells are differentiated effector memory cells with antiviral functions. Blood 104:478–486

Oldenhove G, de Heusch M, Urbain-Vansanten G, Urbain J, Maliszewski C, Leo O, Moser M (2003) CD4+ CD25+ regulatory T cells control T helper cell type 1 responses to foreign antigens induced by mature dendritic cells in vivo. J Exp Med 198:259–266

Pacholczyk R, Kraj P, Ignatowicz L (2002) Peptide specificity of thymic selection of CD4+CD25+ T cells. J Immunol 168:613–620

Papiernik M, de Moraes ML, Pontoux C, Vasseur F, Penit C (1998) Regulatory CD4 T cells: expression of IL-2R alpha chain, resistance to clonal deletion and IL-2 dependency. Int Immunol 10:371–378

Piccirillo CA, Shevach EM (2001) Cutting edge: control of cd8(+) t cell activation by cd4(+)cd25(+) immunoregulatory cells. J Immunol 167:1137–1140

Piccirillo CA, Letterio JJ, Thornton AM, McHugh RS, Mamura M, Mizuhara H, Shevach EM (2002) CD4(+)CD25(+) regulatory T cells can mediate suppressor function in the absence of transforming growth factor beta1 production and responsiveness. J Exp Med 196:237–246

Powrie F, Carlino J, Leach MW, Mauze S, Coffman RL (1996) A critical role for transforming growth factor-beta but not interleukin 4 in the suppression of T helper type 1-mediated colitis by CD45RB(low) CD4+ T cells. J Exp Med 183:2669–2674

Prud'homme GJ, Piccirillo CA (2000) The inhibitory effects of transforming growth factor-beta-1 (TGF-beta1) in autoimmune diseases. J Autoimmun 14:23–42

Read S, Malmstrom V, Powrie F (2000) Cytotoxic T lymphocyte-associated antigen 4 plays an essential role in the function of CD25(+)CD4(+) regulatory cells that control intestinal inflammation. J Exp Med 192:295–302

Romagnoli P, Hudrisier D, van Meerwijk JP (2002) Preferential recognition of self antigens despite normal thymic deletion of CD4(+)CD25(+) regulatory T cells. J Immunol 168:1644–1648

Roncarolo MG, Bacchetta R, Bordignon C, Narula S, Levings MK (2001) Type 1 T regulatory cells. Immunol Rev 182:68–79

Sakaguchi S (2004) Naturally arising CD4+ regulatory T cells for immunologic self-tolerance and negative control of immune responses. Annu Rev Immunol 22:531–562

Sakaguchi S, Sakaguchi N, Asano M, Itoh M, Toda M (1995) Immunologic self-tolerance maintained by activated T cells expressing IL-2 receptor alpha-chains (CD25). Breakdown of a single mechanism of self-tolerance causes various autoimmune diseases. J Immunol 155:1151–1164

Sakaguchi S, Hori S, Fukui Y, Sasazuki T, Sakaguchi N, Takahashi T (2003) Thymic generation and selection of CD25+CD4+ regulatory T cells: implications of their broad repertoire and high self-reactivity for the maintenance of immunological self-tolerance. Novartis Found Symp 252:6–16; discussion 16–23, 106–114

Salomon B, Lenschow DJ, Rhee L, Ashourian N, Singh B, Sharpe A, Bluestone JA (2000) B7/CD28 costimulation is essential for the homeostasis of the CD4+CD25+ immunoregulatory T cells that control autoimmune diabetes. Immunity 12:431–440

Schon MP, Arya A, Murphy EA, Adams CM, Strauch UG, Agace WW, Marsal J, Donohue JP, Her H, Beier DR et al (1999) Mucosal T lymphocyte numbers are selectively reduced in integrin alpha E (CD103)-deficient mice. J Immunol 162:6641–6649

Schon MP, Schon M, Warren HB, Donohue JP, Parker CM (2000) Cutaneous inflammatory disorder in integrin alphaE (CD103)-deficient mice. J Immunol 165:6583–6589

Schwarz A, Maeda A, Wild MK, Kernebeck K, Gross N, Aragane Y, Beissert S, Vestweber D, Schwarz T (2004) Ultraviolet radiation-induced regulatory T cells not only inhibit the induction but can suppress the effector phase of contact hypersensitivity. J Immunol 172:1036–1043

Sebastiani S, Allavena P, Albanesi C, Nasorri F, Biancchi G, Traidl C, Sozzani S, Girolomoni G, Cavani A (2001) Chemokine receptor expression and function in CD4+ T Lymphocytes with regulatory activity 1. J Immunol 166:996–1002

Shevach EM (2002) CD4+ CD25+ suppressor T cells: more questions than answers. Nat Rev Immunol 2:389–400

Shimizu J, Yamazaki S, Takahashi T, Ishida Y, Sakaguchi S (2002) Stimulation of CD25(+)CD4(+) regulatory T cells through GITR breaks immunological self-tolerance. Nat Immunol 3:135–142

Stassen M, Fondel S, Bopp T, Richter C, Müller C, Kubach J, Becker C, Knop J, Enk AH, Schmitt S, Schmitt E, Jonuleit H (2004) Human CD25+ regulatory T cells: two subsets defined by the integrins a4b7 or a4b1 confer distinct suppressive properties upon CD4+ T helper cells. Eur J Immunol 34:1303–1311

Stephens LA, Mason D (2000) CD25 is a marker for CD4+ thymocytes that prevent autoimmune diabetes in rats, but peripheral T cells with this function are found in both CD25+ and CD25– subpopulations. J Immunol 165:3105–3110

Suri-Payer E, Cantor H (2001) Differential cytokine requirements for regulation of autoimmune gastritis and colitis by CD4(+)CD25(+) T cells. J Autoimmun 16:115–123

Suvas S, Kumaraguru U, Pack CD, Lee S, Rouse BT (2003) CD4+CD25+ T cells regulate virus-specific primary and memory CD8+ T cell responses. J Exp Med 198:889–901

Szanya V, Ermann J, Taylor C, Holness C, Fathman CG (2002) The subpopulation of CD4+CD25+ splenocytes that delays adoptive transfer of diabetes expresses L-selectin and high levels of CCR7. J Immunol 169:2461–2465

Takahashi T, Kuniyasu Y, Toda M, Sakaguchi N, Itoh M, Iwata M, Shimizu J, Sakaguchi S (1998) Immunologic self-tolerance maintained by CD25+CD4+ naturally anergic and suppressive T cells: induction of autoimmune disease by breaking their anergic/suppressive state. Int Immunol 10:1969–1980

Takahashi T, Tagami T, Yamazaki S, Uede T, Shimizu J, Sakaguchi N, Mak TW, Sakaguchi S (2000) Immunologic self-tolerance maintained by CD25(+)CD4(+) regulatory T cells constitutively expressing cytotoxic T lymphocyte-associated antigen 4. J Exp Med 192:303–310

Thornton AM, Shevach EM (1998) CD4+CD25+ immunoregulatory T cells suppress polyclonal T cell activation in vitro by inhibiting interleukin 2 production. J Exp Med 188:287–296

Thornton AM, Shevach EM (2000) Suppressor effector function of CD4+CD25+ immunoregulatory T cells is antigen nonspecific. J Immunol 164:183–190

Thorstenson KM, Khoruts A (2001) Generation of anergic and potentially immunoregulatory CD25+CD4 T cells in vivo after induction of peripheral tolerance with intravenous or oral antigen. J Immunol 167:188–195

Tietz W, Allemand Y, Borges E, Laer DV, Hallmann R, Vestweber D, Hamann A (1998) CD4+ T-cells only migrate into inflamed skin if they express ligands for E- and P-selectin. J Immunol 161:963–970

Von Boehmer H (2003) Dynamics of suppressor T cells: in vivo veritas. J Exp Med 198:845–849

Walker LS, Chodos A, Eggena M, Dooms H, Abbas AK (2003) Antigen-dependent proliferation of CD4+ CD25+ regulatory T cells in vivo. J Exp Med 198:249–258

Weiner HL (2001) Oral tolerance: immune mechanisms and the generation of Th3-type TGF-beta-secreting regulatory cells. Microbes Infect 3:947–954

Woo EY, Yeh H, Chu CS, Schlienger K, Carroll RG, Riley JL, Kaiser LR, June CH (2002) Cutting edge: regulatory T cells from lung cancer patients directly inhibit autologous T cell proliferation. J Immunol 168:4272–4276

Yamazaki S, Iyoda T, Tarbell K, Olson K, Velinzon K, Inaba K, Steinman rm (2003) Direct expansion of functional CD25+ CD4+ regulatory T cells by antigen-processing dendritic cells. J Exp Med 198:235–247

Zelenika D, Adams E, Humm S, Graca L, Thompson S, Cobbold SP, Waldmann H (2002) Regulatory T cells overexpress a subset of th2 gene transcripts. J Immunol 168:1069–1079

Peripheral Generation and Function of CD4$^+$CD25$^+$ Regulatory T Cells

L. S. Taams[1] (✉) · A. N. Akbar[2]

[1]Infection and Immunity Research Group, King's College London, Franklin-Wilkins Building, 150 Stamford Street, London SE1 9NN, UK
leonie.taams@kcl.ac.uk

[2]Department Immunology and Molecular Pathology, Windeyer Institute for Medical Sciences, Royal Free and University College Medical School, 46 Cleveland Street, London W1T 4JF, UK

1	CD4$^+$CD25$^+$ Regulatory T Cells	116
2	Thymic Generation of CD4$^+$CD25$^+$ Regulatory T Cells	118
3	Peripheral Generation of CD4$^+$CD25$^+$ Regulatory T Cells	119
4	Suppressive Effects of CD4$^+$CD25$^+$ Regulatory T Cells on the Adaptive Immune Response	121
5	Suppressive Effects of CD4$^+$CD25$^+$ Regulatory T Cells on the Innate Immune Response	123
6	Conclusion	124
	References	125

Abstract The balance between immunity and tolerance is important to maintain immune homeostasis. Several mechanisms are in place to ensure that the immune response is controlled, such as T cell anergy, apoptosis and immune ignorance. A fourth mechanism of peripheral tolerance is the active suppression by regulatory or suppressor T cells. The existence of suppressor T cells was first described in the early 1970s, but these cells became discredited in the 1980s. The work of Shimon Sakaguchi and others, however, has brought these cells back into the limelight and nowadays research into regulatory/suppressor T cells is a very active field of immunology. Different types of regulatory T cells have been described, including CD4$^+$CD25$^+$ T cells that constitutively express CTLA-4, GITR and Foxp3, TGF-β producing Th3 cells, IL-10 producing Tr1 cells, and CD8$^+$CD28$^-$ T cells. This review will focus on the generation and function of CD4$^+$CD25$^+$ regulatory T cells. CD4$^+$CD25$^+$ regulatory cells were originally described as thymus-derived anergic/suppressive T cells. Recent papers, however, indicate that these cells might also be generated in the periphery. CD4$^+$CD25$^+$ regulatory T cells can be activated by self-antigens and non-self-antigens, and once activated can suppress T cells in an antigen nonspecific manner. Interestingly, the suppressive effects of these cells are not restricted to the adaptive immune system (T and B cells) but can also affect the activation and function of innate immune cells (monocytes, macrophages, dendritic cells). These features make the CD4$^+$CD25$^+$ regulatory T cell subset an interesting target for immunotherapy of chronic inflammatory or autoimmune diseases.

Abbreviations

APC	Antigen-presenting cell
CTLA-4	Cytotoxic T lymphocyte associated antigen-4
GITR	Glucocorticoid-induced tumor necrosis factor receptor-family-related gene
IL	Interleukin
mAb	Monoclonal antibody
PBMC	Peripheral blood mononuclear cells
TCR	T cell receptor
TGF-β	Transforming growth factor β
Tregs	Regulatory T cells

1
CD4$^+$CD25$^+$ Regulatory T Cells

Immune tolerance has been a topic of intensive research since the early 1950s. The Nobel Prize winning work of Peter Medawar and colleagues showed that intraembryonic injection of foreign tissue cells into CBA mice resulted in tolerance when skin grafts from the same donor were transplanted into the mice after birth [1]. This immune tolerance was not due to antigenic alteration of the grafts, since injection of lymph node suspensions derived from CBA mice pre-immunized with donor cells led to breakdown of tolerance. Rather it was suggested that active immune tolerance was present. The concept that active tolerance could be mediated by suppressor T cells was introduced in the early 1970s by Gershon and co-workers [2–4]. They showed that the presence of thymocytes during antigen exposure of thymectomized, lethally irradiated and bone marrow-grafted mice resulted in tolerance upon subsequent exposure to the same antigen, even after the addition of fresh thymocytes during the rechallenge. The search for the molecular basis of this phenomenon commenced soon after. Initially, extensive documentation was published on the presence of soluble suppressor factors and suppressor genes such as the I-J gene, which was supposedly located in the mouse MHC locus [5–7]. Subsequent sequencing of this region revealed the absence of the I-J gene and together with a lack of suitable evidence on the existence of soluble suppressor factors, the rapid decline of the suppressor T cell era had begun [8, 9] (Fig. 1). By this stage, many researchers were convinced

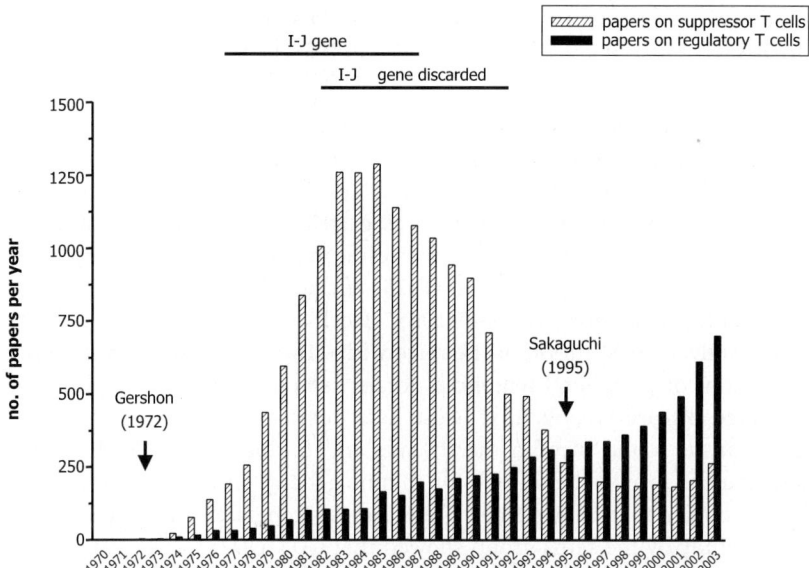

Fig. 1 The rise and fall of suppressor T cells and subsequent rise of regulatory T cells

that using the 'S-word' became a certain way of having one's paper rejected. However, during the mid-1990s this slowly began to change when Sakaguchi and co-workers described a subset of immunosuppressive T cells capable of preventing autoimmune disease in mice. These cells were characterized by the expression of CD4 and CD25, the interleukin-2 (IL-2) receptor α chain [10]. Rather than calling them suppressor T cells, these cells are now referred to as $CD4^+CD25^+$ regulatory T cells (Tregs). When stimulated in vitro, the $CD4^+CD25^+$ Tregs were found to be anergic and suppressive [11]. In vivo depletion of this subset by day-3 thymectomy resulted in the spontaneous development of organ-specific autoimmunity such as gastritis and thyroiditis, and reconstitution of the mice with $CD4^+CD25^+$ Tregs prevented disease [10, 12, 13]. Since then, many groups have investigated the presence and function of these cells in both rodents and humans, and this is accompanied by a steep increase in the number of papers on regulatory T cells (Fig. 1). Perhaps surprisingly though to many of us in the field, we still have not reached the level of output that was seen in the mid-1980s. Despite the activity in the field, many questions concerning the existence and function of $CD4^+CD25^+$ Tregs still exist. In this review we will summarize the current thinking on the generation of $CD4^+CD25^+$ Tregs and their suppressive effects on the adaptive and the innate immune system.

2
Thymic Generation of CD4$^+$CD25$^+$ Regulatory T Cells

Sakaguchi and co-workers demonstrated that CD4$^+$CD25$^+$ regulatory T cells could be detected in the thymus as well as in peripheral lymphoid organs [10, 12, 13]. Thymectomy on day 3 led to the spontaneous development of organ-specific autoimmunity such as gastritis and thyroiditis; however, thymectomy at day 0 or day 7 did not result in disease. This was explained either by a lack of peripheral CD4$^+$CD25$^-$ effector T cells at day 0, or by sufficient influx of suppressive CD4$^+$CD25$^+$ T cells into the periphery at day 7. Importantly, reconstitution of the mice with CD4$^+$CD25$^+$ Tregs from either the thymus or peripheral lymphoid organs such as spleen or lymph nodes prevented disease [10, 12, 13]. These data demonstrated that CD4$^+$CD25$^+$ Tregs can be found in both the thymus and the periphery. Furthermore, these studies provided evidence for thymic generation but did not exclude the possibility that CD4$^+$CD25$^+$ Tregs can be generated in the periphery. A later study by the same group showed that CD4$^+$CD25$^+$ Tregs can indeed be generated in the thymus [14]. Thy-1.2 CD4$^-$CD8$^-$ thymocytes from Balb/c mice were injected into the thymus of Balb/c Thy-1.1 congenic mice and the arising CD4$^+$CD25$^+$ population contained significant numbers of Thy-1.2$^+$ cells. Moreover, CD4$^+$CD25$^+$ T cells developed in vitro from CD4$^-$CD8$^-$ thymocytes in a fetal thymic organ culture. The same paper showed that CD4$^+$CD25$^+$ Tregs acquire their suppressive properties during the thymic selection process. It was shown that anergic/suppressive CD25$^+$CD4$^+$CD8$^-$ thymocytes and CD4$^+$CD25$^+$ T cells developed to a similar extent in ovalbumin (OVA)-specific T cell receptor (TCR) transgenic DO11.10 mice as in nontransgenic mice. However, when DO11.10 mice were crossed on a RAG2-deficient background, the CD4$^+$CD25$^+$ Treg subset was almost absent, indicating that rearrangement of endogenous α chains was required for CD4$^+$CD25$^+$ Treg development. Moreover, the data suggested that during the selection process in the thymus, Tregs interact with MHC class II molecules, albeit complexed with self-peptides. The avidity of this interaction should be high enough to promote an anergic/suppressive phenotype but insufficient to induce deletion. Support for this came from the studies by Caton and co-workers demonstrating that CD4$^+$CD25$^+$ Tregs could be generated upon high-affinity TCR interaction with self-peptides via a process different from positive selection and deletion [15–17]. Further studies indicated that the expression of MHC class II on thymic cortical epithelium was required and sufficient for the development of CD4$^+$CD25$^+$ Tregs [18]. Other groups showed that although regulatory T cells have a preferential recognition of self-peptides, they can be subject to negative selection [19, 20]. It was shown that the total number of

Tregs was dependent on the diversity of the selecting MHC class II:peptide complexes, leading to CD4$^+$CD25$^+$ Tregs with diverse TCR repertoires [19]. Together these findings demonstrate that CD4$^+$CD25$^+$ Tregs can be generated in the thymus, and suggest that they are selected as part of the natural CD4$^+$ T cell repertoire.

3
Peripheral Generation of CD4$^+$CD25$^+$ Regulatory T Cells

The findings above establish that thymic generation of CD4$^+$CD25$^+$ Tregs can take place. However, these data do not explain how CD4$^+$CD25$^+$ Tregs persist in the periphery throughout life taking into account thymic involution. As we have discussed previously [21], CD4$^+$CD25$^+$ Treg numbers should decrease over time as a result of decreased T cell output from the thymus. A relevant question is therefore how are sufficient numbers of effective CD4$^+$CD25$^+$ Tregs maintained throughout life? This is particularly intriguing since CD4$^+$CD25$^+$ Tregs are anergic and susceptible to apoptosis [22, 23]. We have shown that despite their anergic state CD4$^+$CD25$^+$ Tregs are highly differentiated (i.e., CD45RB^{low}) with a memory phenotype (CD45RO$^+$) and short telomeres [22, 23]. This phenotype is indicative of extensive proliferation in vivo, which brings up the important question of how anergic T cells proliferate to such an extent.

One explanation has recently been offered by the demonstration that CD4$^+$CD25$^+$ Tregs can expand in the periphery whilst maintaining their suppressive capacity. Using the DO11 x RIP-mOVA model, Walker et al. found that CD4$^+$CD25$^+$ Tregs were able to expand in vivo in response to OVA/IFA immunization, and even proliferated upon encounter of the antigen in the pancreatic lymph node [24]. Despite the proliferative response, no cytokine production (e.g., IL-2, IL-4, IL-10 or IFN-γ) was detected, suggesting that the Tregs consumed cytokines produced by bystander cells. When tested in vitro, the CD4$^+$CD25$^+$ Tregs were anergic and suppressive. Steinman and co-workers also showed that CD4$^+$CD25$^+$ Tregs are capable of proliferating both in vitro and in vivo upon stimulation with antigen-loaded dendritic cells, which was enhanced by addition of IL-2 [25]. After antigen-specific expansion, CD4$^+$CD25$^+$ Tregs still retained their suppressive activity. These findings indicate that antigen-specific Tregs might be maintained for long periods of time by antigen-specific proliferation in vivo and/or via bystander stimulation with cytokines or APCs.

Besides peripheral expansion, it is also possible that CD4$^+$CD25$^+$ Tregs are actually generated in the periphery [21]. We and others have previously shown that anergic/suppressive T cells can be derived from responsive CD4+ T cell clones upon antigen presentation by nonprofessional antigen-presenting cells. Both rat and human activated T cell clones express MHC class II molecules, thus allowing peptide to be presented to other T cells. Upon this T–T presentation (i.e., presentation of peptide by T cells in the absence of professional APCs), the T cells adopt an anergic and suppressive phenotype [26–29]. Interestingly, the phenotype and function displayed by such anergic T cell clones are very similar to those of the naturally occurring regulatory T cells: the cells have constitutive expression of CD25 and CTLA-4, a highly differentiated phenotype (CD45RO+ and CD45RB^{low}), short telomeres, and suppress in a cell contact-dependent manner [23, 30]. Thus, CD4+CD25+ Tregs might develop in the periphery from existing responder T cells as a consequence of anergy induction. The induction of anergy in these cells could occur under inflammatory conditions when interferon-γ (IFN-γ) production leads to up-regulation of MHC class II molecules on nonprofessional APCs, e.g., epithelial or endothelial cells, keratinocytes or activated T cells [31–34]. These cells can then present self-peptides or protein fragments that are present in the inflammatory milieu in the absence of appropriate costimulation, resulting in the induction of anergic and suppressive T cells. This model implies that CD4+CD25+ Tregs arise that have broad antigen-specificities similar to the CD4+CD25− T cell repertoire. Indeed, we have shown that human CD4+CD25+ Tregs, like their murine counterparts [11], display a broad TCR Vβ repertoire [23]. This has recently been confirmed at the clonal level using the heteroduplex technique. We found that more than 70% of clones that were found in the CD4+CD25+ T cell subset were also found in the CD4+CD25− cells from the same individuals (A.N. Akbar, unpublished observations). In addition, it has been shown that human CD4+CD25+ Tregs do not only suppress T cell proliferation and/or cytokine production in response to self-antigens, e.g., heat shock protein [23] and myelin oligodendrocyte glycoprotein [35], but also in response to non-self proteins such as cow's milk antigen [23], tetanus toxoid or purified protein derivative [23], grass pollen [36], nickel [37] and *Helicobacter pylori* [38]. These experiments are particularly interesting since these latter antigens are normally not expressed in the thymus. Furthermore, recent reports have demonstrated the existence of CD4+CD25+ Tregs specific to foreign or non-self-antigens. Oral administration of β-lactoglobulin to nontransgenic Balb/c mice resulted in the generation of β-lactoglobulin-specific CD4+CD25+ Tregs that suppressed antigen-specific antibody production in a TGF-β-dependent manner [39]. Interestingly, these cells were found in Peyer's patches only, suggesting that the route of antigen administration and/or tissue-specific APC subsets might influence the type of CD4+CD25+ Treg that develops. Recently, further direct evidence for the induction of non-self-peptide-specific Tregs was provided by the demonstration that an allopeptide-specific CD4$^+$CD25$^+$ regulatory T cell line could be generated by repetitive stimulation ex vivo of CD4$^+$CD25$^+$ Tregs [40].

Peripheral generation of CD4$^+$CD25$^+$ Tregs has also been shown in in vivo models. It was shown that adoptive transfer of CD4$^+$ T cells from RAG-2 deficient DO11.10 mice into recipient Balb/c mice T cells resulted in the generation of CD4$^+$CD25$^+$ Tregs from CD4$^+$CD25$^-$ T cells [41]. When antigen was administered either intravenously or orally, the percentage of TCR transgenic CD4$^+$CD25$^+$ Tregs was increased in the periphery. Since RAG-2-deficient mice lack CD4$^+$CD25$^+$ Tregs [14], these CD25$^+$ T cells could only have derived from the CD25$^-$ T cells. Wood et al. also demonstrated peripheral generation of CD4$^+$CD25$^+$ Tregs in mice that were pretreated with donor alloantigen under the cover of anti-CD4 mAb therapy prior to skin grafting. These Tregs could be generated in the absence of a thymus and independent of the expansion of recent thymic emigrants [42]. Horwitz and co-workers demonstrated that CD4$^+$CD25$^+$ Tregs were induced ex vivo from CD4$^+$CD25$^-$ precursors upon stimulation in the presence of transforming growth factor β (TGF-β) [43]. This seems to be due to the induction of the forkhead/winged helix transcription factor Foxp3 by TGF-β [44, 45]. Foxp3 has been proposed to be the crucial switch factor in the induction of CD4$^+$CD25$^+$ Tregs [46–48]. It was demonstrated in mice that Foxp3 is specifically expressed in CD4$^+$CD25$^+$ Tregs and is required for their development and function. Foxp3-deficient mice develop a lethal lymphoproliferative syndrome similar to cytotoxic T lymphocyte associated antigen-4 (CTLA-4)-deficient mice, which appears to be a direct result of a lack of CD4$^+$CD25$^+$ Tregs. Interestingly, overexpression of Foxp3 induces suppressive activity in both CD4$^+$CD25$^-$ and CD4-CD8$^+$ T cells. In humans it was shown that Foxp3 is preferentially expressed on naturally occurring CD4$^+$CD25$^+$ Tregs but can be up-regulated in activated CD4$^+$CD25$^-$ T cells, which correlates with the induction of CD25 and acquisition of suppressive activity [49]. Together these data suggest that CD4$^+$CD25$^+$ Tregs can arise via two different pathways: (a) through selection processes in the thymus, and (b) via peripheral generation from CD4$^+$CD25$^-$ precursor T cells.

4 Suppressive Effects of CD4$^+$CD25$^+$ Regulatory T Cells on the Adaptive Immune Response

It has been well established that CD4$^+$CD25$^+$ Tregs can suppress the adaptive immune response by inhibiting CD4$^+$ and CD8$^+$ T cell proliferation and cytokine production [11, 22, 50–56]. CD4$^+$CD25$^+$ Tregs can also inhibit autoantibody production in vivo, although the direct suppressive effects on B cell immunoglobulin production in vitro have only been marginally investigated [57]. The mechanisms of suppression have mainly been studied in assays of T cell suppression. It has been shown by many groups that cell contact between the Tregs, responder T cells and APCs is required for suppression [11, 50, 58, 59]. CTLA-4, GITR and OX-40 are three candidates named to be involved in this cell-contact-dependent suppression since these molecules are up-regulated on resting and activated $CD4^+CD25^+$ Tregs [60–63]. In mice, the increased levels of CTLA-4 and GITR were shown to have functional consequences, since in vivo blockade of these molecules abrogated suppression [60, 61, 64, 65]. This might have been a result from direct inhibition of the $CD4^+CD25^+$ Tregs or indirectly from stimulatory effects on the responding $CD4^+CD25^-$ T cells [66]. The regulatory role of GITR might not be confined to $CD4^+CD25^+$ Tregs since it was shown that $CD4^+CD25^-GITR^+$ T cells also displayed potent suppressive activity [67]. In humans, the roles of CTLA-4 and GITR are less clear, since $CD4^+CD25^+$ Treg-suppression was still observed when blocking antibodies to either CTLA-4 or GITR were added to in vitro cultures of human blood lymphocytes [53, 55, 63], but not when human thymocytes were used [68].

In accordance with the cell-contact dependency of suppression, a large number of in vitro studies has shown that neutralization of immunosuppressive cytokines such as IL-10, TGF-β and IL-4 did not block suppression [11, 22, 50, 52, 53, 69, 70]. However, soluble factors that work at small range or in high local concentrations might still attribute to the suppressive effects. Indeed a role for IL-10 and/or TGF-β in $CD4^+CD25^+$ Treg-mediated suppression has been described in several in vivo models for transplantation tolerance [71], colitis/inflammatory bowel disease [72–74], superantigen-induced cytokine production [75] and anterior chamber-associated immune deviation [76]. These conflicting data might be explained by differences in regulatory T cell function in vitro and in vivo, but also by recent findings that $CD4^+CD25^+$ Tregs can mediate infectious tolerance [58, 59]. The phrase 'infectious tolerance' was coined by Gershon and co-workers in 1971 [3] and re-introduced by Waldmann and co-workers in the early 1990s [77]. It refers to the induction of an anergic/suppressive phenotype in responder T cells upon interaction with Tregs, thus leading to an amplification of the suppressive effects. Interestingly, the recent findings showed that the 'spreading of suppression' required cell contact between $CD4^+CD25^+$ Tregs and responder cells, whereas the newly generated suppressor T cells suppressed in a cytokine-dependent manner through IL-10 and/or TGF-β [58, 59]. The production of these cytokines could actively induce the de novo generation of $CD4^+CD25^+$ Tregs either from $CD4^+CD25^-$ T cells or via the induction of tolerogenic APCs, thus resulting in a cascade of immunoregulatory events [44, 78, 79]. In addition, it has been suggested that membrane-bound TGF-β might play a role in suppression [57, 80], and that CTLA-4 signaling and TGF-β-mediated suppression are closely associated [68, 81]. Together these data could reconcile the conflicting data on cell contact versus cytokine dependency of CD4$^+$CD25$^+$ Treg-mediated suppression.

5
Suppressive Effects of CD4$^+$CD25$^+$ Regulatory T Cells on the Innate Immune Response

As described above, the investigation of the suppressive mechanism by Tregs showed that T cell suppression was mediated in a cell-contact-dependent manner. However, it was unclear whether this cell contact involved interactions between Tregs APC or between Tregs and responder T cells. In an elegant study Piccirillo and Shevach demonstrated that CD4$^+$CD25$^+$ Tregs that were preactivated anti-with CD3 mAb and APC could suppress CD8$^+$ T cell proliferation and IFN-γ production in response to stimulation with MHC class I/peptide tetramers in the *absence* of APCs [82]. This paper provided direct evidence that CD4$^+$CD25$^+$ Tregs can suppress T cells in the absence of APCs. Nevertheless, this finding did not exclude the possibility that CD4$^+$CD25$^+$ Tregs can exert direct suppressive effects on APCs. Evidence that this might be the case is indeed accumulating. First of all, it has been demonstrated that CD4$^+$CD25$^+$ Tregs require antigen-specific activation before they can exert their suppressive effects [51, 83]. This indicates that CD4$^+$CD25$^+$ Tregs communicate with APCs in vivo through T cell receptor:MHC interactions, raising the possibility that CD4$^+$CD25$^+$ Tregs can influence the APCs. We and others have published previously that anergic/suppressive CD4$^+$ T cells have the ability to suppress the T cell-stimulatory capacity of APCs. These APCs were either spleen-derived B cells and macrophages in Lewis rats [84] or dendritic cells in mice [85]. In these studies, in vitro induced anergic/suppressive T cell clones were used; however, recent studies indicate that also the naturally occurring CD4$^+$CD25$^+$ regulatory T cells can affect the antigen-presenting function of APCs. Cederbom et al. described that CD4$^+$CD25$^+$ Tregs downmodulate CD80 and CD86 on bone marrow-derived DCs in mice, and that this had functional consequences since these DCs were poor inducers of naïve T cell proliferation [86]. Using human DCs, Misra et al. showed that upon coculture with prestimulated CD4$^+$CD25$^+$ Tregs, the expression levels of CD40 and HLA-DR on DCs were reduced and that the percentages of CD86$^+$ and CD83$^+$ DC were decreased relative to untreated DCs [87]. This altered phenotype was associated with a reduction in the T cell-stimulatory capacity during subsequent allogeneic and PPD-specific T cell stimulation assays, even when the DCs were incubated with rhCD40L prior to incubation with $CD4^+CD25^+$ Tregs. The modulatory effect was cell-contact-dependent since virtually no changes in DC phenotype were observed when cells were separated in a transwell system, although some role for IL-10 and TGF-β was suggested. We have found similar data on the capacity of naturally occurring $CD4^+CD25^+$ Tregs to inhibit the activation and function of human monocytes/macrophages (Taams et al., in press). $CD14^+$ monocytes that were cultured with $CD4^+CD25^+$ Tregs displayed lower levels of CD86, and limited up-regulation of MHC class II, CD40 and CD80 relative to monocytes that were precultured without T cells or with $CD4^+CD25^-$ T cells. These Treg-treated monocytes were strongly inhibited in their capacity to produce pro-inflammatory cytokines in response to LPS, and displayed a reduced T cell-stimulatory capacity compared to control monocytes.

Importantly, the regulation of APC function by $CD4^+CD25^+$ Tregs might also occur in vivo. It was shown recently that transfer of antigen-pulsed mature DCs into mice that were depleted for $CD4^+CD25^+$ Tregs resulted in higher Th1 responses compared to nondepleted mice [88]. A different study by Maloy et al. using a T cell-independent mouse model for intestinal inflammation demonstrated that transfer of $CD4^+CD25^+$ Tregs resulted in reduced activation and recruitment of neutrophils, monocytes/macrophages, DCs and NK cells, which was partly mediated by IL-10 and TGF-β [89]. Together these data indicate that both the adaptive and the innate immune system are subject to $CD4^+CD25^+$ Treg-mediated suppression. The ability of Tregs to inhibit the function of many different cell types helps to explain the observations that $CD4^+CD25^+$ Tregs are efficient in suppressing many immune-mediated diseases including autoimmunity [12, 90, 91], transplant rejection [92], tumor immunity [93–95], allergy [96] and infection [38, 97].

6
Conclusion

Two lineages of $CD4^+CD25^+$ Tregs appear to be present. A lineage of thymus-derived Tregs that specifically recognizes self-peptides with high affinity, and a Treg lineage that is generated in the periphery. These peripherally generated cells can be either derived from highly differentiated $CD4^+CD25^-$ effector T cells or develop due to the presence of a specific milieu (e.g., TGF-β, IL-10, nonprofessional APCs) that skews the cells towards an immunosuppressive mode. Importantly $CD4^+CD25^+$ Tregs can suppress the activation and function of cells from the adaptive immune system, i.e., T and B cells, as well as those from the innate immune system, i.e., monocytes/macrophages, dendritic cells and NK cells. Tregs can thus regulate immune responses against self- and alloantigens, (food) allergens and pathogens, hence preventing autoimmunity, chronic inflammation, infection and hypersensitive immune reactions. The current challenge is to understand how we can specifically switch on or enhance the function of CD4$^+$CD25$^+$ Tregs in order to reverse established inflammatory or autoimmune disease.

References

1. Billingham RE, Brent, L Medawar PB (1953) 'Actively acquired tolerance' of foreign cells. Nature 172:603–606
2. Gershon RK, Kondo K (1970) Cell interactions in the induction of tolerance: the role of thymic lymphocytes. Immunology 18:723–737
3. Gershon RK, Kondo K (1971) Infectious immunological tolerance. Immunology 21:903–914
4. Gershon RK, Cohen P, Hencin R, Liebhaber SA (1972) Suppressor T cells. J Immunol 108:586–590
5. Sumida T, Sado T, Kojima M, Ono K, Kamisaku H, Taniguchi M (1985) I-J as an idiotype of the recognition component of antigen-specific suppressor T-cell factor. Nature 316:738–741
6. Uracz W, Asano Y, Abe R, Tada T (1985) I-J epitopes are adaptively acquired by T cells differentiated in the chimaeric condition. Nature 316:741–743
7. Dorf ME, Benacerraf B (1985) I-J as a restriction element in the suppressor T cell system. Immunol Rev 83:23–40
8. Möller G (1988) Do suppressor T cells exist? Scand J Immunol 27:247–250
9. Dorf ME, Kuchroo VK, Collins M (1992) Suppressor T cells: some answers but more questions. Immunol Today 13:241–243
10. Sakaguchi S, Sakaguchi N, Asano M, Itoh M, Toda M (1995) Immunologic self-tolerance maintained by activated T cells expressing IL-2 receptor alpha-chains (CD25). Breakdown of a single mechanism of self-tolerance causes various autoimmune diseases. J Immunol 155:1151–1164
11. Takahashi T, Kuniyasu Y, Toda M, Sakaguchi N, Itoh M, Iwata M, Shimizu J, Sakaguchi S (1998) Immunologic self-tolerance maintained by CD25$^+$CD4$^+$ naturally anergic and suppressive T cells: induction of autoimmune disease by breaking their anergic/suppressive state. Int Immunol 10:1969–1980
12. Asano M, Toda M, Sakaguchi N, Sakaguchi S (1996) Autoimmune disease as a consequence of developmental abnormality of a T cell subpopulation. J Exp Med 184:387–396
13. Sakaguchi S, Sakaguchi N (1990) Thymus and autoimmunity: capacity of the normal thymus to produce pathogenic self-reactive T cells and conditions required for their induction of autoimmune disease. J Exp Med 172:537–545

14. Itoh M, Takahashi T, Sakaguchi N, Kuniyasu Y, Shimizu J, Otsuka F, Sakaguchi S (1999) Thymus and autoimmunity: production of $CD25^+CD4^+$ naturally anergic and suppressive T cells as a key function of the thymus in maintaining immunologic self-tolerance. J Immunol 162:5317–5326
15. Jordan MS, Riley MP, von Boehmer H, Caton AJ (2000) Anergy and suppression regulate $CD4^+$ T cell responses to a self peptide. Eur J Immunol 30:136–144
16. Jordan MS, Boesteanu A, Reed AJ, Petrone AL, Holenbeck AE, Lerman MA, Naji A, Caton AJ (2001) Thymic selection of $CD4^+CD25^+$ regulatory T cells induced by an agonist self-peptide. Nat Immunol 2:301–306
17. Cozzo C, Larkin J, Caton AJ (2003) Self-peptides drive the peripheral expansion of $CD4^+CD25^+$ regulatory T cells. J Immunol 171:5678–5682
18. Bensinger SJ, Bandeira A, Jordan MS, Caton AJ, Laufer TM (2001) Major histocompatibility complex class II-positive cortical epithelium mediates the selection of $CD4^+CD25^+$ immunoregulatory T cells. J Exp Med 194:427–438
19. Pacholczyk R, Kraj P, Ignatowicz L (2001) Peptide specificity of thymic selection of $CD4^+CD25^+$ T cells. J Immunol 168:613–620
20. Romagnoli P, Hudrisier D, van Meerwijk JPM (2002) Preferential recognition of self antigens despite normal thymic deletion of $CD4^+CD25^+$ regulatory T cells. J Immunol 168:1644–1648
21. Akbar AN, Taams LS, Salmon M, Vukmanovic-Stejic M (2003) The peripheral generation of $CD4^+CD25^+$ regulatory T cells. Immunology 109:319–325
22. Taams LS, Smith J, Rustin MH, Salmon M, Poulter LW, Akbar AN (2001) Human anergic/suppressive $CD4^+CD25^+$ T cells: a highly differentiated and apoptosis-prone population. Eur J Immunol 31:1122–1131
23. Taams LS, Vukmanovic-Stejic M, Smith J, Dunne PJ, Fletcher JM, Plunkett FJ, Ebeling SB, Lombardi G, Rustin MH, Bijlsma JWJ, Lafeber FPJG, Salmon M, Akbar AN (2002) Antigen-specific T cell suppression by human $CD4^+CD25^+$ regulatory T cells. Eur J Immunol 32:1621–1630
24. Walker LSK, Chodos A, Eggena M, Dooms H, Abbas AK (2003) Antigen-dependent proliferation of $CD4^+$ $CD25^+$ regulatory T cells in vivo. J Exp Med 198:249–258
25. Yamazaki S, Iyoda T, Tarbell K, Olson K, Velinzon K, Inaba K, Steinman RM (2003) Direct expansion of functional $CD25^+$ $CD4^+$ regulatory T cells by antigen-processing dendritic cells. J Exp Med 198:235–247
26. Lombardi G, Sidhu S, Batchelor R, Lechler R (1994) Anergic T cells as suppressor cells in vitro. Science 264:1587–1589
27. Taams LS, van Rensen AJML, Poelen MCM, van Els CACM, Besseling AC, Wagenaar JPA, van Eden W, Wauben MHM (1998) Anergic T cells actively suppress T cell responses via the antigen presenting cell. Eur J Immunol 28:2902–2912
28. Taams LS, van Eden W, Wauben MHM (1999) Antigen presentation by T cells versus professional APC: differential consequences for T cell activation and subsequent T cell-APC interactions. Eur J Immunol 29:1543–1550
29. Taams LS, van Eden W, Wauben MHM (1999) Dose-dependent induction of distinct anergic phenotypes: multiple levels of T cell anergy. J Immunol 162:1974–1981
30. Taams LS, Wauben MHM (2000) Anergic T cells as active regulators of the immune response. Hum Immunol 61:633–639

31. Bal V, McIndoe A, Denton G, Hudson D, Lombardi G, Lamb J, Lechler R (1990) Antigen presentation by keratinocytes induces tolerance in human T cells. Eur J Immunol 20:1893–1897
32. Lombardi G, Sidhu S, Dodi T, Batchelor R, Lechler R (1994) Failure of correlation between B7 expression and activation of interleukin-2-secreting T cells. Eur J Immunol 24:523–530
33. Marelli-Berg FM, Hargreaves REG, Carmichael P, Dorling A, Lombardi G, Lechler RI (1996) Major histocompatibility complex class II-expressing endothelial cells induce allospecific nonresponsiveness in naive T cells. J Exp Med 183:1603–1612
34. Marelli-Berg FM, Weetman A, Frasca L, Deacock SJ, Imami N, Lombardi G, Lechler RI (1997) Antigen presentation by epithelial cells induces anergic immunoregulatory CD45RO$^+$ T cells and deletion of CD45RA$^+$ T cells. J Immunol 159:5853–5861
35. Wing K, Lindgren S, Kollberg G, Lundgren A, Harris RA, Rudin A, Lundin S, Suri-Payer E (2003) CD4 T cell activation by myelin oligodendrocyte glycoprotein is suppressed by adult but not cord blood CD25$^+$ T cells. Eur J Immunol 33:579–587
36. Tiemessen MM, van Hoffen E, Knulst AC, van der Zee J-A, Knol EF, Taams LS (2002) CD4$^+$CD25$^+$ regulatory T cells are not functionally impaired in adult patients with IgE-mediated cow's milk allergy. J Allergy Clin Immunol 110:934–936
37. Cavani A, Nasorri F, Ottaviani C, Sebastiani S, De Pita O, Girolomoni G (2003) Human CD25$^+$ regulatory T cells maintain immune tolerance to nickel in healthy, nonallergic individuals. J Immunol 171:5760–5768
38. Lundgren A, Suri-Payer E, Enarsson K, Svennerholm A-M, Lundin BS (2003) Helicobacter pylori-specific CD4$^+$ CD25^{high} regulatory T cells suppress memory T-cell responses to H pylori in infected individuals. Infect Immun 71:1755–1762
39. Tsuji NM, Mizumachi K, Kurisaki J-I (2003) Antigen-specific, CD4$^+$CD25$^+$ regulatory T cell clones induced in Peyer's patches. Int Immunol 15:525–534
40. Jiang S, Camara N, Lombardi G, Lechler RI (2003) Induction of allopeptide-specific human CD4$^+$CD25$^+$ regulatory T cells ex vivo. Blood 102:2180–2186
41. Thorstenson KM, Khoruts A (2001) Generation of anergic and potentially immunoregulatory CD25$^+$CD4 T cells in vivo after induction of peripheral tolerance with intravenous or oral antigen. J Immunol 167:188–195
42. Karim M, Kingsley CI, Bushell AR, Sawitzki BS, Wood KJ (2004) Alloantigen-induced CD25$^+$CD4$^+$ regulatory T cells can develop in vivo from CD25$^-$CD4$^+$ precursors in a thymus-independent process. J Immunol 172:923–928
43. Zheng SG, Gray JD, Ohtsuka K, Yamagiwa S, Horwitz DA (2002) Generation ex vivo of TGF-beta-producing regulatory T cells from CD4$^+$CD25$^-$ precursors. J Immunol 169:4183–4189
44. Chen W, Jin W, Hardegen N, Lei KJ, Li L, Marinos N, McGrady G, Wahl SM (2003) Conversion of peripheral CD4$^+$CD25$^-$ naive T cells to CD4$^+$CD25$^+$ regulatory T cells by TGF-beta induction of transcription factor Foxp3. J Exp Med 198:1875–1886
45. Fantini MC, Becker C, Monteleone G, Pallone F, Galle PR, Neurath MF (2004) Cutting edge: TGF-beta Induces a regulatory phenotype in CD4$^+$CD25- T cells through Foxp3 Induction DOWN-Regulation of Smad7. J Immunol 172:5149–5153
46. Fontenot JD, Gavin MA, Rudensky AY (2003) Foxp3 programs the development and function of CD4$^+$CD25$^+$ regulatory T cells. Natue Immunol 4:330–336

47. Hori S, Nomura T, Sakaguchi S (2003) Control of regulatory T cell development by the transcription factor FOXP3. Science:1057–1061
48. Khattri R, Cox T, Yasayko S-A, Ramsdell F (2003) An essential role for Scurfin in CD4+CD25+ T regulatory cells. Nature Immunol 4:337–342
49. Walker MR, Kasprowicz DJ, Gersuk VH, Benard A, Van Landeghen M, Buckner JH, Ziegler SF (2003) Induction of FoxP3 and acquisition of T regulatory activity by stimulated human CD4+CD25− T cells. J Clin Invest 112:1437–1443
50. Thornton AM, Shevach EM (1998) CD4+CD25+ immunoregulatory T cells suppress polyclonal T cell activation in vitro by inhibiting interleukin 2 production. J Exp Med 188:287–296
51. Thornton AM, Shevach EM (2000) Suppressor effector function of CD4+CD25+ immunoregulatory T cells is antigen nonspecific. J Immunol 164:183–190
52. Stephens LA, Mottet C, Mason D, Powrie F (2001) Human CD4+CD25+ thymocytes and peripheral T cells have immune suppressive activity in vitro. Eur J Immunol 31:1247–1254
53. Levings MK, Sangregorio R, Roncarolo M-G (2001) Human CD25+CD4+ T regulatory cells suppress naive and memory T cell proliferation and can be expanded in vitro without loss of function. J Exp Med 193:1295–1301
54. Ng WF, Duggan PJ, Ponchel F, Matarese G, Lombardi G, Edwards AD, Isaacs JD, Lechler RI (2001) Human CD4+CD25+ cells: a naturally occurring population of regulatory T cells. Blood 98:2736–2744
55. Baecher-Allan C, Brown JA, Freeman GJ, Hafler DA (2001) CD4+CD25^{high} regulatory T cells in human peripheral blood. J Immunol 167:1245–1253
56. Baecher-Allan C, Viglietta V, Hafler DA (2002) Inhibition of human CD4+CD25+high regulatory T cell function. J Immunol 169:6210–6217
57. Nakamura K, Kitani A, Strober W (2001) Cell contact-dependent immunosuppression by CD4+CD25+ regulatory T cells is mediated by cell surface-bound transforming growth factor β. J Exp Med 194:629–644
58. Dieckmann D, Bruett CH, Ploettner H, Lutz MB, Schuler G (2002) Human CD4+CD25+ regulatory, contact-dependent T cells induce interleukin 10-producing, contact-independent type 1-like regulatory T cells. J Exp Med 196:247–253
59. Jonuleit H, Schmitt E, Kakirman H, Stassen M, Knop J, Enk AH (2002) Infectious tolerance: human CD25+ regulatory T cells convey suppressor activity to conventional CD4+ T helper cells. J Exp Med 196:255–260
60. McHugh RS, Whitters MJ, Piccirillo CA, Young DA, Shevach EM, Collins M, Byrne MC (2002) CD4+CD25+ immunoregulatory T cells: gene expression analysis reveals a functional role for the glucocorticoid-induced TNF receptor. Immunity 16:311–323
61. Shimizu J, Yamazaki S, Takahashi T, Ishida Y, Sakaguchi S (2002) Stimulation of CD25+CD4+ regulatory T cells through GITR breaks immunological self-tolerance. Nature Immunol 3:135–142
62. Van Amelsfort JMR, Jacobs KMG, Bijlsma JWJ, Lafeber FPJG, Taams LS (2004) CD4+CD25+ regulatory T cells in rheumatoid arthritis: differences in presence, phenotype and function between peripheral blood and synovial fluid. Arthritis Rheum 50:2775–2785

63. Levings MK, Sangregorio R, Sartirana C, Moschin AL, Battaglia M, Orban PC, Roncarolo M-G (2002) Human CD25$^+$CD4$^+$ T suppressor cell clones produce transforming growth factor beta, but not interleukin 10, and are distinct from type 1 T regulatory cells. J Exp Med 196:1335–1346
64. Read S, Malmstrom V, Powrie F (2000) Cytotoxic T lymphocyte-associated antigen 4 plays an essential role in the function of CD25$^+$CD4$^+$ regulatory cells that control intestinal inflammation. J Exp Med 192:295–302
65. Takahashi T, Tagami T, Yamazaki S, Uede T, Shimizu J, Sakaguchi N, Mak TW, Sakaguchi S (2000) Immunologic self-tolerance maintained by CD25$^+$CD4$^+$ regulatory T cells constitutively expressing cytotoxic T lymphocyte-associated antigen 4. J Exp Med 192:303–309
66. Sutmuller RPM, van Duivenvoorde LM, van Elsas A, Schumacher TNM, Wildenberg ME, Allison JP, Toes REM, Offringa R, Melief CJM (2001) Synergism of cytotoxic T lymphocyte-associated antigen 4 blockade and depletion of CD25$^+$ regulatory T cells in antitumor therapy reveals alternative pathways for suppression of autoreactive cytotoxic T lymphocyte responses. J Exp Med 194:823–832
67. Uraushihara K, Kanai T, Ko K, Totsuka T, Makita S, Iiyama R, Nakamura T, Watanabe M (2003) Regulation of murine inflammatory bowel disease by CD25$^+$ CD25$^-$ CD4$^+$ Glucocorticoid-Induced TNF receptor family-related gene+ regulatory T cells. J Immunol 171:708–716
68. Annunziato F, Cosmi L, Liotta F, Lazzeri E, Manetti R, Vanini V, Romagnani P, Maggi E, Romagnani S (2002) Phenotype, localization, and mechanism of suppression of CD4$^+$CD25$^+$ human thymocytes. J Exp Med 196:379–387
69. Jonuleit H, Schmitt E, Stassen M, Tuettenberg A, Knop J, Enk AH (2001) Identification and functional characterization of human CD4$^+$CD25$^+$ T cells with regulatory properties isolated from peripheral blood. J Exp Med 193:1285–1294
70. Dieckmann D, Plottner H, Berchtold S, Berger T, Schuler G (2001) Ex vivo isolation and characterization of CD4$^+$CD25$^+$ T cells with regulatory properties from human blood. J Exp Med 193:1303–1310
71. Kingsley CI, Karim M, Bushell AR, Wood KJ (2002) CD25$^+$CD4$^+$ regulatory T cells prevent graft rejection: CTLA-4$^-$ IL-10-dependent immunoregulation of alloresponses. J Immunol 168:1080–1086
72. Annacker O, Pimenta-Araujo R, Burlen-Defranoux O, Barbosa TC, Cumano A, Bandeira A (2001) CD25$^+$ CD4$^+$ T cells regulate the expansion of peripheral CD4 T cells through the production of IL-10. J Immunol 166:3008–3018
73. Nakamura K, Kitani A, Fuss I, Pedersen A, Harada N, Nawata H, Strober W (2004) TGF-beta1 plays an important role in the mechanism of CD4$^+$CD25$^+$ regulatory T cell activity in both humans and mice. J Immunol 172:834–842
74. Liu H, Hu B, Xu D, Liew FY (2003) CD4$^+$CD25$^+$ regulatory T cells cure murine colitis: the role of IL-10, TGF-β, CTLA4. J Immunol 171:5012–5017
75. Pontoux C, Banz A, Papiernik M (2002) Natural CD4 CD25$^+$ regulatory T cells control the burst of superantigen-induced cytokine production: the role of IL-10. Int Immunol 14:233–239
76. Skelsey ME, Mayhew E, Niederkorn JY (2003) CD25$^+$, interleukin-10-producing CD4$^+$ T cells are required for suppressor cell production and immune privilege in the anterior chamber of the eye. Immunology 110:18–29

77. Qin S, Cobbold SP, Pope H, Elliott J, Kioussis D, Davies J, Waldmann H (1993) "Infectious" transplantation tolerance. Science 259:974–977
78. Goudy KS, Burkhardt BR, Wasserfall C, Song S, Campbell-Thompson ML, Brusko T, Powers MA, Clare-Salzler MJ, Sobel ES, Ellis TM, Flotte TR, Atkinson MA (2003) Systemic overexpression of IL-10 induces $CD4^+CD25^+$ cell populations in vivo and ameliorates type 1 diabetes in nonobese diabetic mice in a dose-dependent fashion. J Immunol 171:2270–2278
79. Jonuleit H, Schmitt E, Schuler G, Knop J, Enk AH (2000) Induction of interleukin 10-producing, nonproliferating $CD4^+$ T cells with regulatory properties by repetitive stimulation with allogeneic immature human dendritic cells. J Exp Med 192:1213–1222
80. Oida T, Zhang X, Goto M, Hachimura S, Totsuka M, Kaminogawa S, Weiner HL (2003) $CD4^+CD25^-$ T cells that express latency-associated peptide on the surface suppress $CD4^+CD45RB^{high}$-induced colitis by a TGF-beta-dependent mechanism. J Immunol 170:2516–2522
81. Chen W, Jin W, Wahl SM (1998) Engagement of cytotoxic T lymphocyte-associated antigen 4 (CTLA-4) induces transforming growth factor β (TGF-β) production by murine $CD4^+$ T cells. J Exp Med 188:1849–1857
82. Piccirillo CA, Letterio JJ, Thornton AM, McHugh RS, Mamura M, Mizuhara H, Shevach EM (2002) $CD4^+CD25^+$ regulatory T cells can mediate suppressor function in the absence of transforming growth factor $\beta 1$ production and responsiveness. J Exp Med 196:237–245
83. Piccirillo CA, Shevach EM (2001) Control of $CD8^+$ T cell activation by $CD4^+CD25^+$ immunoregulatory cells. J Immunol 167:1137–1140
84. Taams LS, Boot EPJ, van Eden W, Wauben MHM (2000) "Anergic" T cells modulate the T-cell activating capacity of antigen-presenting cells. J Autoimmunity 14:335–341
85. Vendetti S, Chai J-G, Dyson J, Simpson E, Lombardi G, Lechler R (2000) Anergic T cells inhibit the antigen-presenting function of dendritic cells. J Immunol 165:1175–1181
86. Cederbom L, Hall H, Ivars F (2000) $CD4^+CD25^+$ regulatory T cells down-regulate co-stimulatory molecules on antigen-presenting cells. Eur J Immunol 30:1538–1543
87. Misra N, Bayry J, Lacroix-Desmazes S, Kazatchkine MD, Kaveri SV (2004) Cutting edge: human $CD4^+CD25^+$ T cells restrain the maturation and antigen-presenting function of dendritic cells. J Immunol 172:4676–4680
88. Oldenhove G, de Heusch M, Urbain-Vansanten G, Urbain J, Maliszewski C, Leo O, Moser M (2003) $CD4^+$ $CD25^+$ regulatory T cells control T helper cell type 1 responses to foreign antigens induced by mature dendritic cells in vivo. J Exp Med 198:259–266
89. Maloy KJ, Salaun L, Cahill R, Dougan G, Saunders NJ, Powrie F (2003) $CD4^+CD25^+$ Tr cells suppress innate immune pathology through cytokine-dependent mechanisms. J Exp Med 197:111–119
90. Suri-Payer E, Amar AZ, Thornton AM, Shevach EM (1998) $CD4^+CD25^+$ T cells inhibit both the induction and effector function of autoreactive T cells and represent a unique lineage of immunoregulatory cells. J Immunol 160:1212–1218

91. Viglietta V, Baecher-Allan C, Weiner HL, Hafler DA (2004) Loss of functional suppression by CD4$^+$CD25$^+$ regulatory T cells in patients with multiple sclerosis. J Exp Med 199:971–979
92. Wood KJ, Sakaguchi S (2003) Regulatory T cells in transplantation tolerance. Nature Rev Immunol 3:199–210
93. Shimizu J, Yamazaki S, Sakaguchi S (1999) Induction of tumor immunity by removing CD25$^+$CD4$^+$ T cells: a common basis between tumor immunity and autoimmunity. J Immunol 163:5211–5218
94. Gallimore A, Sakaguchi S (2002) Regulation of tumour immunity by CD25$^+$ T cells. Immunology 107:5–9
95. Woo EY, Yeh H, Chu CS, Schlienger K, Carroll RG, Riley JL, Kaiser LR, June CH (2002) Regulatory T cells from lung cancer patients directly inhibit autologous T cell proliferation. J Immunol 168:4272–4276
96. Ling EM, Smith T, Nguyen XD, Pridgeon C, Dallman M, Arbery J, Carr VA, Robinson DS (2004) Relation of CD4$^+$CD25$^+$ regulatory T-cell suppression of allergen-driven T-cell activation to atopic status and expression of allergic disease. Lancet 363:608–615
97. Belkaid Y, CA Piccirillo, Mendez S, Shevach EM, Sacks DL (2002) CD4$^+$CD25$^+$ regulatory T cells control Leishmania major persistence and immunity. Nature 420:502–507

Dendritic Cells: Key Cells for the Induction of Regulatory T Cells?

K. Mahnke (✉) · A. H. Enk

Department of Dermatology, University of Heidelberg, Voßstrasse 2,
69115 Heidelberg, Germany
Karsten.mahnke@med.uni-heidelberg.de

1	Introduction	134
2	Activation and Maturation Status of DCs Determines the Outcome of an Immune Response	135
2.1	Immature DCs as Inducers of Treg	135
3	Cytokines and Pharmaceuticals Affect the Ability of DCs to Induce Regulatory T Cells	138
3.1	TNFα and Semi-mature DCs	138
3.2	Interleukin-10 Modulates DCs for Tolerance Induction	138
3.3	Pharmaceuticals Interfere with DC Maturation	139
3.4	RelB Translocation is Crucial for DC Maturation	140
4	Subsets of DCs That Induce Regulatory T Cells	141
4.1	CD8$^-$ Versus CD8$^+$	141
4.2	Plasmacytoid DCs	142
5	Spatial Distribution of Tolerogenic DC Phenotypes	143
6	Feedback Mechanisms Between Treg and DCs	144
7	Conclusion	145
	References	145

Abstract Even though dendritic cells (DCs) are well known for their capacity to induce immune responses, recent results show that they are also involved in the induction of tolerance. These two contrary effects of otherwise homologous DCs on a developing immune response may be explained by different DC developmental stages, i.e., different subsets of DCs may exist and/or different spatial distribution of DCs in the body might influence their function. However, independently from the subtype(s), it is obvious that the ability of DCs to act in a tolerogenic fashion depends on the maturation status, since immature DCs are prone to induce regulatory T cells and hence promote tolerance, whereas mature DCs stimulate effector T cells, facilitating immunity. The means by which DCs convey tolerance are not entirely clear yet, but secretion of suppressive cytokines such as IL-10 and induction of regulatory lymphocytes are involved. In this review we focus on the interaction between DCs and T cells and highlight some mechanisms in the decision-making process of whether immunity or tolerance is induced.

1
Introduction

Dendritic cells (DCs) were originally characterized by their strong immunostimulatory properties. They express large amounts of MHC class II molecules and T cell costimulatory molecules of the B7 family on their surface. Therefore DCs, as compared to other types of antigen-presenting cells, posses the unique feature of inducing immune reactions de novo.

Recently several results emerged showing that DCs are also key cells in induction of tolerance, most likely by the means of induction of regulatory T cells. At first glance, these two opposite functions of one and the same DC, i.e., induction of effector T cells on one hand and Treg on the other hand, are hard to reconcile. However, different DC developmental stages or different subsets of DCs as well as different spatial distribution of DCs may explain these opposite functions. The main focus of this report is to review different pathways utilized by DCs to induce or stimulate regulatory T cells (Treg).

Regulatory T cells (Treg), in broader terms, consist of different subsets of T cells that are characterized by their ability to suppress proliferation of conventional effector T cells by various means. To date, three main groups of Treg can de distinguished, mainly by their functional properties (for review, see [1]) Briefly, T regulatory (Tr)-1 cells as well as T helper (Th)-3 T cells express common T cell markers such as CD4 and are characterized by secretion of IL-10 and TGF-β, which provides a means by which proliferation of conventional CD4$^+$ cells is blocked. In contrast, genuine Treg, which are characterized by their expression of CD25, block T cell proliferation by an unknown cell-to-cell contact-dependent mechanism.

However, there are many overlapping features shared by the different subtypes of regulatory T cells (i.e., production of IL-10) and some of the reports reviewed here do not further characterize the subtype of Treg. Therefore we use the term "regulatory T cells" in a broader sense, without necessarily implying that Treg generated by DCs are naturally occurring "genuine Treg," as originally described by Shevach and Sakagucchi [2, 3].

2
Activation and Maturation Status of DCs Determines the Outcome of an Immune Response

2.1
Immature DCs as Inducers of Treg

After initial protocols were published describing the in vitro generation of DCs either from bone marrow (in mouse) or from $CD14^+$ monocytes (human), numerous experiments addressing the immunostimulatory function of DCs were conducted. These experiments used either in vitro generated or in vitro cultivated DCs, hence all of these DCs were manipulated ex vivo as opposed to the in situ situation. Accordingly, most of the experiments conducted demonstrated the superior ability of these activated DCs to stimulate T cell proliferation and to induce T effector functions. In retrospect, it is now conceivable that the in vitro cultivation of the DCs most likely lead to activation and/or maturation of the DCs, and obviously this status differs significantly from the steady-state DCs, which reside in situ in uninflamed tissues.

A first hint that the resting DCs in vivo may be different from in vitro matured DCs can be deducted from early experiments of Schuler et al. [4]. These reports showed that freshly prepared Langerhans cells (skin-derived DCs) required maturation before they were able to stimulate T cell proliferation in a mixed lymphocyte reaction (MLR). Thus, the immunostimulatory capacity of DCs seems strongly connected with a mature and/or activated phenotype.

However, since the main readout for DC function was their immunostimulatory capacity as determined by MLRs, immature or resting DCs were long regarded as inactive cells that needed proper stimulation (e.g., by invading microorganisms or infectious stimuli) in order to execute their function.

First evidence that these immature DCs are not just inactive, but instead are able to induce tolerance, derived from results obtained with in vitro differentiated immature human DCs. Jonuleit et al. could show that peripheral $CD4^+$ T cells acquire regulatory properties after repeated in vitro stimulation with immature DCs [5]. In these experiments, DCs were generated from peripheral blood monocytes by incubation with GMCSF and IL-4, but terminal differentiation with proinflammatory agents such as interleukin (IL)-1, IL-6 and prostaglandin E2 was omitted. Thereafter, $CD4^+$ T cells were repeatedly incubated with these in vitro generated immature DCs, and after three periods of co-incubation, the T cells were co-cultured with freshly isolated $CD4^+$ T cells and stimulated with anti-CD3 and anti-CD28 antibodies. Normally, incubation of T cells with CD3/CD28 induces vigorous T cell proliferation, but when T cells precultivated with immature DCs were present, no T cell proliferation could be recorded, i.e., the precultivated T cells were able to block proliferation of conventional effector T cells. This inhibition was mediated by cell–cell contact and was independent of soluble mediators. Moreover, the precultured T cells themselves were hyporesponsive to anti-CD3/CD28 stimulation, did not produce IL-2 and expressed the surface molecule CD25. Therefore, these T cells induced by repeated stimulation with immature DC fulfill the criteria for genuine regulatory T cells (Treg), as first described by Shevach and Sakaguchi in the murine system [2, 6]. That these Treg do indeed also play a role in vivo in humans was further substantiated by results showing that trace amounts of $CD4^+/CD25^+$ Treg are present in the peripheral blood of healthy volunteers (approx. 5% of all $CD4^+$ T cells) and that these cells posses similar immunosuppressive capacities as compared to their in vitro generated counterparts [7]. In aggregate, these results have demonstrated that immature DCs are able to induce Treg in vitro; however, in search of an in vivo correlate experiments in mice had to be conducted.

In these experiments, DCs were loaded with antigens in situ by antibody targeting, thus avoiding further activation of the DCs by isolation or cultivation methods. As described by Hawiger and Mahnke, model antigens such as Ovalbumin (OVA) or hen egg lysozyme (HEL) were biochemically coupled with anti-DEC-205 antibodies and injected into mice [8–10]. These antigen-antibody conjugates target to the DC-specific antigen receptor DEC-205 that mediates uptake and presentation without further activating the DCs in situ. The following analysis of the immune response revealed that presentation of OVA to T cell by DCs in the steady state in vivo led to induction of $CD4^+CD25^+$ T cells. These T cells had regulatory properties, as they were able to inhibit proliferation of conventional $CD4^+$ T cells in MLR assays in a cell–cell contact-dependent manner.

In contrast, the induction of Treg as well as the deletion of antigen-specific $CD4^+$ T cells was abolished when DCs activating stimuli such as anti-CD40 antibodies or CpGs were injected simultaneously with the antigen–antibody conjugates. Thus, these findings underline that immature DCs are mandatory for the induction of Treg and lead to the concept that steady-state DCs show how peripheral tolerance is maintained (Fig. 1).

In this concept, it is conceivable that the maturation status of DCs determines whether immunity or tolerance is induced [11]. For example, in the absence of pathogens and inflammation, DCs residing in the periphery mainly pick up self-peptides and cell detritus without being activated. Therefore DCs remain immature and upon antigen presentation to T cells tolerance ensues. In contrast, during inflammation, DCs become activated via their pattern recognition receptors and toll-like receptors (TLRs), which are engaged by the pathogens. This leads to upregulation of T cell stimulatory molecules such as B7-1, B7-2, MHC-class II and CD40, and results in T cell activation. This

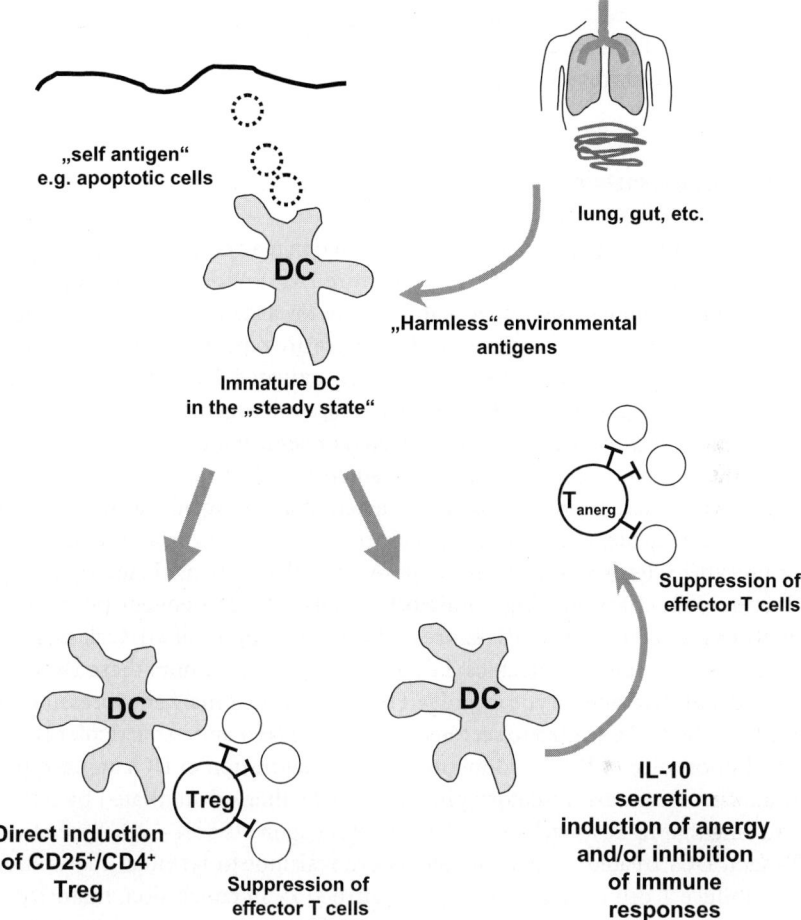

Fig. 1 DCs in peripheral tissues as sentinels for Treg induction. DCs residing in peripheral tissues take up self-antigens, e.g., via apoptotic vesicles or cellular debris. Also subsets of specialized DCs are located in areas that are exposed to innocuous environmental antigens, e.g., the gut and the lung. In the absence of inflammation, these steady-state DCs migrate towards lymphoid organs and induce CD4+/CD25+ regulatory T cells by direct contact or develop into IL-10-producing DCs that anergize T cells. Either way, these DC-induced Treg cells are able to curb proliferation of effector T cells and thus contribute to maintenance of peripheral tolerance

hypothesis is attractive since it explains observations that the DCs in the periphery possess tolerogenic as well as stimulatory capacities under different physiological circumstances [12].

3
Cytokines and Pharmaceuticals Affect the Ability of DCs to Induce Regulatory T Cells

3.1
TNFα and Semi-mature DCs

The term "immature" is not accurately defined in many aspects and according to a long-standing definition true immature DCs are only found in peripheral tissues, whereas the impetus to migrate towards regional lymph nodes requires at least some activation. Indeed there are reports showing that lung-derived migratory DCs (and hence partly activated DCs) account for the induction of regulatory T cells [13]. Therefore tolerogenic DCs found in the lymph node may be differentially activated or semi-mature.

In this regard, TNFα may play a role, since it has been shown that injection of DCs cultivated in presence of TNFα acted in a tolerogenic fashion [14]. In these experiments, DCs were able to block autoimmunity in a murine model of multiple sclerosis (EAE). This suppressive effect was mediated by the induction of IL-10-producing regulatory T cells. The subsequent phenotypic analysis revealed that the DCs expressed regular amounts of MHC class II and T cell co-stimulatory molecules, i.e., according to the authors these DCs displayed a mature phenotype as judged by their surface-marker expression. In contrast, these DCs failed to secrete IL-1β, IL-6, TNFα and in particular IL-12. The importance of IL-12 production for full maturation of DCs and acquisition of an immunostimulatory phenotype is further substantiated by results showing that IL-10 as well as cAMP are potent agonists of IL-12p70 secretion. In fact, DCs treated with these agents are resistant to terminal maturation and induce T cell unresponsiveness in vitro [15]. In conclusion, maturity of DCs may not merely be judged by their surface-marker expression; instead cytokine expression also has to be taken into account and only upregulation of several different indicators warrant a fully activated phenotype of DCs.

3.2
Interleukin-10 Modulates DCs for Tolerance Induction

IL-10 was originally described as cytokine-synthesis-inhibiting factor (CSIF) with regard to its effects exerted on IFNγ production of TH1 T cells. Meanwhile, it has been found to exert suppressive effects on a wide range of different populations of lymphocytes. When human or murine DCs are exposed to IL-10 in in vitro culture systems, the cells display reduced surface expression of MHC class I and MHC class II molecules and reduced expression of T cell co-stimulatory molecules of the B7 family. In addition, the release of pro-inflammatory cytokines, i.e., IL-1β, IL-6, TNFα and most markedly IL-12, is abolished after IL-10 treatment [16, 17]. However, all of these effects could only be recorded when immature DCs were exposed to IL-10. In contrast, mature DCs are insensitive to IL-10 and display a stable phenotype in the presence of IL-10 once they have matured [18, 19].

According to their reduced MHC and B7 expression, the IL-10-treated DCs are inferior in T cell stimulation as opposed to their fully activated counterparts, but IL-10 does not merely keep DCs in an immature state, instead there is evidence that IL-10 modulates DC maturation enabling DCs to induce T cells with regulatory properties. For example, freshly isolated Langerhans cells inhibit proliferation of TH1 cells after exposure to IL-10 but had no effect on TH2 cells [20]. Moreover, it has been shown that IL-10-modulated DCs from peripheral blood induce alloantigen-specific anergy or anergy in melanoma-specific $CD4^+$ and $CD8^+$ T cells [21, 22]. Further analysis of these anergic T cells revealed reduced IL-2 and IFN-γ production and in contrast to genuine Treg, reduced expression of the IL-2 receptor α-chain CD25. However, in addition to these anergic T cells, some authors have also observed the emergence of genuine Treg after injection of IL-10 as indicated by $CD25^+$ upregulation and cell–cell contact requirement for their suppressive activity [23].

The therapeutic use of these IL-10-modulated DCs is under investigation since injection of in vitro generated, IL-10-modified DCs can prevent autoimmunity in a murine model of multiple sclerosis (EAE) and prolonged graft survival significantly in a murine GVHD model [24, 25]. Although most of these protocols involved in vitro exposure of DCs to IL-10, there is recent evidence that IL-10-driven DC modulation may also play a role in generation of regulatory T cells in vivo. For instance, Wakkach et al. not only confirmed previous in vitro results showing that addition of IL-10 to in vitro cultures differentiated DCs to a $CD45^{high}$ tolerogenic phenotype, but also demonstrated that this tolerogenic phenotype, along with regulatory Tr1 cells, is significantly enriched in spleens of IL-10 transgenic mice [23]. Thus these data show that IL-10 plays an important role in rendering DCs not merely immature but also modifies their ability to induce regulatory T cells in vivo.

3.3
Pharmaceuticals Interfere with DC Maturation

In accordance with the concept that immature DCs induce Treg rather then effector T cells, several pharmaceuticals have been tested for their ability to induce Treg by affecting the maturation status of DCs. Among them are the vitamin D3 methobolite $1\alpha,25\text{-}(OH)_2D_3$, N-acetyl-L-cysteine and common immunosuppressive drugs such as corticosteroids, cyclosporin A, rapamycin and aspirin [26–31]. All of them have been shown to suppress DC maturation and as a consequence, anergy and/or regulatory T cells were induced. The effects are numerous and in the following examples are only outlined.

Direct induction of Treg in vitro by pharmacologically treated DCs has been observed after exposure of DCs to *N*-acetyl-L-cysteine, and injection of DCs exposed to a mixture of vitamin-D3 and mycophenolate mofetil induced full tolerance in a murine allograft model [32]. Interestingly, adoptive transfer of T cells from such tolerant mice into previously untreated mice prevented the rejection of respective allografts, thus indicating that probably regulatory T cells had been induced by vitamin D3 treated DCs in vivo. Furthermore, administration of rapamycin in clinically relevant doses prevented the full maturation of DCs and downregulated their IL-12 secretion and their capacity to induce T cell proliferation in vitro. Upon adoptive transfer of these rapamycin-treated DCs, an allo-antigen specific T cell hyporesponsiveness could be observed in the recipients [33]. In conclusion, there is plenty of evidence showing that drugs affecting DC maturation by the means of preventing DC maturation are also most likely inducers of Treg in vivo.

3.4
RelB Translocation is Crucial for DC Maturation

Although most pharmaceuticals mentioned above have no structural similarities, it is most likely that their suppressive effects were mediated by the same mechanism, namely inhibition of maturation of DCs. On a molecular level, DC maturation is guided by relB, a subunit of the NFκB transcription factor. RelB has been shown to play a major role in DC function by regulating CD40 and MHC expression. Upon stimuli exerted by TNFα, LPS or virus-derived IL-1, relB translocates to the nucleus and promotes transcription of CD40, CD80/86 and MHC genes, all of which are indicators of DC activation [34, 35]. Accordingly, blockage of this translocation can lock DCs in an immature state, as indicated by results using RelB-deficient mice. However, most of the pharmaceuticals that inhibit DC maturation as discussed above, also interact with the relB pathway. For instance there is evidence that mycophenolate mofetil, glucocorticoids and vitamin D3 all downregulate NFκB expression. After exposure of DCs to these drugs, their function is indeed modulated in a way that induction of regulatory T cells is promoted [32, 36–38].

In addition to IL-10 secretion and surface-marker expression, relB may also be a useful marker to qualify DC as Treg-inducing DCs. Evidence derives from observations showing that nuclear relB is absent in steady-state DCs located in peripheral tissues, whereas relB becomes upregulated in the nucleus in DCs residing in inflamed or lymphoid tissues [39]. Overall, nuclear translocation of relB in DC is a reliable marker for DC activation and application of pharmaceuticals preventing or delaying nuclear relB expression in vivo may provide a tool by which regulatory T cells are induced via immature DCs.

4
Subsets of DCs That Induce Regulatory T Cells

4.1
CD8⁻ Versus CD8⁺

Teleologically it seems plausible that in the absence of microbial infection and inflammation the induction of regulatory T cells is the default function of DCs. Because in the steady state, the majority of foreign antigens to which DCs are exposed are innocuous and are derived from cell detritus or harmless environmental antigens [40].

Since DCs are constantly sampling the tissue environment, presentation of these self-antigens followed by induction of regulatory T cells might provide a means by which peripheral tolerance is maintained (Fig. 1). However, it cannot be excluded that beyond the immature vs. mature phenotype, different subsets of DCs exist that are intrinsically programmed to induce regulatory T cells regardless of their activation status.

A great deal of work has been done to distinguish specialized subsets of DCs by surface-marker expression and their capacity to induce or prevent immune reactions. CD8 was among the first molecules that defined DC subsets and these subsets have indeed a differential impact on tolerance vs. immunity. Ken Shortman's laboratory has found early evidence that different lineages of DCs, as determined by the CD8 expression in mice, may exist [41,42]. A subset of $CD8\alpha^+$ DCs were identified in thymus and in spleen, and it has been suggested to be of lymphoid origin as opposed to conventional, CD8⁻ DCs that presumably are derived from myeloid precursors. Similarly, so-called lymphoid DCs were also identified in humans.

Initial experiments pointed towards tolerizing properties of these DCs, as they were inferior in inducing T cell proliferation and were able to limit IL-2 production [43, 44]. Moreover, further results from Suess et al. showed enhanced FasL expression by these cell, allowing the killing of potentially autoreactive lymphocytes [45]. However, recent results show that CD8⁺ DCs are not exclusively involved in induction of regulatory T cells but are also able to stimulate T cell responses [46, 47]. Accordingly, in that context the characterization of CD8⁺ DCs as "veto cells" was too bold [48, 49].

However, although not all CD8$^+$ DCs are assigned to a tolerogenic phenotype, current results suggest that at least CD8$^+$ DCs residing in lymphoid tissues are responsible for induction self-tolerance to tissue-associated antigens. For instance, it has been shown that a CD8$^+$ subset presents self-antigens and apoptotic bodies to CD4$^+$ as well as CD8$^+$ T cells, resulting in tolerance [44, 50]. In addition to these direct suppressive effects, it has also been shown that CD8$^+$ DCs are involved in direct induction of regulatory T cells in vivo [51].

Although the CD8 marker has not been proven to be an exclusive marker for Treg-inducing DCs, its value to characterize and isolate possibly tolerizing DCs for clinical applications has formally been established. For example, O'Connel et al. [52] selectively expanded CD8$^+$ DCs in mice by injection of Flt3L and after adoptive transfer of these purified DCs into syngeneic mice, increased allograft survival was recorded. Interestingly, this effect was independent of the maturation status of the transferred DCs, since in vitro matured CD8$^+$ DCs exerted similar tolerogenic effects. Moreover, even early precursors of DCs expressing the CD8 marker promote the engraftment of allogeneic hematopoietic stem cells in mice [53].

Thus these data show that in vivo among CD8$^+$ DCs (a) subpopulation(s) exist, which induce Treg and future investigations have to elucidate these tolerogenic phenotype(s) in particular.

4.2
Plasmacytoid DCs

Recently a novel subset of DCs has been characterized, so-called plasmacytoid DCs (pDCs). They are the main source of IFN type I and upon viral infection these cells presumably prime naive T cells to produce IFNγ and IL-10. However, pDCs also have the capacity to induce T cell anergy. For instance, Kuwana et al. reported that freshly isolated pDCs induced Ag-specific anergy in CD4$^+$ T cells [54]. Although pDCs are able to secrete IL-10, soluble factors do not seem to play a role in anergy induction; instead inhibitory cell surface molecules such as the Ig-like transcript (ILT) 3 and 4 are involved [55]. It has also been reported that pDCs induce naive human CD8$^+$ T cells into IL-10^{high}IFN^{lo} producing T cells that were able to suppress bystander proliferation of conventional CD8$^+$ T cells. Interestingly, these pDCs had to be activated with CD40L, hence immaturity of pDC does not seem to be required in order to induce regulatory T cells [56].

Although most of the data regarding tolerogenic properties of pDCs was generated using in vitro culture systems, there is limited evidence that pDCs might be a useful tool for therapeutical regimens. In Rhesus macaques, large numbers of potentially tolerogenic pDCs can be found in the blood stream after treatment with Flt3L or G-CSF [57, 58], and in parallel it has been shown that G-CSF-treated blood cells from humans reduced severity of human GVHD upon infusion [59, 60]. However, the impact of in vivo mobilized pDCs on immunity and whether they provide a tool for tolerance induction in therapeutic settings remains to be determined in further trials.

5
Spatial Distribution of Tolerogenic DC Phenotypes

The search for specialized subsets of DCs that are able to induce regulatory T cells remains complex since several markers overlap between immature DCs and possibly tolerogenic subsets, and refined characterization of DCs of different spatial origin complicates reliable classification as tolerogenic or immunostimulatory subsets. For instance, Wakkach et al. [23] isolated $CD11c^{low}$, $CD45^{high}$ DCs from the lymph nodes and the spleen of mice that secrete high levels of IL-10 and induce Tr1 regulatory T cells in vitro and in vivo. In comparison to other DCs, these DCs are characterized by their weak expression of CD11c, their expression of CD45 (normally expressed by T cells) and their plasmacytoid morphology. Further nonclassical DC markers, such as B220 and CD8 were identified on a subset of thymic and peripheral DCs [61]. These DCs secrete measurable amounts of type 1 interferon and are able to induce Treg in vitro. In addition to thymic DCs, another $B220^+$ DC subset that may take part in peripheral tolerance was identified by Lu et al. They were able to isolate a $B220^+$, $CD19^-$, $DEC-205^+$ subset of DCs that even after activation with IL-3 and CD40 induces Tr1 cells [62]. Given that thymus and liver are intrinsically tolerizing organs, one can speculate that these organs contain high amounts of Treg-inducing DCs and the mere activation status of the DCs is not the crucial factor deciding tolerance vs. immunity.

The notion that the anatomical side might have an impact on whether regulatory T cells or T effector cells are induced by the DCs is corroborated by results obtained with DCs residing in mucosal surfaces. For example, in the lung and in the gut DCs are constantly exposed to numerous innocuous antigens and thus regulatory T cells that curb overboarding immune reactions have to be present. Accordingly, lung [13] as well as Peyer's patch DCs [63] have been shown to produce large amounts of IL-10 that in turn can promote differentiation of Tr1 cells by either keeping incoming DCs in an immature status or by direct effects on Tr1 differentiation [51, 64].

6
Feedback Mechanisms Between Treg and DCs

Many results support the concept that DCs are inducers of Treg under certain circumstances. However, recent results imply that Treg, on the other hand, also affect DC functions [65]. For example, Misra et al. have shown that DC cocultured with Treg remain in an immature state as judged by surface-marker expression [19]. These Treg-exposed DCs were inferior in induction of T cell proliferation and produced significant amounts of IL-10. In another murine cardiac transplantation model, increased numbers of splenic $CD4^+/CD25^+$ Treg and immature DC were observed after treatment of the recipients with 15-deoxyspergualin, a commonly used anti-rejection drug [66]. As expected, these immature DC purified from tolerant recipients induced the generation of $CD4^+/CD25^+$ Treg when incubated with naive T cells. Surprisingly, when these Treg isolated from tolerant recipients were incubated with DC progenitors, generation of DCs with tolerogenic properties, i.e., inferior T cell stimulatory capacity and IL-10 production was observed. In conclusion, these results

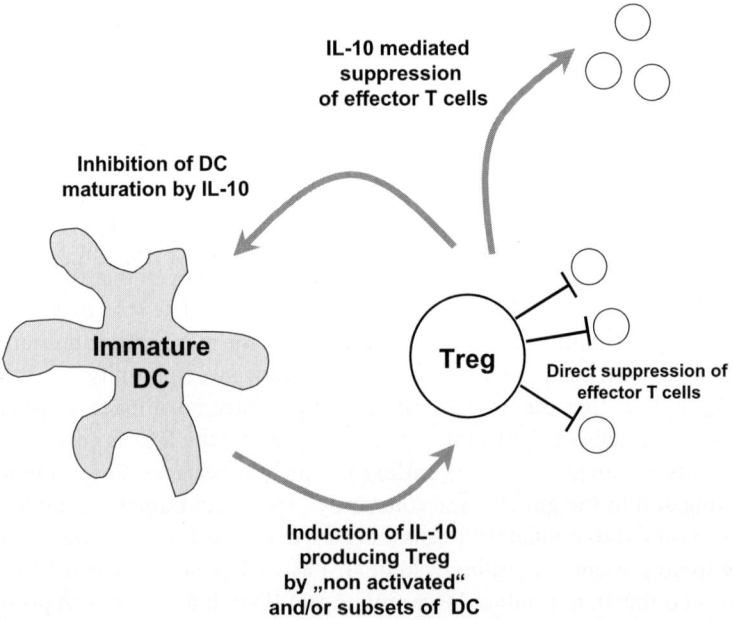

Fig. 2 DCs as part of a self-maintaining regulatory loop. DCs induce regulatory T cells either by cell–cell contact or by cytokine secretion. Treg, on the other hand, produce IL-10 and/or TGF-β, which in turn keeps DCs in an immature tolerogenic state that further promotes Treg induction

support the notion that IL-10 is a critical factor in a self-maintaining feed back loop, i.e., IL-10 derived from regulatory T cells has been shown to play a role in locking immature DCs in a tolerogenic state, which in turn induces further regulatory T cells that may contribute to IL-10 production [19]. However, this positive feed back loop can ensure prolonged immunosuppression and does not only rely on the cell–cell contact required by genuine Treg (Fig. 2).

7
Conclusion

There is strong evidence that DCs have immunosuppressive properties mainly by inducing regulatory T cells. Although the exact mechanisms are not clear yet, a number of reports support the notion that the activation and/or maturation status is crucial for the decision on whether tolerance or immunity is induced. In the absence of inflammatory stimuli, DCs remain in the steady state, which allows them to induce regulatory T cells.

Although many different T cell subpopulations are induced (reports ranging from Treg to Tr1 to TH3-like T cells), the common denominator is their capacity to curb T cell activation. Their impact for tolerance is indeed substantiated by results, showing that removal of different subpopulations of Treg commonly results in autoimmune diseases in different animal models. Therefore steady-state DCs seem crucial for maintenance of peripheral tolerance, since they may serve as sentinels for self-antigens in the peripheral tissues. In the steady state, DCs in noninfected peripheral tissues mainly encounter self-antigens (e.g., cell detritus, apoptotic bodies) or harmless environmental antigens that are transported to regional lymph nodes. Upon contact with T cells, these nonactivated DCs induce regulatory T cells, which in turn suppress potentially self-reactive effector T cells.

Therefore, the constant generation of Treg by nonactivated DCs may be a way to maintain peripheral tolerance.

In the future, biological agents that increase and/or mobilize immature DCs in vivo or block maturation of DCs may be suitable candidates for the development of novel therapeutics to treat allergic and autoimmune diseases.

References

1. Jonuleit H, Schmitt E (2003) The regulatory T cell family: distinct subsets and their interrelations. J Immunol 171:6323–6327
2. Thornton AM, Shevach EM (1998) CD4+CD25+ immunoregulatory T cells suppress polyclonal T cell activation in vitro by inhibiting interleukin 2 production. J Exp Med 188:287–296

3. Sakaguchi S, Sakaguchi N, Asano M, Itoh M, Toda M (1995) Immunologic self-tolerance maintained by activated T cells expressing IL-2 receptor alpha-chains (CD25). Breakdown of a single mechanism of self-tolerance causes various autoimmune diseases. J Immunol 155:1151–1164
4. Schuler G Steinman RM (1985) Murine epidermal Langerhans cells mature into potent immunostimulatory dendritic cells in vitro. J Exp Med 161:526–546
5. Jonuleit H, Schmitt E, Schuler G, Knop J, Enk AH (2000) Induction of interleukin 10-producing, nonproliferating CD4(+) T cells with regulatory properties by repetitive stimulation with allogeneic immature human dendritic cells. J Exp Med 192:1213–1222
6. Sakaguchi S, Fukuma K, Kuribayashi K, Masuda T (1985) Organ-specific autoimmune diseases induced in mice by elimination of T cell subset. I. Evidence for the active participation of T cells in natural self-tolerance; deficit of a T cell subset as a possible cause of autoimmune disease. J Exp Med 161:72–87
7. Jonuleit H, Schmitt E, Stassen M, Tuettenberg A, Knop J, Enk AH (2001) Identification and functional characterization of human CD4(+)CD25(+) T cells with regulatory properties isolated from peripheral blood. J Exp Med 193:1285–1294
8. Bonifaz L, Bonnyay D, Mahnke K, Rivera M, Nussenzweig MC, Steinman RM (2002) Efficient targeting of protein antigen to the dendritic cell receptor DEC-205 in the steady state leads to antigen presentation on major histocompatibility complex class I products and peripheral CD8(+) T cell tolerance. J Exp Med 196:1627–1638
9. Hawiger D, Inaba K, Dorsett Y, Guo M, Mahnke K, Rivera M, Ravetch JV, Steinman RM, Nussenzweig MC (2001) Dendritic cells induce peripheral T cell unresponsiveness under steady state conditions in vivo. J Exp Med 194:769–779
10. Mahnke K, Qian Y, Knop J, Enk AH (2003) Induction of CD4+/CD25+ regulatory T cells by targeting of antigens to immature dendritic cells. Blood 101:4862–4869
11. Mahnke K, Knop J, Enk AH (2003) Induction of tolerogenic DCs: 'you are what you eat'. Trends Immunol 24:646–651
12. Mahnke K, Schmitt E, Bonifaz L, Enk AH, Jonuleit H (2002) Immature, but not inactive: the tolerogenic function of immature dendritic cells. Immunol Cell Biol 80:477–483
13. Akbari O, DeKruyff RH, Umetsu DT (2001) Pulmonary dendritic cells producing IL-10 mediate tolerance induced by respiratory exposure to antigen. Nat Immunol 2:725–731
14. Menges M, Rossner S, Voigtlander C, Schindler H, Kukutsch NA, Bogdan C, Erb K, Schuler G, Lutz MB (2002) Repetitive injections of dendritic cells matured with tumor necrosis factor alpha induce antigen-specific protection of mice from autoimmunity. J Exp Med 195:15–21
15. Griffin MD, Lutz W, Phan VA, Bachman LA, McKean DJ, Kumar R (2001) Dendritic cell modulation by 1alpha,25 dihydroxyvitamin D3 and its analogs: a vitamin D receptor-dependent pathway that promotes a persistent state of immaturity in vitro and in vivo. Proc Natl Acad Sci U S A 98:6800–6805
16. Chang CH, Furue M, Tamaki K (1995) B7-1 expression of Langerhans cells is up-regulated by proinflammatory cytokines, and is down-regulated by interferon-gamma or by interleukin-10. Eur J Immunol 25:394–398

17. Koch F, Stanzl U, Jennewein P, Janke K, Heufler C, Kampgen E, Romani N, Schuler G (1996) High level IL-12 production by murine dendritic cells: upregulation via MHC class II and CD40 molecules and downregulation by IL-4 and IL-10. J Exp Med 184:741–746
18. Steinbrink K, Graulich E, Kubsch S, Knop J, Enk AH (2002) CD4(+) and CD8(+) anergic T cells induced by interleukin-10-treated human dendritic cells display antigen-specific suppressor activity. Blood 99:2468–2476
19. Misra N, Bayry J, Lacroix-Desmazes S, Kazatchkine MD, Kaveri SV (2004) Cutting edge: human CD4+CD25+ T cells restrain the maturation and antigen-presenting function of dendritic cells. J Immunol 172:4676–4680
20. Enk AH, Angeloni VL, Udey MC, Katz SI (1993) Inhibition of Langerhans cell antigen-presenting function by IL-10. A role for IL-10 in induction of tolerance. J Immunol 151:2390–2398
21. Sato K, Yamashita N, Matsuyama T (2002) Human peripheral blood monocyte-derived interleukin-10-induced semi-mature dendritic cells induce anergic CD4(+) and CD8(+) T cells via presentation of the internalized soluble antigen and cross-presentation of the phagocytosed necrotic cellular fragments. Cell Immunol 215:186–194
22. Steinbrink K, Jonuleit H, Muller G, Schuler G, Knop J, Enk AH (1999) Interleukin-10-treated human dendritic cells induce a melanoma-antigen-specific anergy in CD8(+) T cells resulting in a failure to lyse tumor cells. Blood 93:1634–1642
23. Wakkach A, Fournier N, Brun V, Breittmayer JP, Cottrez F, Groux H (2003) Characterization of dendritic cells that induce tolerance and T regulatory 1 cell differentiation in vivo. Immunity 18:605–617
24. Muller G, Muller A, Tuting T, Steinbrink K, Saloga J, Szalma C, Knop J, Enk AH (2002) Interleukin-10-treated dendritic cells modulate immune responses of naive and sensitized T cells in vivo. J Invest Dermatol 119:836–841
25. Sato K, Yamashita N, Baba M, Matsuyama T (2003) Modified myeloid dendritic cells act as regulatory dendritic cells to induce anergic and regulatory T cells. Blood 101:3581–3589
26. Piemonti L, Monti P, Allavena P, Sironi M, Soldini L, Leone BE, Socci C, Di Carlo V (1999) Glucocorticoids affect human dendritic cell differentiation and maturation. J Immunol 162:6473–6481
27. Piemonti L, Monti P, Sironi M, Fraticelli P, Leone BE, Dal Cin E, Allavena P, Di Carlo V (2000) Vitamin D3 affects differentiation, maturation, and function of human monocyte-derived dendritic cells. J Immunol 164:4443–4451
28. Hackstein H, Morelli AE, Larregina AT, Ganster RW, Papworth GD, Logar AJ, Watkins SC, Falo LD, Thomson AW (2001) Aspirin inhibits in vitro maturation and in vivo immunostimulatory function of murine myeloid dendritic cells. J Immunol 166:7053–7062
29. Matyszak MK, Citterio S, Rescigno M, Ricciardi-Castagnoli P (2000) Differential effects of corticosteroids during different stages of dendritic cell maturation. Eur J Immunol 30:1233–1242
30. Verhasselt V, Vanden Berghe W, Vanderheyde N, Willems F, Haegeman G, Goldman M (1999) N-acetyl-L-cysteine inhibits primary human T cell responses at the dendritic cell level: association with NF-kappaB inhibition. J Immunol 162:2569–2574

31. Vosters O, Neve J, De Wit D, Willems F, Goldman M, Verhasselt V (2003) Dendritic cells exposed to nacystelyn are refractory to maturation and promote the emergence of alloreactive regulatory t cells. Transplantation 75:383–389
32. Gregori S, Casorati M, Amuchastegui S, Smiroldo S, Davalli AM, Adorini L (2001) Regulatory T cells induced by 1 alpha,25-dihydroxyvitamin D3 and mycophenolate mofetil treatment mediate transplantation tolerance. J Immunol 167:1945–1953
33. Hackstein H, Taner T, Zahorchak AF, Morelli AE, Logar AJ, Gessner A, Thomson AW (2003) Rapamycin inhibits IL-4-induced dendritic cell maturation in vitro and dendritic cell mobilization and function in vivo. Blood 101:4457–4463
34. O'Sullivan BJ, MacDonald KP, Pettit AR, Thomas R (2000) RelB nuclear translocation regulates B cell MHC molecule, CD40 expression, and antigen-presenting cell function. Proc Natl Acad Sci U S A 97:11421–11426
35. Pettit AR, Quinn C, MacDonald KP, Cavanagh LL, Thomas G, Townsend W, Handel M, Thomas R (1997) Nuclear localization of RelB is associated with effective antigen-presenting cell function. J Immunol 159:3681–3691
36. Dong X, Craig T, Xing N, Bachman LA, Paya CV, Weih F, McKean DJ, Kumar R, Griffin MD (2003) Direct transcriptional regulation of RelB by 1alpha,25-dihydroxyvitamin D3 and its analogs: physiologic and therapeutic implications for dendritic cell function. J Biol Chem 278:49378–49385
37. Penna G, Adorini L (2000) 1 Alpha,25-dihydroxyvitamin D3 inhibits differentiation, maturation, activation, and survival of dendritic cells leading to impaired alloreactive T cell activation. J Immunol 164:2405–2411
38. Mehling A, Grabbe S, Voskort M, Schwarz T, Luger TA, Beissert S (2000) Mycophenolate mofetil impairs the maturation and function of murine dendritic cells. J Immunol 165:2374–2381
39. Thompson AG, Pettit AR, Padmanabha J, Mansfield H, Frazer IH, Strutton GM, Thomas R (2002) Nuclear RelB+ cells are found in normal lymphoid organs and in peripheral tissue in the context of inflammation, but not under normal resting conditions. Immunol Cell Biol 80:164–169
40. Wilson NS, El Sukkari D, Belz GT, Smith CM, Steptoe RJ, Heath WR, Shortman K, Villadangos JA (2003) Most lymphoid organ dendritic cell types are phenotypically and functionally immature. Blood 102:2187–2194
41. Henri S, Vremec D, Kamath A, Waithman J, Williams S, Benoist C, Burnham K, Saeland S, Handman E, Shortman K (2001) The dendritic cell populations of mouse lymph nodes. J Immunol 167:741–748
42. Wu L, D'Amico A, Hochrein H, O'Keeffe M, Shortman K, Lucas K (2001) Development of thymic and splenic dendritic cell populations from different hemopoietic precursors. Blood 98:3376–3382
43. Kronin V, Fitzmaurice CJ, Caminschi I, Shortman K, Jackson DC, Brown LE (2001) Differential effect of CD8(+) and CD8(-) dendritic cells in the stimulation of secondary CD4(+) T cells. Int Immunol 13:465–473
44. Belz GT, Behrens GM, Smith CM, Miller JF, Jones C, Lejon K, Fathman CG, Mueller SN, Shortman K, Carbone FR, Heath WR (2002) The CD8alpha(+) dendritic cell is responsible for inducing peripheral self-tolerance to tissue-associated antigens. J Exp Med 196:1099–1104
45. Suss G, Shortman K (1996) A subclass of dendritic cells kills CD4 T cells via Fas/Fas-ligand-induced apoptosis. J Exp Med 183:1789–1796

46. Maldonado-Lopez R, De Smedt T, Michel P, Godfroid J, Pajak B, Heirman C, Thielemans K, Leo O, Urbain J, Moser M (1999) CD8alpha+ and CD8alpha− subclasses of dendritic cells direct the development of distinct T helper cells in vivo. J Exp Med 189:587–592
47. Smith AL, Fazekas de St Groth B (1999) Antigen-pulsed CD8alpha+ dendritic cells generate an immune response after subcutaneous injection without homing to the draining lymph node. J Exp Med 189:593–598
48. Kronin V, Vremec D, Winkel K, Classon BJ, Miller RG, Mak TW, Shortman K, Suss G (1997) Are CD8+ dendritic cells (DC) veto cells? The role of CD8 on DC in DC development and in the regulation of CD4 and CD8 T cell responses. Int Immunol 9:1061–1064
49. Martin P, del Hoyo GM, Anjuere F, Ruiz SR, Arias CF, Marin AR, Ardavin C (2000) Concept of lymphoid versus myeloid dendritic cell lineages revisited: both CD8alpha(−) and CD8alpha(+) dendritic cells are generated from CD4(low) lymphoid-committed precursors. Blood 96:2511–2519
50. Valdez Y, Mah W, Winslow MM, Xu L, Ling P, Townsend SE (2002) Major histocompatibility complex class II presentation of cell-associated antigen is mediated by CD8alpha+ dendritic cells in vivo. J Exp Med 195:683–694
51. Bilsborough J, George TC, Norment A, Viney JL (2003) Mucosal CD8alpha+ DC, with a plasmacytoid phenotype, induce differentiation and support function of T cells with regulatory properties. Immunology 108:481–492
52. O'Connell PJ, Li W, Wang Z, Specht SM, Logar AJ, Thomson AW (2002) Immature and mature CD8alpha+ dendritic cells prolong the survival of vascularized heart allografts. J Immunol 168:143–154
53. Gandy KL, Domen J, Aguila H, Weissman IL (1999) CD8+TCR+ and CD8+TCR− cells in whole bone marrow facilitate the engraftment of hematopoietic stem cells across allogeneic barriers. Immunity 11:579–590
54. Kuwana M (2002) Induction of anergic and regulatory T cells by plasmacytoid dendritic cells and other dendritic cell subsets. Hum Immunol 63:1156–1163
55. Robinson SP, Patterson S, English N, Davies D, Knight SC, Reid CD (1999) Human peripheral blood contains two distinct lineages of dendritic cells. Eur J Immunol 29:2769–2778
56. Gilliet M, Liu YJ (2002) Generation of human CD8 T regulatory cells by CD40 ligand-activated plasmacytoid dendritic cells. J Exp Med 195:695–704
57. Coates PT, Barratt-Boyes SM, Zhang L, Donnenberg VS, O'Connell PJ, Logar AJ, Duncan FJ, Murphey-Corb M, Donnenberg AD, Morelli AE, Maliszewski CR, Thomson AW (2003) Dendritic cell subsets in blood and lymphoid tissue of rhesus monkeys and their mobilization with Flt3 ligand. Blood 102:2513–2521
58. Coates PT, Duncan FJ, Colvin BL, Wang Z, Zahorchak AF, Shufesky WJ, Morelli AE, Thomson AW (2004) In vivo-mobilized kidney dendritic cells are functionally immature, subvert alloreactive T-cell responses, and prolong organ allograft survival. Transplantation 77:1080–1089
59. Arpinati M, Green CL, Heimfeld S, Heuser JE, Anasetti C (2000) Granulocyte-colony stimulating factor mobilizes T helper 2-inducing dendritic cells. Blood 95:2484–2490

60. Arpinati M, Chirumbolo G, Urbini B, Bonifazi F, Bandini G, Saunthararajah Y, Zagnoli A, Stanzani M, Falcioni S, Perrone G, Tura S, Baccarani M, Rondelli D (2004) Acute graft-versus-host disease and steroid treatment impair CD11c+ and CD123+ dendritic cell reconstitution after allogeneic peripheral blood stem cell transplantation. Biol Blood Marrow Transplant 10:106–115
61. Martin P, del Hoyo GM, Anjuere F, Arias CF, Vargas HH, Fernandez L, Parrillas V, Ardavin C (2002) Characterization of a new subpopulation of mouse CD8alpha+ B220+ dendritic cells endowed with type 1 interferon production capacity and tolerogenic potential. Blood 100:383–390
62. Lu L, Bonham CA, Liang X, Chen Z, Li W, Wang L, Watkins SC, Nalesnik MA, Schlissel MS, Demestris AJ, Fung JJ, Qian S (2001) Liver-derived DEC205+B220+CD19- dendritic cells regulate T cell responses. J Immunol 166:7042–7052
63. Iwasaki A, Kelsall BL (1999) Freshly isolated Peyer's patch, but not spleen, dendritic cells produce interleukin 10 and induce the differentiation of T helper type 2 cells. J Exp Med 190:229–239
64. Levings MK, Sangregorio R, Galbiati F, Squadrone S, de Waal MR, Roncarolo MG (2001) IFN-alpha and IL-10 induce the differentiation of human type 1 T regulatory cells. J Immunol 166:5530–5539
65. Serra P, Amrani A, Yamanouchi J, Han B, Thiessen S, Utsugi T, Verdaguer J, Santamaria P (2003) CD40 ligation releases immature dendritic cells from the control of regulatory CD4+CD25+ T cells. Immunity 19:877–889
66. Min WP, Zhou D, Ichim TE, Strejan GH, Xia X, Yang J, Huang X, Garcia B, White D, Dutartre P, Jevnikar AM, Zhong R (2003) Inhibitory feedback loop between tolerogenic dendritic cells and regulatory T cells in transplant tolerance. J Immunol 170:1304–1312

Part II
Involvement of Disease Models

Autoimmune Gastritis Is a Well-Defined Autoimmune Disease Model for the Study of $CD4^+CD25^+$ T Cell-Mediated Suppression

R. S. McHugh (✉)

Malaghan Institute of Medical Research, 6001 Wellington, New Zealand
rmchugh@malaghan.org.nz

1	Introduction	154
2	Milestones in $CD4^+CD25^+$ In Vitro Characterization	155
2.1	Development of an In Vitro Assay System of Suppression	155
2.2	Genetic Analysis of $CD4^+CD25^+$ T Cells	157
3	Autoimmune Gastritis Model of $CD4^+CD25^+$ T Cell-Mediated Suppression	159
3.1	Immunopathology of AIG	160
3.2	The H/K ATPase Autoantigen	160
3.3	Pathogenic $CD4^+$ T Cells	161
3.4	Dendritic Cells Presenting H/K ATPase	163
3.5	Models of AIG Induction	164
4	$CD4^+CD25^+$ T Cell-Mediated Suppression of AIG	165
4.1	Involvement of Lymphopenia	165
4.2	Involvement of Immunosuppressive Cytokines	166
4.3	Involvement of Co-stimulatory Molecules	169
5	Concluding Remarks	170
	References	171

Abstract Autoimmune gastritis (AIG) is an experimental model that closely resembles human autoimmune gastritis, the underlying pathology of pernicious anemia. Pathogenic $CD4^+$ T cells are reactive to the parietal cell autoantigen, H/K ATPase, and are controlled by $CD4^+CD25^+$ T cells in an immunosuppressive cytokine-independent manner. Comparison of $CD4^+CD25^+$ T cell-mediated suppression in other autoimmune models shows inconsistencies with respect to requirements of cytokines for immunosuppression. More recent data, however, indicate that the evidence for requirement of IL-10 and TGF-β could be due to the complex nature of the T cells causing the disease as well as the role of induced regulatory T cell populations. AIG provides a well-defined model that may allow for better analysis of $CD4^+CD25^+$ T cell in vivo biology. Evidence from this model indicates that immune responses must be initiated and then $CD4^+CD25^+$ T cells are recruited to control the quality of the immune response.

Abbreviations

AIG	Autoimmune gastritis
IBD	Inflammatory bowel disease
d3Tx	Thymectomy on day 3 of life
Treg	Regulatory T cell
GITR	Glucocorticoid-induced TNF receptor
gLN	Gastric LN
DC	Dendritic cell

1
Introduction

It is now approaching 10 years since the identification of a naturally occurring $CD4^+$ T cell with constitutive expression of CD25 (IL-2Rα) as a potent suppressor T cell population capable of controlling immune pathology (Sakaguchi et al. 1995). Initial in vivo phenomena centered around their ability to suppress the induction of organ-specific autoimmune disease induced by day 3 thymectomy (d3Tx) of certain mouse strains (Asano et al. 1996; Suri-Payer et al. 1998) or by transfer of autoeffector T cells to immunocompromised animals (Sakaguchi et al. 1995). Today, these cells are recognized as major players in immune responses to not only autoantigens, but also allo, tumor- and bacteria/viral/parasitic-antigens (McHugh and Shevach 2002b).

Following in vitro characterization of $CD4^+CD25^+$ T cells from mice, it was confirmed that there was a homologous population of $CD4^+CD25^+$ T suppressor cells in humans with in vitro characteristics similar to those of mice (Shevach 2001). Recently, investigators have begun analysis of this cell population in various human disease states. Indeed, there has been a correlation between the frequency or functional reduction of $CD4^+CD25^+$ T cells and various autoimmune and allergic disorders (Kukreja et al. 2002; Ling et al. 2004; Salama et al. 2003; Viglietta et al. 2004).

Although first described by their control over immune responses in vivo, the greatest characterization of these cells has been carried out in vitro. Recent work is now dedicated to elucidating their activities in vivo, trying to translate their in vitro activities to in vivo therapy. Interestingly, some of the outcomes of in vivo biology of $CD4^+CD25^+$ T cells have not been predicted by their in vitro functions. As well, their in vivo activity in controlling various diseases has also shown some inconsistencies.

Since the discovery of the $CD4^+CD25^+$ T suppressor cell population, many different types of $CD4^+$ regulatory cells (Tr1, Th3), mainly induced in vitro, have been reported (Shevach 2002). Additionally, the number of immune models used to define these cell types has grown exponentially. These in vivo models differ in requirements for induction of disease, cell types involved and the contribution of environmental and genetic factors. It has recently been put forth that some of the inconsistencies could lie with confusion between the involvement of naturally occurring Tregs and induced Tregs in these disease models (Piccirillo and Shevach 2004). As well, the various immune models may require different modes of suppressive activity, therefore leading to controversy over the $CD4^+CD25^+$ T cell mechanism of suppression.

The purpose of this review is twofold. It is becoming well established that $CD4^+CD25^+$ T cells play a role in a variety of immune responses. With so many variables that complicate an in vivo system, combined with the heterogeneity and complexity of a polyclonal $CD4^+CD25^+$ T cell population, it is difficult to control every parameter. Autoimmune gastritis (AIG) presents a well-characterized in vivo model for elucidation of $CD4^+CD25^+$ T cell in vivo biology. AIG has a known autoantigen, H/K ATPase, and strict requirement for disease induction by $CD4^+$ T cells and disease suppression by $CD4^+CD25^+$ T cells. H/K ATPase-specific TCR transgenic mice have been generated and are able to induce severe AIG, therefore eliminating the need for a polyclonal autoeffector population ($CD4^+CD45Rb^{hi}$ or $CD4^+CD25^-$). Secondly, I would like to describe a model where $CD4^+CD25^+$ T cell-mediated suppression does not occur in the steady state, but requires appropriate immune activation of autoaggressive effectors to manifest.

2
Milestones in $CD4^+CD25^+$ In Vitro Characterization

Recently, $CD4^+CD25^+$ T cells have been expertly reviewed elsewhere summarizing their origin, in vitro activity and possible therapeutic potential (Sakaguchi 2004). I would like to highlight some of the landmarks of in vitro characterization and how these aspects of $CD4^+CD25^+$ biology may relate to the in vivo model of autoimmune suppression.

2.1
Development of an In Vitro Assay System of Suppression

With the demonstration that $CD4^+CD25^+$ T cells were capable of inhibiting the induction of autoimmune disease, several groups set out to purify this subset and develop an in vitro assay system to test the suppressive function of these cells. It was shown that soluble anti-CD3-induced $CD4^+$ T cell proliferation could be inhibited when increasing numbers of $CD4^+CD25^+$ T cells were added

(Takahashi et al. 1998; Thornton and Shevach 1998). Unlike CD4$^+$CD25$^-$ cells, the CD25$^+$ subset was unable to proliferate to TCR stimulation alone and required IL-2 or IL-4 for growth. These cells were subsequently classified as anergic; however, this term should be classified as their strict need for exogenous IL-2, as CD4$^+$CD25$^+$ T cells, as a population, are highly responsive to TCR stimulation (see Sect. 2.2).

The ability of CD4$^+$CD25$^+$ T cells to inhibit proliferation of the responding T cell population lay in their ability to inhibit the transcription of IL-2 in the responding population. Indeed, reagents such as IL-2 and agonistic anti-CD28 were able to restore the proliferative capacity of the responding T cells (Takahashi et al. 1998; Thornton and Shevach 1998). Some investigators hypothesized that the anergic state of the CD4$^+$CD25$^+$ subset was important for their suppressive activity, and breaking this state, by such reagents, would subsequently turn off their suppressive activity (Takahashi et al. 1998). Recently, Thornton et al. (2004b) have shown that stimulation of CD4$^+$CD25$^+$ T cells with IL-2 or IL-4 is crucial to arm these cells with their suppressive activity. In this study, both T cell proliferation and IL-2 mRNA levels were analyzed during the in vitro suppression assay. As expected, if anti-IL-2 was added during the suppressive co-culture, all proliferation was blocked, but CD4$^+$CD25$^+$ cells were unable to suppress IL-2 message in the responding T cells. This demonstrated that CD4$^+$CD25$^+$ T cells need both a TCR stimulus and IL-2 signaling to suppress the continued production of IL-2 by responding T cells.

This study (Thornton et al. 2004b) was interesting because it looked at a block in IL-2 message as a read-out of suppression rather than proliferation of the co-culture. As mentioned above, if IL-2 is added to the suppressive co-culture, proliferation is restored and therefore thought to overcome suppression. When IL-2 message was analyzed in the same co-culture, however, it was suppressed. This indicates, along with the above data, that addition of IL-2 does not overcome suppression, but is rather necessary for full suppressor function.

In vivo, mice deficient in IL-2, IL-2 signaling and co-stimulatory molecules, have low to no CD4$^+$CD25$^+$ T cells demonstrating a need for responsiveness to IL-2 for their generation (Sakaguchi 2004). It is also a possibility that low levels of IL-2, in addition to affecting their generation and maintenance, may also influence their suppressive abilities. Translating this data into an in vivo hypothesis, this could indicate that an immune response, inducing local production of IL-2 by responding cells must occur before CD4$^+$CD25$^+$ T cells can suppress the effector cells.

The in vitro assay system also demonstrated a requirement for TCR ligation in the induction of suppressive activity. It was shown that CD4$^+$CD25$^+$ T cells needed to be activated through their TCR and the resulting suppression was cell-contact-dependent (Thornton and Shevach 1998). Once activated, this suppressive activity no longer depended on antigen and could suppress any T cell nonspecifically (Thornton and Shevach 2000). Additionally, there was no requirement for the same MHC:peptide complexes presented on the same APC for suppression to occur. These studies indicate the potential for any immune response to be suppressed as long as $CD4^+CD25^+$ T cells receive a TCR and IL-2R stimulus. This preactivation also increased the suppressive potency of the cells by up to fourfold. With such potent nonspecific suppression following activation of $CD4^+CD25^+$ T cells, it is difficult to imagine that any immune response would be induced. Therefore regulation of $CD4^+CD25^+$ T cell activity and its timing during an immune response is critical.

2.2
Genetic Analysis of $CD4^+CD25^+$ T Cells

This activation requirement for suppressive activity led to the hypothesis that molecules, most likely cell surface, needed to be induced and once expressed would allow for nonspecific suppression. Several investigators began analysis of genes specifically upregulated by $CD4^+CD25^+$ subsets (Gavin et al. 2002; McHugh et al. 2002; Zelenika et al. 2002). $CD4^+CD25^+$ T cells were highly responsive to this stimulation, upregulating approximately four times as many genes as their $CD25^-$ counterparts. This analysis tried to answer several questions.

1. What is the suppressive molecule?
2. How do $CD4^+CD25^+$ cells maintain their anergic state?
3. Can $CD4^+CD25^+$ T cells be further subdivided into suppressive and non-suppressive subsets?

Although none of these questions were fully answered, a more detailed phenotype of these cells was delineated. Since this analysis, even more molecules (Bruder et al. 2004), such as the transcription factor FoxP3 (Fontenot et al. 2003; Hori et al. 2003; Khattri et al. 2003), have been identified as markers for $CD4^+CD25^+$ T cells. By identifying more cell surface molecules on $CD4^+CD25^+$ T cells, certain subsets, mainly based on bimodal expression of CD62L (Szanya et al. 2002) and CD103 (Lehmann et al. 2002), and recently other integrins (Stassen et al. 2004), were shown to have distinct suppressive activity in vivo or altered function in vitro. Although CD25 still remains the most reliable marker in terms of suppressive activity in vitro, subsets expressing CD103 or CD62L have been shown to more efficiently suppress colitis or diabetes, respectively. It is interesting to note that $CD103^+$ $CD4^+CD25^+$ T cells have a greater number of $CD62L^{lo}$ cells (R.S.M., unpublished observation). Could this indicate that in different tissues and with different diseases, subsets within the $CD4^+CD25^+$ T cell population can display different functions?

Analysis of freshly isolated $CD4^+CD25^+$ T cells revealed the constitutive expression of the glucocorticoid-induced TNF receptor (GITR), a member of the TNFR superfamily (McHugh et al. 2002; Shimizu et al. 2002). Two groups independently determined that antibodies to this molecule were able to restore proliferation of the responding cells in an in vitro suppression assay. This receptor was not found to be the suppressor effector molecule, but engagement of GITR on $CD4^+CD25^+$ T cells was thought to downregulate their ability to suppress. Although anti-GITR negated the suppressive activity of $CD4^+CD25^+$ T cells, its stimulation of $CD4^+CD25^+$ T cells increased their responsiveness to IL-2 (McHugh et al. 2002).

Several groups have now cloned the ligand for GITR and have shown that engagement of GITR with its natural ligand will also overcome suppressive activity of $CD4^+CD25^+$ T cells (Kim et al. 2003; Stephens et al. 2004; Tone et al. 2003). Many of these reports demonstrate that GITR engagement on $CD4^+CD25^-$ T cells is co-stimulatory and one study actually demonstrates, utilizing $GITR^{-/-}$ mice, that engagement of GITR on the responding T cells, but not $CD4^+CD25^+$ T cells as previously hypothesized, is required for reversal of suppression (Stephens et al. 2004).

Consistently, interactions of GITR with its ligand are shown to overcome the ability of $CD4^+CD25^+$ mediated suppression in vitro and in some instances in vivo (Kohm et al. 2004; Shimizu et al. 2002); therefore it is necessary to determine where, when and how GITR-L is expressed during an immune response. Several groups have shown that GITR-L is constitutively expressed on various APCs and this expression is down-regulated with activation signals, such as engagement of TLRs in vitro (Stephens et al. 2004; Tone et al. 2003). This timing of expression is important, indicating that at the initial stages of APC activation and T cell priming, GITR is possibly engaging GITR-L, and therefore $CD4^+CD25^+$ T cells are unable to suppress (Fig. 1). But with further maturation of APCs, GITR-L is down-regulated, no longer having a hold on suppression. While responding T cells are being stimulated by APCs, $CD4^+CD25^+$ T cells can expand by stimulation through their TCR, GITR and local IL-2 production. Once GITR-L is down-regulated, $CD4^+CD25^+$ T cells are at sufficient numbers to begin quelling the immune response. The nature of the T cell response, whether self-antigen or foreign-antigen, may additionally influence how easily $CD4^+CD25^+$ T cells can suppress a response. A careful analysis of the pattern and timing of GITR-L expression in vivo during various immune responses is necessary to determine the possible roles these interactions play in activation of T cell responses as well as their suppression.

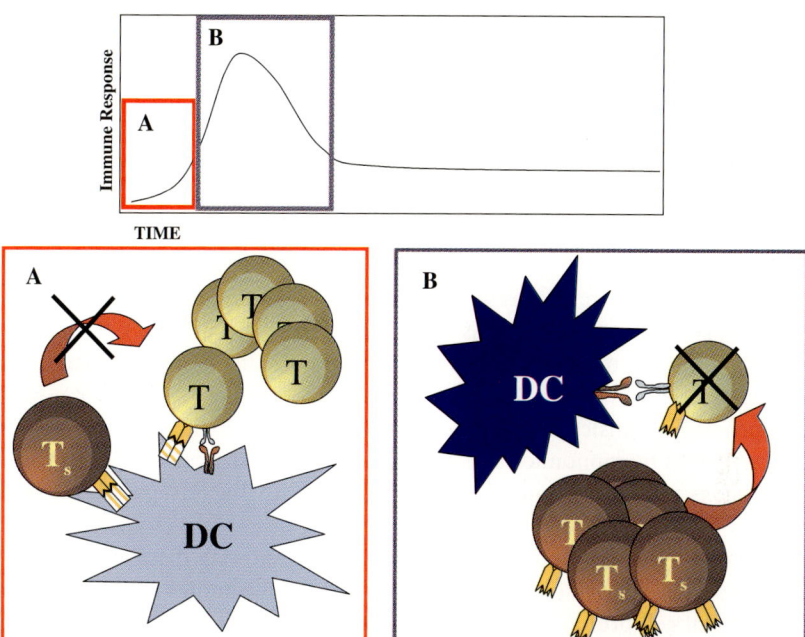

Fig. 1A, B Model of GITR/GITR-L interactions for the control of immunosuppression. At the initiation of the immune response (**A**), DCs are able to present antigen to effector T cells (T_e). Interactions with GITR-L enable Te to overcome regulation by T_s and therefore have an advantage in activation. At this same time GITR-L stimulation of $CD4^+CD25^+$ T cells allow for increased sensitivity to IL-2 and proliferation. As the immune response progresses, GITR-L is downregulated on the DCs, allowing $CD4^+CD25^+$ T cells to control activation of naïve T_e as well as effector T_e. As $CD4^+CD25^+$ T cells have expanded, they are in sufficient numbers to control the immune response

3
Autoimmune Gastritis Model of $CD4^+CD25^+$ T Cell-Mediated Suppression

Over the years, many autoimmune models have been employed to investigate the in vivo biology of suppressor T cells (Shevach 2000). One of the original autoimmune models used in the study of $CD4^+CD25^+$ biology is AIG induced by thymectomy on day 3 of life (d3Tx) or $CD25^-$ T cell transfer to immunocompromised animals. Another widely utilized autoimmune disease model is inflammatory bowel disease (IBD) or colitis. Transfer of $CD4^+CD45Rb^{hi}$ (Powrie et al. 1994) or $CD4^+CD25^-$ T cells (Liu et al. 2003;

Suri-Payer and Cantor 2001) into SCID or RAG$^{-/-}$ mice will induce this wasting disease. This model is comprehensively reviewed in this issue, but will be discussed in comparison with AIG as two model systems used to elucidate CD4$^+$CD25$^+$ T cell suppressive activity in vivo.

3.1
Immunopathology of AIG

Experimental AIG in mice resembles human autoimmune gastritis, the underlying pathology of pernicious anemia (Alderuccio et al. 2002). Pernicious anemia is one of the more prevalent autoimmune diseases and is the most common cause of vitamin B_{12} deficiency, as antibodies and T cells target cells that produce intrinsic factor (Toh et al. 1997). Gastritis in humans and mice is characterized by mononuclear cell infiltrates within the gastric mucosa and submucosa and production of autoantibodies reactive against gastric parietal cells.

Circulating autoantibodies are closely associated with disease pathology in both humans and mice, with the majority of the antibodies reactive against the parietal cell proton pump, H/K ATPase (Jones et al. 1991). Autoreactive T cell clones identified in humans (Bergman et al. 2003; D'Elios et al. 2001) and mice (De Silva et al. 1999; Katakai et al. 1997; Suri-Payer et al. 1999) have been found specific for H/K ATPase as well, and common peptide epitopes are shared between the species (Bergman et al. 2003).

Severe AIG results in loss of parietal and chief cells. This destruction of the gastric mucosa cellular architecture has been suggested to be FasL-dependent (Marshall et al. 2002; Nishio et al. 1996). A role for IFN-γ(Barrett et al. 1996), but not TNF-α(Marshall et al. 2004), in the initiation of disease has been demonstrated as anti-IFN-γ antibody treatment early in disease induction blocks AIG. Loss of parietal cell production of intrinsic factor results in vitamin B_{12} deficiency leading to gastric, blood and neurological disorders (Toh et al. 1997).

3.2
The H/K ATPase Autoantigen

The cellular and humoral immune response has been seen to both chains of the H/K ATPase heterodimer (Toh et al. 2000), but the majority of reported CD4$^+$ T cells are seen to be reactive to alpha chain peptides. There is still controversy over which chain, if any, of H/K ATPase is important in the initiation of AIG. Studies using mice transgenic for α (H/Kα:I-E) or β (H/Kβ:I-E) chain under the control of a class II promoter targeting expression to the thymus indicates the β chain is the critical autoantigen target (Alderuccio et al. 1997). The d3Tx of H/Kβ:I-E mice did not result in AIG, suggesting that β chain expression in the thymus negatively selects autoreactive T cells. Interestingly, α chain message is naturally expressed in the thymus during gestation and after birth, but is insufficient for complete deletion of all α chain reactive TCRs (Alderuccio et al. 1997). Actually, H/K ATPase reactive TCR transgenic thymocytes from A23 mice (see Sect. 3.3) are well selected and skewed toward CD4 single positive cells (McHugh et al. 2001b).

An alternate explanation as why *H/Kβ*: I-E transgenic mice do not develop AIG after d3Tx is that β chain expression is required for full protein expression and assembly of both chains (Gottardi and Caplan 1993). Therefore β chain rescues α chain expression, leading to subsequent deletion of α and β reactive T cells. This possibility is actively being investigated.

3.3
Pathogenic CD4$^+$ T Cells

Several groups have demonstrated that CD4$^+$ T cells are the pathogenic cells in AIG (Alderuccio et al. 2002). Autoantibodies are insufficient to transfer disease and there have been no requirements for B cells or CD8$^+$ T cells for induction of disease. Within the chronic lesions of AIG, T cells, B cells and APCs associate in an organized tertiary lymphoid structure possibly supported by CXCL13, CCL4, CCL5, CXCL9 and CXCL10 production (Katakai et al. 2003). Although the expression of these chemokines may indicate a Th1-biased environment, many cytokines associated with a Th2 profile have been detected in the gastric mucosa of AIG$^+$ mice (Martinelli et al. 1996). These include IL-5 and IL-10; however, there is a notable absence of IL-4 production. Indeed, both Th1- and Th2-skewed CD4$^+$ gastric clones have been isolated from the gastric LN of AIG$^+$ mice (Suri-Payer et al. 1999).

Several H/K ATPase reactive T cell clones have been characterized. Two clones reactive to the α chain isolated from AIG$^+$ animals after d3Tx have been described (Suri-Payer et al. 1999). TxA23 (α630–641) has a typical Th1 profile secreting IFNγ and TNFα. Upon transfer to immunocompromised mice, they induce severe AIG with the characteristic mononuclear cell infiltrate. TxA51 (α889–900) displays a Th2 pattern of differentiation, producing IL-4, IL-10 (Suri-Payer et al. 1999) and IL-5 (S. Chegini and E. Shevach, unpublished observations). These cells also induced a severe pathology upon transfer to immunocompromised mice; however, infiltrate into the gastric mucosa primarily consisted of eosinophils. Although the polyclonal lesion seems to be significantly Th1-influenced, Th2 cells are capable of differentiation and causing disease pathology. Both these clones are controlled with co-transfer of

CD4⁺CD25⁺ T cells, demonstrating suppression of both naïve (CD4⁺CD25⁻) and effector T cells (gastric clones).

A23 (McHugh et al. 2001b) and A51 (Candon et al. 2004) transgenic mice have been developed from the cloned TCRs of TxA23 (Vα2.6/Vβ2) and TxA51 (Vα17.3/Vβ4), respectively. A23 mice display 100% penetrance of disease on susceptible backgrounds. The T cells isolated from A23 mice display a Th1 cytokine profile and show strong activation within the draining gastric lymph node (gLN). Signs of disease and activation are seen as early as day 10 of life. These animals are capable of generating CD4⁺CD25⁺ T cells that can be activated by the H/K ATPase self-antigen; however, these cells are not capable of controlling the immune pathology in the transgenic mice. This inability of CD4⁺CD25⁺ suppressor activity could be secondary to the overall increase in autoreactive T cell precursors. Other TCR transgenics reactive to self-antigens, especially those specific for myelin proteins (Lafaille et al. 1994), however, do seem to be controlled by regulatory T cells. The disease incidence in these mice remains low and usually requires immunization with myelin proteins or crossing to a RAG$^{-/-}$ background to induce disease.

AIG has been described in mice carrying a single TCR α chain transgene (Sakaguchi et al. 1994). These mice spontaneously develop AIG, but also have CD4⁺CD25⁺ cells present in the periphery of an adult (A. Thornton, unpublished observation). One hypothesis is that introduction of atypical gene expression within the thymus could delay the development of CD4⁺CD25⁺ cells, which generally begin to emigrate on day 3-4 of life. This delay, in combination with neonatal lymphopenia and early, localized expression of autoantigen, could result in autoimmune disease. All these circumstances, as well as increased autoreactive T cells, could lead to this fulminant disease.

A51 mice also displayed signs of AIG, however at a lower incidence, 50%-80%, and it is manifested later in life, around 10 weeks (Candon et al. 2004). TCR transgenic T cells isolated from the gLN were primed to produce Th2 cytokines. Similar to transfer of TxA51 clone, the A51 mice had a polymorphonuclear cell infiltrate composed of mostly eosinophils. Interestingly, the H/K ATPase peptide that A51 TCR transgenic T cells are reactive against is not efficiently presented by APC in vitro. This may account for the lower incidence and delay in disease onset.

A third TCR transgenic mouse with T cells reactive to H/K ATPase has been described by Alderuccio et al. (2000). The TCR was cloned from a T cell hybridoma generated from AIG⁺ mice immunized with H/K ATPase β chain$_{253-277}$ peptide. However, disease only developed spontaneously in about 20% of the mice. The T cells in these mice were not selected well in the thymus, perhaps indicating the TCR affinity for this peptide is not efficient for positive selection. Furthermore, the low incidence of spontaneous disease could be because these autoreactive T cells were only revealed following immunization of peptide in CFA. Therefore it is possible that this form of stimulation is required for their disease-inducing potential.

3.4
Dendritic Cells Presenting H/K ATPase

How autoreactive $CD4^+$ T cells become activated to initiate autoimmune disease is an actively investigated area of the pathophysiology of many autoimmune diseases. In the peripheral tissues, dendritic cells (DCs) sample the environment, acquiring self-antigens from tissue sites, perhaps by the phagocytosis of apoptotic cells (Steinman et al. 2003). These DCs migrate to the draining lymph nodes where they present the antigen in the context of MHC to specific T cells. It has recently been shown that the autoantigen H/K ATPase is processed and presented in the gastric LN of unmanipulated BALB/c mice (Scheinecker et al. 2002). DCs likely pick up this antigen in the gastric mucosa, ingesting naturally apoptotic parietal cells. In this regard, close contact between DCs and parietal cells in the gastric mucosa has been observed.

Purifying $CD8\alpha^+$ and $CD8\alpha^{lo/-}$ DCs from gLN demonstrated direct presentation of an in situ processed autoantigen to H/K ATPase reactive clones. This was confirmed in vivo with proliferation of A23 T cells exclusively within the gLN of unmanipulated BALB/c mice (Scheinecker et al. 2002). A23 T cells adoptively transferred into BALB/c mice, like other self-reactive T cells, expanded and then subsequently contracted and could not be detected 3 weeks after adoptive transfer (R. DiPaolo and E. Shevach, unpublished observation).

Although there is constant turnover and presentation of the autoantigen in the steady state, this does not lead to spontaneous autoimmunity. There are several possibilities to explain why there is not a progression to autoaggression. First, the presence of $CD4^+CD25^+$ T cells could continually suppress DC activation of autoreactive T cells. Depletion of $CD25^+$ cells, however, with anti-CD25 antibody, rarely leads to the induction of autoimmunity (McHugh and Shevach 2002a). This indicates that another level of peripheral tolerance is possibly involved. The DCs may present H/K ATPase in a tolerogenic manner, as previously reported with the presentation of other self-antigens within the draining LN (Steinman et al. 2000, 2003). Therefore, $CD4^+CD25^+$ T cells may not be necessary to control presentation of self-antigen in this context. For autoimmunity to manifest, autoreactive T cells would need to be activated with mature DCs capable of immune stimulation. AIG can be induced after H/K ATPase immunization (Scarff et al. 1997) or localized transgenic-production of GM-CSF (Biondo et al. 2001).

3.5
Models of AIG Induction

AIG can be induced by various means. These models have been separated into four main categories: (1) lymphopenic, (2) nonlymphopenic, (3) transgenic, and (4) spontaneous (Alderuccio et al. 2002). The most common model is thymectomy on day 3 of life (d3Tx). In susceptible strains of mice, such as BALB/c, d3Tx resulted in AIG as well as several other organ-specific autoimmune diseases (Kojima and Prehn 1981). The underlying cause of this was the early removal of $CD25^+$ suppressor cells in combination with a state of lymphopenia. The role of $CD25^+$ cells was confirmed when Sakaguchi et al. could reproduce the same autoimmune profile in immunocompromised mice upon transfer of $CD25^-$ T cells (Sakaguchi et al. 1995).

The autoimmune diseases induced by both methods, as well as by gastritis-inducing clones, could be completely suppressed with co-transfer of $CD25^+$ T cells if given within 1 week of induction of disease (McHugh et al. 2001a). The suppression was less effective if $CD25^+$ T cells were transferred after that time point, indicating that $CD25^+$ T cell suppression may not be efficient once a certain level of T cell activation or pathology has begun. This contrasts $CD25^+$ T cell control of IBD. Pathology in the colon would eventually subside if $CD4^+CD25^+$ T cells were given 4 weeks after disease induction (Mottet et al. 2003); however, transfer of Tr1 clones were able to immediately halt disease progression (Foussat et al. 2003). It is interesting that in both AIG and

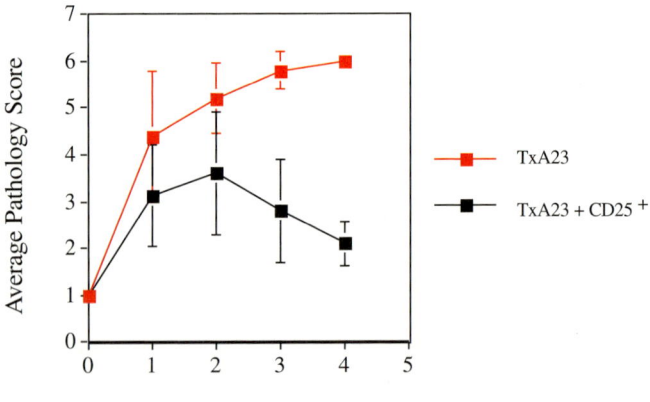

Fig. 2 Autoimmune pathology is initiated in the presence of $CD4^+CD25^+$ T cells. TxA23, an H/K ATPase-specific clone, was co-injected with $CD4^+CD25^+$ T cells into BALB/c$^{nu/nu}$ mice. Every week after adoptive transfer, stomachs were harvested, H&E stained and scored for AIG pathology

IBD, $CD4^+CD25^+$ T cell suppression is not immediate. Analysis of the gastric mucosa at early time points after adoptive transfer of effector cells revealed a transient lymphocytic infiltrate into the tissue even in the presence of suppressor cells (Fig. 2). $CD4^+CD25^+$ T cells, if co-transferred would eventually suppress AIG and infiltration would clear by 4 weeks.

4
$CD4^+CD25^+$ T Cell-Mediated Suppression of AIG

4.1
Involvement of Lymphopenia

Although not categorized as lymphopenic, all the models known to induce AIG involve a certain degree of lymphopenia, either due to thymectomy, the use of T cell-deficient animals or the neonatal period of life (Min et al. 2004). An initial hypothesis as to how $CD25^+$ T cells were controlling induction of disease was by inhibiting or limiting the homeostatic/lymphopenia-induced proliferation of the effector cells. There have been data for and against $CD4^+CD25^+$ T cell control of lymphopenia-induced proliferation. Annacker et al. (2001) demonstrated that co-transfer of $CD4^+CD25^+$ T cells would decrease the early proliferation of $CFSE^+CD4^+CD25^-$ T cells and could control peripheral T cell numbers at later time points. Other groups (Martin et al. 2004; McHugh and Shevach 2002a) have failed to see this same effect on the early proliferation of effector cells, and the modest inhibition seen by Annacker et al. (2001) might be due to an overall increase in T cells transferred. As previously mentioned, in immunodeficient animals receiving $CD25^-$ and $CD4^+CD25^+$ T cells, the overall accumulation of T cells in the periphery is significantly reduced compared to $CD4^+CD25^-$ T cell transfer alone. This must be interpreted with caution, however, as immunodeficient mice receiving $CD4^+CD25^-$ cells alone develop severe immunopathology, which can lead to a greater expansion of peripheral T cells.

Suppression of IBD has recently been shown to be controlled by not only known suppressor cell populations ($CD4^+CD25^+$ and $CD4^+CD45Rb^{lo}$), but by T cells in the naïve cell pool (Barthlott et al. 2003). By transfer of increasing numbers of $CD4^+CD45Rb^{hi}$ cells, or even monoclonal TCR transgenic T cells, to immunocompromised mice, the incidence of IBD declined. This regulatory activity was associated with high proliferation potential upon transfer, indicating that rapid expansion, and therefore, filling of the empty space would lead to control of immunopathology. In contrast to this model, transfer of high numbers of $CD4^+CD25^-$ T cells did not inhibit the induction of AIG

(R.S.M., unpublished observations), again indicating that different disease models may be controlled by different mechanisms of suppression.

To attempt to separate depletion of CD25$^+$ T cells and lymphopenia, McHugh and Shevach (2002a) set out to induce AIG by antibody depletion of CD25$^+$ cells in vivo. Contrary to previous data (Taguchi and Takahashi 1996), AIG was rarely induced by CD25$^+$ T cell depletion. This observation has been confirmed by several groups looking to induce autoimmune disease (Laurie et al. 2002) or tumor immunity (Onizuka et al. 1999; Shimizu et al. 1999; Sutmuller et al. 2001). The depletion in vivo was effective as splenocytes from these mice were able to transfer AIG to immunocompromised animals (McHugh and Shevach 2002a). CD25$^+$ cells do eventually reconstitute the animals, but in our hands CD25$^+$ T cell levels were still depleted 6 weeks after antibody treatment. It is possible that AIG is controlled by the reconstituting CD25$^+$ cells, but it is also possible that in the steady state there are other tolerance-inducing mechanisms that control autoaggressive T cells.

Although CD25$^+$ cell depletion alone was insufficient to induce AIG, depletion in combination with immunization of H/K ATPase in IFA induced chronic severe AIG (McHugh and Shevach 2002a). H/K ATPase immunization in CFA will induce a limited amount of pathology; however, once the immunization is ceased, pathology will recede (Scarff et al. 1997). In total, these observations lead to a model where AIG requires both depletion of CD25$^+$ T cells and a strong stimulus for autoreactive cells, such as immunization, inflammation of the tissue, or lymphopenia (Fig. 3). CD4$^+$CD25$^+$ T cells play a role in control of autoimmune activation in this context, but in the steady state, other tolerogenic mechanisms, such as immature DCs may control autoeffector cells (Steinman et al. 2003).

4.2
Involvement of Immunosuppressive Cytokines

Within the biology of CD4$^+$CD25$^+$ T cells, there has yet to be anything more controversial than the role of immunosuppressive cytokines. The in vitro suppression assay system allowed for a model of CD4$^+$CD25$^+$ T cells that mediated suppression in an activation-dependent, contact-dependent, and cytokine-independent manner (Thornton and Shevach 1998). Most researchers investigating CD4$^+$CD25$^+$ cells in the mouse and human system have not been able to overcome suppression by adding antibodies to immunoregulatory cytokines IL-4, IL-10 or TGFβ (Shevach 2002). Additionally, CD4$^+$CD25$^+$ cells from IL-4-, IL-10- (Thornton and Shevach 2000) or TGFβ- (Piccirillo et al. 2002) deficient animals were as equally suppressive as wild-type CD4$^+$CD25$^+$ T cells in vitro. In vivo data from IBD (Asseman et al. 1999; Powrie et al. 1996)

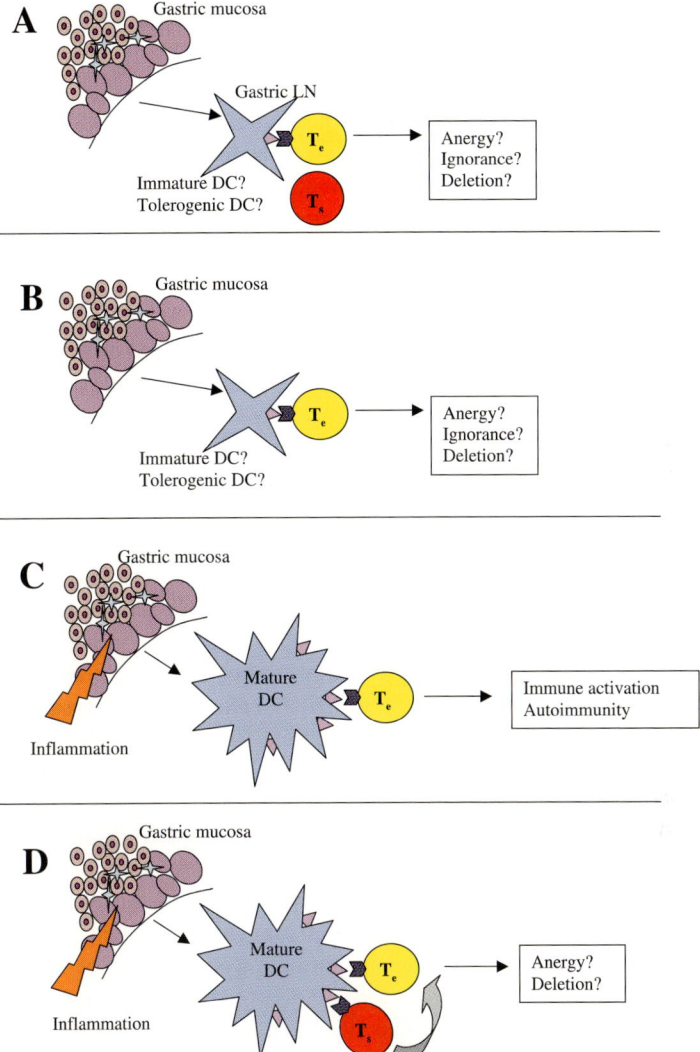

Fig. 3A–D In the absence of CD4+CD25+ T cells, additional signals are needed to initiate autoimmunity. In the steady state (**A**), autoreactive effector cells are kept in check by multiple mechanisms, CD4+CD25+ T cells or tolerogenic DCs. Depletion of CD4+CD25+ T cells does not lead to autoimmunity, indicating another mechanism for control of autoreactive T cells (**B**). Depletion of CD4+CD25+ T cells in combination with tissue inflammation, or immunization, leads to autoimmunity that is not controlled by other tolerance mechanisms (**C**). In the presence of CD4+CD25+ T cells, inflammation may activate the autoreactive T cells, but there autoactivity is kept in check by CD4+CD25+ T cells (**D**)

and other models (Cameron et al. 1997; Homann et al. 1999; Krause et al. 2000; Seddon and Mason 1999) have indicated a role for IL-4, IL-10 and/or TGFβ in suppression of autoimmune disease. Antibodies blocking either IL-10 or TGF-β were able to reverse suppression mediated by CD4$^+$CD45Rb^{lo} cells. As well, IL-10$^{-/-}$ mice on susceptible backgrounds developed IBD. Interestingly, these same animals did not develop gastritis (Suri-Payer and Cantor 2001).

When Nakamura et al. (2001) published their study identifying membrane-bound TGF-β on the surface of resting and activated CD4$^+$CD25$^+$ T cells, this seemed to be a link between the necessity for cell contact and the dependency of TGF-β in in vivo model systems. Although TGF-β may play a role in CD4$^+$CD25$^+$ T cell-mediated suppression or activation, it is not essential for their activity in vitro (Piccirillo et al. 2002). It has been demonstrated that CD4$^+$CD25$^+$ T cells purified from the thymus of TGF-β-deficient mice are fully functional suppressors. Moreover, several genetically modified responder T cells incapable of inhibition by TGF-β are equally suppressible by CD4$^+$CD25$^+$ T cells.

To address whether immunosuppressive cytokines played a role in AIG, splenocytes from IL-4- or IL-10-deficient animals were used as a source of suppressor cells in the d3Tx or CD25- T cell transfer model. IL-4 and IL-10$^{-/-}$ CD4$^+$CD25$^+$ were as efficient as wild-type BALB/c in suppression of AIG (McHugh et al. 2001a; Suri-Payer and Cantor 2001). This indicates that IL-4 or IL-10 production by CD4$^+$CD25$^+$ T cells is not necessary for the inhibition of AIG. This lack of a requirement for IL-10 in AIG suppression is in contrast to previous studies with IBD. Recently, however, long-lived autoreactive memory cells have been identified within the CD4$^+$CD45Rb^{lo} or CD4$^+$CD25$^+$ suppressor cell pool, especially if purified from the mesenteric LN (Asseman et al. 2003). Adoptive transfer of these suppressor populations in combination with anti-IL-10R antibody revealed pathogenic cells capable of inducing IBD. In the same study, it was also reported that splenic CD4$^+$CD25$^+$ T cells purified from IL-10-deficient animals were capable of suppressing naïve CD45Rb^{hi} cells. Therefore it seems that control of memory effectors (CD45Rb^{lo}) is IL-10-dependent, but suppression of naïve cells (CD45Rb^{hi}) is less dependent on IL-10.

CD4$^+$CD25$^+$ T cells are capable of suppressing AIG induced by naïve (CD25$^-$) and effector (clones) T cells (Suri-Payer et al. 1998). It has not been determined, however, whether IL-10 production is required for inhibition of AIG induced by the fully differentiated gastritic clones. It is possible that IL-10 is necessary for suppression of these autoaggressive effectors. Unlike IBD, it has not been demonstrated that within the CD4$^+$CD25$^-$ pool of cells resides previously activated H/K ATPase reactive memory T cells. It is actively being investigated whether potential H/K ATPase reactive T cells are anergized, deleted or just kept in check by CD4$^+$CD25$^+$ T cells. A recent report utilizing the IBD model indicates that CD4$^+$CD45Rbhi cells that have been suppressed by co-transfer of CD4$^+$CD25$^+$ T cells are still capable of inducing IBD if transferred alone to another immunodeficient mouse (Martin et al. 2004).

Use of anti-IL-10R indicates that perhaps cell types, other than CD4$^+$CD25$^+$ cells, produce IL-10 necessary for suppression of immunopathology. In vitro work using human CD4$^+$CD25$^+$ T cells has identified their potential for infectious tolerance, instructing CD25$^-$ T cells to make IL-10 (Dieckmann et al. 2002) or TGF-β (Jonuleit et al. 2002). Moreover, in vivo work by Foussat et al. (2003) has hinted at such a mechanism where CD4$^+$CD25$^+$ T cells may play a role inducing other cells to produce IL-10.

TGF-β is another candidate immunosuppressive cytokine that has been implicated in control of autoimmune disease. In the CD25$^-$ T cell adoptive transfer model of AIG, we employed anti-TGF-β antibodies with co-transfer of CD4$^+$CD25$^+$ cells and saw no decrease in efficiency of suppression (Piccirillo et al. 2002). Again, this is a difference between suppression requirements of AIG and IBD. Experiments using anti-TGF-β antibodies, however, cannot distinguish between CD4$^+$CD25$^+$ production of TGF-β and other cells' production. Therefore, one conclusion of this data is that CD25$^+$ T cells can instruct another cell, perhaps an induced Treg to produce TGF-β that can subsequently have an effect. Indeed this may be the case as recent data has shown that CD4$^+$CD25$^+$ T cells isolated from TGF-$\beta^{-/-}$ mice are able to suppress IBD, but in a TGF-β dependent manner (F. Powrie, personal communication).

4.3
Involvement of Co-stimulatory Molecules

CD4$^+$CD25$^+$ T cells constitutively express CTLA-4 (Read et al. 2000; Takahashi et al. 2000), the B7 counter-receptor responsible for downregulation of T cell responses (Walunas et al. 1994). CTLA-4-deficient mice suffer from massive lymphoproliferation and autoimmune pathology, leading to death within at a few weeks of life (Waterhouse et al. 1995). This defect in CTLA-4 was found to not be cell autonomous as a mixture of CTLA-4$^{+/+}$ and CTLA-4$^{-/-}$ bone marrow was able to control the immunopathology normally seen in a CTLA-4-deficient mouse (Bachmann et al. 1999). It was additionally demonstrated that in vitro and in vivo treatment with a blocking anti-CTLA-4 antibody would result in a lack of CD4$^+$CD25$^+$ T cell-mediated suppression (Read et al. 2000; Takahashi et al. 2000).

The role of CTLA-4 in AIG was addressed by anti-CTLA-4 treatment of immunocompromised mice that had received CD4$^+$CD25$^-$ cells alone or with CD4$^+$CD25$^+$ T cells. These experiments did not reveal any effect on CD4$^+$CD25$^+$ T cells ability to inhibit AIG (McHugh et al. 2001a). Again, this suggests that individual models of disease have different requirements for suppression. In vitro analysis of the role of CTLA-4 has revealed that activation of the responding cell can influence the requirements for CTLA-4 signaling in CD4$^+$CD25$^+$ T cell-mediated suppression (Thornton et al. 2004a). Perhaps pathogenic T cells involved in IBD receive greater stimulation than those inducing AIG, and therefore the suppression is more reliant on CTLA-4 signals.

As mentioned in Sect. 2.1, mice deficient in IL-2, IL-2R and co-stimulatory molecules, such as CD28, have few to no CD4$^+$CD25$^+$ T cells. CD28-deficient mice have about 40%–50% of the CD25$^+$ cells found in wild-type BALB/c (McHugh et al. 2001a; Salomon et al. 2000). Although, CD4$^+$CD25$^+$ T cells from CD28$^{-/-}$ mice display suppressive activity, these cells were less efficient in suppressing AIG (McHugh et al. 2001a) and IBD (de Jong et al. 2004). It is not clear what the in vivo deficiency of these cells is, but may possibly be secondary to survival. Another possibility is the requirement CD4$^+$CD25$^+$ cells have for IL-2 signaling to support full suppressor functions.

It has recently been noted that GITR expression is not upregulated in the absence of CD28 signaling (Stephens et al. 2004). As previously demonstrated, GITR signaling increases IL-2 responsiveness (McHugh et al. 2002). Perhaps in CD28$^{-/-}$ mice, GITR levels are low, which lowers IL-2 responsiveness in vivo. Therefore, CD28$^{-/-}$ CD4$^+$CD25$^+$ T cells do not receive sufficient IL-2 stimulation for full suppressive activity.

5
Concluding Remarks

Throughout this review, several lines of in vitro and in vivo evidence have been compiled indicating the timing of CD4$^+$CD25$^+$ T cell suppression. First, CD4$^+$CD25$^+$ T cells require TCR and IL-2 stimulation for suppression. Second, lymphocytic infiltrate transiently occurs in the presence of CD4$^+$CD25$^+$ cells and may take up to 4 weeks to clear. Next, absence of CD4$^+$CD25$^+$ T cells does not alter tolerance to self-antigens in the steady state, but are essential following strong autoreactive stimulation. Lastly, GITR-L, whose engagement of GITR can prevent CD4$^+$CD25$^+$ T cell suppression of responding T cells, is expressed constitutively by APCs and is only down-regulated with APC maturation by TLR and other stimulations. Taken together, this suggests that CD4$^+$CD25$^+$ T cell suppression of self-reactivity does not come into play until DCs have had appropriate maturation to present self-antigen in an immunostimulatory manner. Recent analysis of in vivo immune responses to immature or mature DCs demonstrates that the presence of CD4$^+$CD25$^+$ T cells only controls responses to mature DCs (Oldenhove et al. 2003). In the context of presentation of self-antigen by immature DCs, other tolerogenic mechanisms or other regulatory cells may play a role. As well, GITR-L could be expressed by immature DCs and therefore negate any suppressive mechanisms of CD4$^+$CD25$^+$ T cells. Such strong stimulatory signals from inflammation or lymphopenia would initial autoimmunity and subsequently its control.

With their therapeutic potential, it is becoming increasingly important to work out the suppressive mechanism of CD4$^+$CD25$^+$ T cells in vivo. The various cell types involved and requirements for disease induction, however, can complicate analysis in vivo. Indeed, the nature of the immune response or the state of T cell activation may require various means of control. The autoimmune disease AIG presents a well-defined in vivo model for the analysis of CD4$^+$CD25$^+$ T cell biology. A monoclonal CD4$^+$ T cell reactive to the known self-antigen, H/K ATPase, is solely capable of disease induction. Additional tools such as H/K ATPase transgenics and knockouts allow for analysis of the role of antigen-specificity of autoimmune suppression. In being able to control the initiating effector population as well as being able to visualize the DCs presenting the self-antigen, AIG provides an excellent tool for elucidating the in vivo mechanisms of CD4$^+$CD25$^+$ T cell suppression.

References

Alderuccio F, Gleeson PA, Berzins SP, Martin M, VanDriel IR, Toh BH (1997) Expression of the gastric H/K-ATPase alpha-subunit in the thymus may explain the dominant role of the beta-subunit in the pathogenesis of autoimmune gastritis. Autoimmunity 25:167–175

Alderuccio F, Cataldo V, van Driel IR, Gleeson PA, Toh BH (2000) Tolerance and autoimmunity to a gastritogenic peptide in TCR transgenic mice. Int Immunol 12:343–352

Alderuccio F, Sentry JW, Marshall AC J., Biondo M, Toh BH (2002) Animal models of human disease: Exp autoimmune gastritis- A model for autoimmune gastritis and pernicious anemia. Clinical Immunol 102:48–58

Annacker O, Pimenta-Araujo R, Burlen-Defranoux O, Barbosa TC, Cumano A, Bandeira A (2001) CD25($^+$) CD4($^+$) T cells regulate the expansion of peripheral CD4 T cells through the production of IL-10. J Immunol 166 3008–3018

Asano M, Toda M, Sakaguchi N, Sakaguchi S (1996) Autoimmune disease as a consequence of developmental abnormality of a T cell subpopulation. J Exp Med 184:387–396

Asseman C, Mauze S, Leach MW, Coffman RL, Powrie F (1999) An essential role for interleukin 10 in the function of regulatory T cells that inhibit intestinal inflammation. J Exp Med 190:995–1003

Asseman C, Read S, Powrie F (2003) Colitogenic Th1 cells are present in the antigen-experienced T cell pool in normal mice: control by CD4$^+$ regulatory T cells and IL-10. J Immunol 171:971–978

Bachmann MF, Kohler G, Ecabert B, Mak TW, Kopf M (1999) Cutting edge: Lymphoproliferative disease in the absence of CTLA-4 is not T cell autonomous. J Immunol 163 1128–1131

Barrett SP, Gleeson PA, deSilva H, Toh BH, vanDriel IR (1996) Interferon-gamma is required during the initiation of an organ-specific autoimmune disease. Eur J Immunol 26 1652–1655

Barthlott T, Kassiotis G, Stockinger B (2003) T cell regulation as a side effect of homeostasis and competition. J Exp Med 197:451–460

Bergman MP, Amedei A, D'Elios MM, Azzurri A, Benagiano M, Tamburini C, van der Zee R, Vandenbroucke-Grauls CM, Appelmelk BJ, Del Prete G (2003) Characterization of H$^+$,K$^+$-ATPase T cell epitopes in human autoimmune gastritis. Eur J Immunol 33:539–545

Biondo M, Nasa Z, Marshall A, Toh BH, Alderuccio F (2001) Local transgenic expression of granulocyte macrophage-colony stimulating factor initiates autoimmunity. J Immunol 166 2090–2099

Bruder D, Probst-Kepper M, Westendorf AM, Geffers R, Beissert S, Loser K, von Boehmer H, Buer J, Hansen W (2004) Neuropilin-1: a surface marker of regulatory T cells. Eur J Immunol 34:623–630

Cameron MJ, Arreaza GA, Zucker P, Chensue SW, Strieter RM, Chakrabarti S, Delovitch TL (1997) IL-4 prevents insulitis and insulin-dependent diabetes mellitus in nonobese diabetic mice by potentiation of regulatory T helper-2 cell function. J Immunol 159:4686–4692

Candon S, Mchugh RS, Foucras G, Natarajan K, Shevach EM, Margulies DH (2004) Spontaneous organ specific Th2-mediated autoimmunity in TCR transgenic mice. J Immunol 172:2917–2924

D'Elios MM, Bergman MP, Azzurri A, Amedei A, Benagiano M, De Pont JJ, Cianchi F, Vandenbroucke-Grauls CM, Romagnani S, Appelmelk BJ, Del Prete G (2001) H$^+$,K$^+$-ATPase (proton pump) is the target autoantigen of Th1-type cytotoxic T cells in autoimmune gastritis. Gastroenterology 120:377–386

De Jong YP, Rietdijk ST, Faubion WA, Abadia-Molina AC, Clarke K, Mizoguchi E, Tian J, Delaney T, Manning S, Gutierrez-Ramos J-C. et al (2004) Blocking inducible co-stimulator in the absence of CD28 impairs Th1 and CD25$^+$ regulatory T cells in murine colitis. Int Immunol 16:205–213

De Silva HD, Gleeson PA, Toh BH, Van Driel IR, Carbone FR (1999) Identification of a gastritogenic epitope of the H/K ATPase beta-subunit. Immunology 96:145–151

Dieckmann D, Bruett CH, Ploettner H, Lutz MB, Schuler G (2002) Human CD4$^+$CD25$^+$ regulatory, contact-dependent T cells induce interleukin 10-producing, contact-independent type 1-like regulatory T cells. J Exp Med 196:247–253

Fontenot JD, Gavin MA, Rudensky AY (2003) Foxp3 programs the development and function of CD4($^+$)CD25($^+$) regulatory T cells. Nat Immunol 4:330–336

Foussat A, Cottrez F, Brun V, Fournier N, Breittmayer J-P, Groux H (2003) A comparative study between T regulatory type 1 and CD4$^+$CD25$^+$ T cells in the control of inflammation. J Immunol 171:5018–5026

Gavin MA, Clarke SR, Negrou E, Gallegos A, Rudensky A (2002) Homeostasis and anergy of CD4+CD25+ suppressor T cells in vivo. Nature Immunol 3:33–41

Gottardi CJ, Caplan MJ (1993) Molecular requirements for the cell-surface expression of multisubunit ion-transport ATPase. Identification of protein domains that participate in Na, K-ATPase and H, K-ATPase subunit assembly. J Biol Chem 268:14342–14347

Homann D, Holz A, Bot A, Coon B, Wolfe T, Petersen J, Dyrberg TP, Grusby MJ, von Herrath MG (1999) Autoreactive CD4(+) T cells protect from autoimmune diabetes via bystander suppression using the IL-4/stat6 pathway. Immunity 11:463–472

Hori S, Nomura T, Sakaguchi S (2003) Control of regulatory T cell development by the transcription factor Foxp3. Science 299:1057–1061

Jones CM, Callaghan JM, Gleeson PA, Mori Y, Masuda T, Toh BH (1991) The parietal-cell autoantibodies recognized in neonatal thymectomy-induced murine gastritis are the alpha-subunit and beta-subunit of the gastric proton pump. Gastroenterology 101:287–294

Jonuleit H, Schmitt E, Kakirman H, Stassen M, Knop J, Enk AH (2002) Infectious tolerance: human CD25+ regulatory T cells convey suppressor activity to conventional CD4+ T helper cells. J Exp Med 196:255–260

Katakai T, Agata Y, Shimizu A, Ohshima C, Nishio A, Inaba M, Kasakura S, Mori KJ, Masuda T (1997) Structure of the TCR expressed on a gastritogenic T cell clone, Il-6, frequent appearance of similar clonotypes in mice bearing autoimmune gastritis. Int Immunol 9:1849–1855

Katakai T, Hara T, Sugai M, Gonda H, Shimizu A (2003) Th1-biased tertiary lymphoid tissue supported by CXC chemokine ligand 13-producing stromal network in chronic lesions of autoimmune gastritis. J Immunol 171 4359–4368

Khattri R, Cox T, Yasayko SA, Ramsdell F (2003) An essential role for Scurfin in CD4(+)CD25(+) T regulatory cells. Nature Immunol 4:337–342

Kim JD, Choi BK, Bae JS, Lee UH, Han IS, Lee HW, Youn BS, Vinay DS, Kwon B (2003) Cloning and characterization of GITR ligand. Genes Immun 4:564–569

Kohm AP, Williams JS, Miller SD (2004) Cutting edge: ligation of the glucocorticoid-induced TNF receptor enhances autoreactive CD4(+) T cell activation and experimental autoimmune encephalomyelitis. J Immunol 172:4686–4690

Kojima A, Prehn RT (1981) Genetic susceptibility to post-thymectomy autoimmune-diseases in mice. Immunogenetics 14:15–27

Krause I, Blank M, Shoenfeld Y (2000) Immunomodulation of experimental autoimmune diseases via oral tolerance. Crit Rev Immunol 20:1–16

Kukreja A, Cost G, Marker J, Zhang CH, Sun Z, Lin-Su K, Ten S, Sanz M, Exley M, Wilson B et al (2002) Multiple immuno-regulatory defects in type-1 diabetes. J Clin Invest 109:131–140

Lafaille JJ, Nagashima K, Katsuki M, Tonegawa S (1994) High incidence of spontaneous autoimmune encephalomyelitis in immunodeficient antimyelin basic-protein T-cell receptor transgenic mice. Cell 78:399–408

Laurie KL, Van Driel IR, Gleeson PA (2002) Role of CD4(+)CD25(+) immunoregulatory T cells in the induction of autoimmune gastritis. Immunol Cell Biol 80:567–573

Lehmann J, Huehn J, de la Rosa M, Maszyna F, Kretschmer U, Krenn V, Brunner M, Scheffold A, Hamann A (2002) Expression of the integrin alpha (E)beta (7) identifies unique subsets of CD25(+) as well as CD25(−) regulatory T cells. Proc Natl Acad Sci U S America 99:13031–13036

Ling EM, Smith T, Nguyen XD, Pridgeon C, Dallman M, Arbery J, Carr VA, Robinson DS (2004) Relation of CD4$^+$CD25$^+$ regulatory T-cell suppression of allergen-driven T-cell activation to atopic status and expression of allergic disease. Lancet 363:608–615

Liu H, Hu B, Xu D, Liew FY (2003) CD4$^+$CD25$^+$ regulatory T cells cure murine colitis: the role of IL-10, TGF-β, CTLA-4. J Immunol 171:5012–5017

Marshall ACJ, Alderuccio F, Toh BH (2002) Fas/CD95 is required for gastric mucosal damage in autoimmune gastritis. Gastroenterology 123:780–789

Marshall ACJ, Toh BH, Alderuccio F (2004) Tumor necrosis factor alpha is not implicated in the genesis of experimental autoimmune gastritis. J Autoimmunity 22:1–11

Martin B, Banz A, Bienvenu B, Cordier C, Dautigny N, Becourt C, Lucas B (2004) Suppression of CD4$^+$ T lymphocyte effector functions by CD4$^+$CD25$^+$ cells in vivo. J Immunol 172:3391–3398

Martinelli TM, vanDriel IR, Alderuccio F, Gleeson PA, Toh BH (1996) Analysis of mononuclear cell infiltrate and cytokine production in murine autoimmune gastritis. Gastroenterology 110:1791–1802

McHugh RS, Shevach EM (2002a) Cutting edge: depletion of CD4$^+$CD25$^+$ regulatory T cells is necessary, but not sufficient, for induction of organ-specific autoimmune disease. J Immunol 168:5979–5983

McHugh RS, Shevach EM (2002b) The role of suppressor T cells in regulation of immune responses. J Allergy Clin Immunol 110:693–702

McHugh R, Shevach E, Thornton A (2001a) Control of organ-specific autoimmunity by immunoregulatory CD4$^+$CD25$^+$ T cells. Microb Infect 3:919–927

McHugh RS, Shevach EM, Margulies DH, Natarajan K (2001b) A T cell receptor transgenic model of severe, spontaneous organ-specific autoimmunity. Eur J Immunol 31:2094–2103

McHugh RS, Whitters MJ, Piccirillo CA, Young DA, Shevach EM, Collins M, Byrne MC (2002) CD4$^+$CD25$^+$ Immunoregulatory T cells: gene expression analysis reveals a functional role for the glucocorticoid-induced TNF receptor. Immunity 16:311–323

Min B, McHugh R, Sempowski GD, Mackall C, Foucras G, Paul WE (2004) Neonates support lymphopenia-induced proliferation. Immunity 18:131–140

Mottet C, Uhlig HH, Powrie F (2003) Cutting edge: cure of colitis by CD4$^+$CD25$^+$ regulatory T cells. J Immunol 170 3939–3943

Nakamura K, Kitani A, Strober W (2001) Cell contact-dependent immunosuppression by CD4($^+$)CD25($^+$) regulatory T cells is mediated by cell surface-bound transforming growth factor beta. J Exp Med 194:629–644

Nishio A, Katakai T, Oshima C, Kasakura S, Sakai M, Yonehara S, Suda T, Nagata S, Masuda T (1996) A possible involvement of Fas-Fas ligand signaling in the pathogenesis of murine autoimmune gastritis. Gastroenterology 111:959–967

Oldenhove G, de Heusch M, Urbain-Vansanten G, Urbain J, Maliszewski C, Leo O, Moser M (2003) CD4($^+$) CD25($^+$) regulatory T cells control T helper cell type 1 responses to foreign antigens induced by mature dendritic cells in vivo. J Exp Med 198:259–266

Onizuka S, Tawara I, Shimizu J, Sakaguchi S, Fujita T, Nakayama E (1999) Tumor rejection by in vivo administration of anti-CD25 (interleukin-2 receptor alpha) monoclonal antibody. Cancer Res 59:3128–3133

Piccirillo CA, Shevach EM (2004) Naturally-occurring CD4+CD25+ immunoregulatory T cells: central players in the arena of peripheral tolerance. Semin Immunol 16:81–88

Piccirillo CA, Letterio JJ, Thornton AM, Mchugh RS, Mamura M, Mizuhara H, Shevach EM (2002) CD4+CD25+ regulatory T cells can mediate suppressor function in the absence of transforming growth factor beta1 production and responsiveness. J Exp Med 196:237–246

Powrie F, Leach M, Coffman RL (1994) CD45Rbhigh Cd4+ T-cells induce a pathogenic Th1 response in the colon when transferred to C-B-17 Scid mice which is prevented by co-transfer of the Cd45rblow population. J Cell Biochem 418–425

Powrie F, Carlino J, Leach MW, Mauze S, Coffman RL (1996) A critical role for transforming growth factor-beta but not interleukin 4 in the suppression of T helper type 1-mediated colitis by CD45RB(low) CD4(+) T cells. J Exp Med 183:2669–2674

Read S, Malmstrom V, Powrie F (2000) Cytotoxic T lymphocyte-associated antigen 4 plays an essential role in the function of CD25(+)CD4(+) regulatory cells that control intestinal inflammation. J Exp Med 192:295–302

Sakaguchi S (2004) Naturally arising CD4+ regulatory T cells for immunologic self-tolerance and negative control of immune responses. Ann Rev Immunol 22:531–562

Sakaguchi S, Ermak TH, Toda M, Berg LJ, Ho W, Destgroth BF, Peterson PA, Sakaguchi N, Davis MM (1994) Induction of autoimmune-disease in mice by germline alteration of the T-cell receptor gene-expression. J Immunol 152:1471–1484

Sakaguchi S, Sakaguchi N, Asano M, Itoh M, Toda M (1995) Immunological self-tolerance maintained by activated T-cells expressing IL-2 receptor alpha-chains (CD25): breakdown of a single mechanism of self-tolerance causes various autoimmune diseases. J Immunol 155:1151–1164

Salama AD, Chaudhry AN, Holthaus KA, Mosley K, Kalluri R, Sayegh MH, Lechler RI, Pusey CD, Lightstone L (2003) Regulation by CD25(+) lymphocytes of autoantigen-specific T-cell responses in Goodpasture's (anti-GBM) disease. Kidney Int 64:1685–1694

Salomon B, Lenschow DJ, Rhee L, Ashourian N, Singh B, Sharpe A, Bluestone JA (2000) B7/CD28 costimulation is essential for the homeostasis of the CD4(+)CD25(+) immunoregulatory T cells that control autoimmune diabetes. Immunity 12:431–440

Scarff KJ, Pettitt JM, VanDriel IR, Gleeson PA, Toh BH (1997) Immunization with gastric H^+/K^+-ATPase induces a reversible autoimmune gastritis. Immunol 92:91–98

Scheinecker C, McHugh R, Shevach EM, Germain RN (2002) Constitutive presentation of a natural tissue autoantigen exclusively by dendritic cells in the draining lymph node. J Exp Med 196:1079–1090

Seddon B, Mason D (1999) Regulatory T cells in the control of autoimmunity: the essential role of transforming growth factor beta and interleukin 4 in the prevention of autoimmune thyroiditis in rats by peripheral CD4(+)CD45RC(−) cells and CD4(+)CD8(−) thymocytes. J Exp Med 189:279–288

Shevach EM (2000) Regulatory T cells in autoimmmunity. Ann Rev Immunol 18:423–449

Shevach EM (2001) Certified professionals: CD4(+)CD25(+) suppressor T cells. J Exp Med 193:F41–F45

Shevach EM (2002) CD4+CD25+ suppressor T cells: more questions than answers. Nat Rev Immunol 2:389–400

Shimizu J, Yamazaki S, Sakaguchi S (1999) Induction of tumor immunity by removing CD25($^+$)CD4($^+$) T cells: a common basis between tumor immunity and autoimmunity. J Immunol 163:5211–5218

Shimizu J, Yamazaki S, Takahashi T, Ishida Y, Sakaguchi S (2002) Stimulation of CD25+CD4+ regulatory T cells through GITR breaks immunological self-tolerance. Nat Immunol 3:135–142

Stassen M, Fondel S, Bopp R, Richter C, Muller C, Kubach J, Becker C, Knop J, Enk AH, Schmitt S et al (2004) Human CD25+ regulatory T cells: two subsets defined by the integrins $\alpha 4\beta 7$ or $\alpha 4\beta 1$ confer distinct suppressive properties upon CD4+ T helper cells. Eur J Immunol 34:1303–1311

Steinman RM, Turley S, Mellman I, Inaba K (2000) The induction of tolerance by dendritic cells that have captured apoptotic cells. J Exp Med 191:411–416

Steinman RM, Hawiger D, Nussenzweig MC (2003) Tolerogenic dendritic cells. Ann Rev Immunol 21:685–711

Stephens GL, McHugh RS, Whitters MJ, Young DA, Collins M, Shevach EM (2004) Engagement of GITR on effector T cells by its ligand mediates resistance to suppression by CD4+CD25+ T cells. J Immunol 173:5008–5020

Suri-Payer E, Cantor H (2001) Differential cytokine requirements for regulation of autoimmune gastritis and colitis by CD4($^+$)CD25($^+$) T cells. J Autoimmunity 16:115–123

Suri-Payer E, Amar AZ, Thornton AM, Shevach EM (1998) CD4($^+$)CD25($^+$) T cells inhibit both the induction and effector function of autoreactive T cells and represent a unique lineage of immunoregulatory cells. J Immunol 160:1212–1218

Suri-Payer E, Amar AZ, McHugh R, Natarajan K, Margulies DH, Shevach EM (1999) Post-thymectomy autoimmune gastritis: fine specificity and pathogenicity of anti-H/K ATPase-reactive T cells. Eur J Immunol 29:669–677

Sutmuller RPM, van Duivenvoorde LM, van Elsas A, Schumacher TNM, Wildenberg ME, Allison JP, Toes REM, Offringa R, Melief CJM (2001) Synergism of cytotoxic T lymphocyte-associated antigen 4 blockade and depletion of CD25+ regulatory T cells in antitumor therapy reveals alternative pathways for suppression of autoreactive cytotoxic T lymphocyte responses. J Exp Med 194:823–832

Szanya V, Ermann J, Taylor C, Holness C, Fathman CG (2002) The Subpopulation of CD4($^+$) CD25($^+$) splenocytes that delays adoptive transfer of diabetes expresses L-selectin and high levels of CCR7. J Immunol 169:2461–2465

Taguchi O, Takahashi T (1996) Administration of anti-interleukin-2 receptor alpha antibody in vivo induces localized autoimmune disease. Eur J Immunol 26:1608–1612

Takahashi T, Kuniyasu Y, Toda M, Sakaguchi N, Itoh M, Iwata M, Shimizu J, Sakaguchi S (1998) Immunologic self-tolerance maintained by CD25($^+$)CD4($^+$) naturally anergic and suppressive T cells: induction of autoimmune disease by breaking their anergic/suppressive state. Int Immunol 10:1969–1980

Takahashi T, Tagami T, Yamazaki S, Uede T, Shimizu J, Sakaguchi N, Mak TW, Sakaguchi S (2000) Immunologic self-tolerance maintained by CD25($^+$)CD4($^+$) regulatory T cells constitutively expressing cytotoxic T lymphocyte-associated antigen 4. J Exp Med 192:303–309

Thornton AM, Shevach EM (1998) CD4($^+$)CD25($^+$) immunoregulatory T cells suppress polyclonal T cell activation in vitro by inhibiting interleukin 2 production. J Exp Med 188:287–296

Thornton AM, Shevach EM (2000) Suppressor effector function of CD4($^+$)CD25($^+$) immunoregulatory T cells is antigen nonspecific. J Immunol 164:183–190

Thornton A, Piccirillo CA, Shevach EM (2004a) Activation requirements for the induction of CD4$^+$CD25$^+$ T cells suppressor function. Eur J Immunol 34:366–376

Thornton AM, Donovan EE, Piccirillo CA, Shevach EM (2004b) Cutting edge: IL-2 is critically required for the in vitro activation of CD4$^+$CD25$^+$ T cell suppressor function. J Immunol 172:6519–6523

Toh BH, vanDriel IR, Gleeson PA (1997) Mechanisms of disease: pernicious anemia. New Engl J Med 337:1441–1448

Toh BH, Sentry JW, Alderuccio F (2000) The causative H$^+$/K$^+$ ATPase antigen in the pathogenesis of autoimmune gastritis. Immunol Today 21:348–354

Tone M, Tone Y, Adams E, Yates SF, Frewin MR, Cobbold SP, Waldmann H (2003) Mouse glucocorticoid-induced tumor necrosis factor receptor ligand is costimulatory for T cells. Proc Natl Acad Sci U S A 100:15059–15064

Viglietta V, Baecher-Allan C, Weiner HL, Hafler DA (2004) Loss of functional suppression by CD4($^+$)CD25($^+$) regulatory T cells in patients with multiple sclerosis. J Exp Med 199:971–979

Walunas TL, Lenschow DJ, Bakker CY, Linsley PS, Freeman GJ, Green JM, Thompson CB, Bluestone JA (1994) CTLA-4 can function as a negative regulator of T-cell activation. Immunity 1:405–413

Waterhouse P, Penninger JM, Timms E, Wakeham A, Shahinian A, Lee KP, Thompson CB, Griesser H, Mak TW (1995) Lymphoproliferative disorders with early lethality in mice deficient in Ctla-4. Science 270:985–988

Zelenika D, Adams E, Humm S, Graca L, Thompson S, Cobbold SP, Waldmann H (2002) Regulatory T cells overexpress a subset of Th2 gene transcripts. J Immunol 168:1069–1079

Regulatory T Cells in Experimental Colitis

M. Gad (✉)

Department of Medical Anatomy, The Panum Institute,
The University of Copenhagen, Blegdamsvej 3 C, 2200N Copenhagen, Denmark
m.gad@mai.ku.dk

1	Introduction	180
2	Inflammatory Bowel Diseases	180
3	Bacterial Flora in Inflammatory Bowel Disease	181
4	Animal Models of Inflammatory Bowel Disease	182
4.1	The SCID Transfer Model of Colitis	183
4.2	Other Models of Colitis Caused by a Dysregulated Immune System	185
5	Regulatory T Cells Prevent Colitis	185
6	Naturally Occurring Regulatory T Cells	186
7	Mechanisms of $CD4^+CD25^+$ Treg Cell-Mediated Immunosuppressive Functions	188
7.1	Cytokine Requirements for the Control of Colitis by $CD4^+CD25^+$ Treg	188
7.2	Cellular Requirements for the Regulation of Colitis by $CD4^+CD25^+$ Treg	192
8	Other Subsets of Regulatory T Cells Involved in the Control of Colitis	194
9	Where Do the Treg Cells Localize and What Do They Target?	195
10	Antigen Specificity for Regulatory T Cells in Colitis	198
11	Regulatory T Cells as a Therapeutic Agent for Inflammatory Bowel Disease	199
12	Conclusion	200
	References	201

Abstract Induction and maintenance of peripheral tolerance are important mechanisms to maintain the balance of the immune system. Growing evidence indicates that dysregulation of mucosal T cell responses may lead to loss of tolerance to commensal flora and to the development of inflammatory bowel diseases (IBD). Many studies suggest that active suppression of enteroantigen reactive cells mediated by regulatory

T cells contributes to the maintenance of natural intestinal immune homeostasis. The use of the multiple animal models has not only improved our understanding of IBD, but also contributed to new suggestions of treatment strategies involving the use of regulatory T cells. The present review summarizes our current knowledge of regulatory T cells and their involvement in experimental IBD. The well-characterized SCID T cell transfer model and the naturally occurring regulatory $CD4^+CD25^+$ T cells are highlighted.

1
Introduction

The intestinal immune system is a very large and complex part of the immune system, which interfaces with a variety of endogenous and exogenous stimuli. The gut mucosal immune system encounters more antigens than any other part of the body and must discriminate clearly between invasive organisms and harmless antigens, such as food antigens and commensal bacteria. The mechanisms controlling the balance between tolerance and active immunity are therefore very critical, although not well understood. If the immune control mechanisms break down the consequences can be very devastating. Loss of tolerance to food antigens or commensal flora may lead to inflammatory disorders such as food allergies and inflammatory bowel disease (IBD), respectively (Bilsborough et al. 2002; Wittig et al. 2003). Induction and maintenance of peripheral tolerance are important mechanisms to maintain the balance of the immune system. Accumulating evidence suggests that apart from T cell anergy and clonal deletion by apoptosis, active suppression mediated by regulatory T cells contribute to the maintenance of natural immunological self-tolerance as well as of tolerance towards enteroantigens.

2
Inflammatory Bowel Diseases

The inflammatory bowel diseases (IBD), which include Crohn's disease (CD) and ulcerative colitis (UC), are chronic inflammatory disorders effecting 0.3% of the Western population (Podolsky 2002). CD can affect any part of the gastrointestinal tract, from the oral cavity to the anus, whereas UC is limited to the colon and rectum. The etiology of CD and UC remains unknown, but it probably involves a combination of genetic predisposition, environmental conditions, and abnormalities in immune regulation (Chutkan 2001; Farrell et al. 2001; Podolsky 2002). In particular, the intestinal mucosal immune system has been a major focus of research, as IBD is characterized by a hyper-reactive immune system, underlined by a heavy influx of T cells, B cells, monocytes, and neutrophils into the intestinal mucosa. On the simplest level, an imbalance between pro- and anti-inflammatory mediators leads to chronic inflammation in the gastrointestinal tract of patients with IBD. Specific cytokines important for the induction of mucosal immunity and regulation of the mucosal immune responses include the pro-inflammatory mediators IL-1, IL-6, IL-12 and TNF-α, produced by monocytes and macrophages. In addition, the CD4$^+$ T cells infiltrating the lamina propria (LP) of IBD patients display an altered cytokine profile as compared with healthy individuals. LP-derived CD4$^+$ T cells from CD patients produce increased levels of IFN-γ and IL-2, whereas LP-derived CD4$^+$ T cells from UC patients produce increased levels of IL-4 and IL-5 (Farrell et al. 2001). These observations suggest that that the immune responses are Th1 and Th2 screwed in CD and UC patients, respectively.

3
Bacterial Flora in Inflammatory Bowel Disease

Although the etiology of IBD has not been clearly linked to any specific infectious agent, it is well known from experimental models of IBD that colitis cannot be induced in animals raised under germ-free conditions (Sartor 1997; Schultz et al. 1999; Sellon et al. 1998). In the SCID transfer model of colitis, only a mild form of IBD developed after transfer of CD4$^+$CD45RB^{high} T cells into recipients with a restricted enteric flora (Aranda et al. 1997). In addition, treatment with broad spectrum antibiotics reduces the severity of IBD (Madsen et al. 2000). These studies are consistent with a study by Duchmann et al. (1999) reporting a colonic mucosal T cell reactivity to endogenous flora in IBD patients, not present in healthy individuals. We have previously demonstrated that CD4$^+$ T cells from SCID mice with IBD, in contrast to CD4$^+$ T cells from normal BALB/c mice, respond by proliferation and cytokine secretion when exposed to enteric bacterial extracts (Brimnes et al. 2001; Gad et al. 2003). In addition, CD4$^+$ T cells from normal mice depleted in vivo or in vitro of CD4$^+$CD25$^+$ T cells proliferate extensively in the presence of enterobacterial antigens but are refractory to enteroantigens from the feces of germfree mice (Gad et al. 2004).

However, although the enteric flora necessary for IBD to develop has not been well characterized, a number of different bacterial species have been identified as being able to trigger the development of colitis in murine models (Rath et al. 1996; Sellon et al. 1998). One such species is the Gram-negative bacterium *Helicobacter hepaticus*. It has been shown that *H. hepaticus* can cause colitis in immunodeficient mice (Li et al. 1998; Ward et al. 1996) and intensify colitis in immunodeficient mice reconstituted with naïve CD45RB^{high} CD4$^+$ T cells (Cahill et al. 1997). In addition, transfer of CD4$^+$ T cells from IL-10$^{-/-}$ mice into RAG$^{-/-}$ mice results in colitis in *H. hepaticus*-infected but not in uninfected recipients (Kullberg et al. 2002). In human studies *Mycobacteria* (Sanderson et al. 1992) and a subtype of *Escherichia coli* (Darfeuille-Michaud et al. 1998) have been found to play a pathogenic role in CD, whereas the presence of *Shingella*, *Salmonella* and *Yersinia* (Sartor et al. 1996) have been investigated as potential causal agents in UC.

Recent studies have tried to manipulate the intestinal microflora by treating with potentially protective bacteria such as lactobacilli and bifidobacteria species (Campieri et al. 2001), which are harmless components of the normal human and murine gastrointestinal microflora. It has been shown that certain probiotics can induce specific anti-inflammatory effects and they have been proposed as a therapy of colitis (Borruel et al. 2002, 2003). Consistent with this, treatment with *Lactobacillus* has shown to prevent the development of spontaneous colitis in IL-10-deficient mice (Madsen et al. 1999). The role of lactobacilli and bifidobacteria in human colitis is still not well characterized, although a significant decrease in the number of lactobacilli was found in colonic biopsies from patients with UC (Fabia et al. 1993). Clinical trials with the use of probiotics to treat patients with IBD or pouchitis proved to be quite effective (Gionchetti et al. 2000; Rembacken et al. 1999). Together, many independent studies suggest that enteric bacteria may trigger IBD, although the nature of these bacterially derived antigen(s) is unknown.

4
Animal Models of Inflammatory Bowel Disease

Studies in experimental models of mucosal inflammation have led to major new insights into the abnormalities present in human IBD as well as to new approaches in the therapy of these diseases (Hoffmann et al. 2002; Singh et al. 2001a; Strober et al. 2002). Models, based on knockout and transgenic animals, have generated the greatest interest and are commonly used. In particular, the adoptive transfer of T cells into immunodeficient mice as severe combined immune deficient (SCID) mice and recombination activation gene (RAG) deficient mice, which lack functional T and B cells, has been used to induce colitis in the recipients. The SCID transfer model will be described in more detail below, as it is one of the most widely used immunological models of inflammatory bowel disease and of major importance for the study of regulatory T cells.

4.1
The SCID Transfer Model of Colitis

In the transfer models of colitis, transfer of low numbers of CD4$^+$ T cells (Claesson et al. 1996) or a subpopulation hereof from an immunocompetent syngeneic donor mouse to an immunodeficient animal (SCID or RAG$^{-/-}$) leads to chronic and lethal colitis in the recipient. In addition, transplantation of a full gut wall graft from a normal donor mouse into the skin of a histocompatible SCID induces IBD (Rudolphi et al. 1994). While the original studies suggested that only adoptive transfer of sorted CD45RB^{high} T cells leads to colitis (Morrissey et al. 1993; Powrie et al. 1993), we have repeatedly shown development of colitis following transfer to SCID mice of nonfractionated CD4$^+$ T cells (Claesson et al. 1996) and even after transfer of CD45RB^{low} T cells (Claesson et al. 1999), although the onset of disease in these cases started relatively late at 12–16 weeks after transfer. In particular, in vitro activated CD4$^+$ T cells stimulated with Concanavalin A for 3 days or freshly derived CD4$^+$CD25$^-$ T cells are highly effective with regards to induction of colitis, which develops 6–8 weeks after transfer (Claesson et al. 1999; Liu et al. 2003; M. Gad et al., submitted). Until now transfer of naïve CD45RB^{high} or Con A activated unfractionated CD4$^+$ T cells have been the best described models of colitis. However, recently the colitogenic potential of the cells within the antigen experienced CD45RB^{low} T cell pool was thoroughly investigated (Asseman et al. 2003). Consistent with studies from our laboratory (Claesson et al. 1999), it was revealed that colitogenic Th1 cells are present in the antigen experienced CD4$^+$CD45RB^{low} T cell population enriched within the CD25$^-$ subset but that the pathogenicity of these cells is controlled by IL-10. Thus, development of colitis was only seen in SCID mice after transfer of CD4$^+$CD45RB^{low} T cells if the recipients were treated with anti-IL-10R mAb or if transferred CD4$^+$CD45RB^{low}CD25$^-$ T cells were derived from IL-10$^{-/-}$ mice. The pathogenic reactivity of the CD45RB^{low} population was reduced when donor cells were isolated from germfree mice, indicating that the pathogenic T cells in the CD4$^+$CD45RB^{low} T cell population represent an antigen experienced population of T cells driven by enteric bacteria in the donor mice (Asseman et al. 2003). In contrast, transfer of CD4$^+$CD45RB^{high} T cells isolated from germfree mice to SCID mice is still able to induce colitis, suggesting that these naïve T cells differentiate into colitogenic Th1 cells upon exposure to the resident bacteria in the recipient. Attempts to induce colitis in immunodeficient animals using transfer of CD4$^+$CD45RB^{low}CD25$^+$ T cells have failed. However, in the absence of IL-10, pathogenic T cells have been revealed within the CD25$^+$ T cell population isolated from MLN but not from the spleen (Asseman et al. 2003), probably reflecting a higher frequency of bacteria-reactive

Table 1 The colitis inducing potency of different preparations or subsets of $CD4^+$ T cells in the $SCID/RAG^{-/-}$ transfer model

Transfer	Cytokine addition	🐭
$CD45RB^{high}$ T cells	–	IBD
$CD4^+CD25^-$ T cells	–	IBD
$CD4^+$ T cells	–	IBD
Con A activated $CD4^+$ T cells	–	IBD
Gut wall graft	–	IBD
$CD4^+CD45RB^{low}$ T cells	–	IBD/No IBD
$CD4^+CD45RB^{low}$ T cells	Anti IL-10R	IBD
$IL-10^{-/-}CD45RB^{low}CD25^-$ cells	–	IBD
$CD45RB^{low}CD25^+$	–	No IBD
$CD45RB^{low}CD25^+$	Anti-IL-10R	MLN: IBD, spleen: No IBD

IBD can be induced in $SCID/RAG^{-/-}$ mice by transfer of different subsets of $CD4^+$ T cells, although with different kinetics. Thus mice transplanted with $CD45RB^{high}$ or $CD25^-$ T cells develop colitis after 6–8 weeks, whereas transfer of Con A activated $CD4^+$ T cells induces colitis within 8–10 weeks, and transfer of unfractionated $CD4^+$ or $CD4^+CD45RB^{low}$ T cells induces colitis 12–18 weeks after transplantation. In addition, colitis is induced in SCID mice by a gut wall graft from an immunocompetent syngeneic donor. See text for references.

activated $CD25^+$ T cells in the MLN than in the spleen. In addition, different modifications of the SCID transfer model have been developed to induce colitis (Kullberg et al. 2002; Liu et al. 2003). For an overview see Table 1.

In the SCID transfer model, the transferred $CD4^+$ T cells repopulate the spleen, the mesenteric lymph nodes and the intestinal mucosa of the SCID mouse, whereas neither the thymus nor the peripheral distal lymph nodes are repopulated (Reimann et al. 1995). Subsequently, the recipients develop a lethal inflammatory bowel disease, with the main symptoms being weight loss, diarrhea and rectal prolapse (Claesson et al. 1996; Leach et al. 1996). In addition, the disease is characterized by mucosal hypertrophy, epithelial hyperplasia, decreased number of goblet cells and infiltration of the intestinal lamina propria (LP) and spleen with mononuclear cells. In severely diseased mice, transmural cell infiltration, epithelial ulceration and crypt abscesses are also seen. The histological changes are mainly found in the colon and occasionally in the small intestine (Claesson et al. 1996; Leach et al. 1996). The infiltrating mononuclear cells are dominated by the pathogenic, donor-derived $CD4^+$ T cells. These cells display surface markers consistent with a mucosa seeking and activated memory phenotype, i.e., they are CD69$^+$, CD25$^+$, CD44$^+$, CD45RB^{low}, $\alpha 4\beta 7^+$ and L-selectin^{low} (Reimann et al. 1993). The LP CD4$^+$ T cells in SCID mice with colitis have a high turnover indicated by increased levels of both proliferation and apoptosis compared with CD4$^+$ T cells from normal mice (Bregenholt et al. 1998). In addition, these cells express a Th1 cytokine phenotype and secrete IFN-γ, TNF-α, and IL-2 (Bregenholt and Claesson 1998a).

4.2
Other Models of Colitis Caused by a Dysregulated Immune System

Genetic models as deletion of either the cytokines IL-10 (IL-10$^{-/-}$) (Rennick et al. 2000), IL-2 (IL-2$^{-/-}$) (Ehrhardt et al. 1997) or their receptors, CRFB4$^{-/-}$ (Spencer et al. 1998) and IL-2$\alpha^{-/-}$ results in colitis. Also, TCR-$\alpha^{-/-}$ (Mizoguchi et al. 1996), MHC class II$^{-/-}$ (Mombaerts et al. 1993), G$\alpha_{12}{}^{-/-}$ (Rudolph et al. 1995) as well as the HLA-B27 transgenic rat model (Taurog et al. 1994) develop mucosal inflammation.

In addition, it should be mentioned that although the role of T cells in the induction of intestinal inflammation has received much attention, it has recently been shown that innate immune mechanisms alone are able to mediate intestinal inflammation as demonstrated in Rag$^{-/-}$ mice in which exposure to *H. Hepaticus* leads to chronic colitis (Maloy et al. 2003).

5
Regulatory T Cells Prevent Colitis

General mechanisms are believed to be of importance for the prevention of autoaggression, including protection against intestinal inflammation such as T cell deletion, T cell anergy and immunological ignorance. Moreover, it appears that the lymphocyte homeostasis in normal mice is under active control by the activity of a distinct subset of regulatory T cells, which in addition may play an important role in the prevention of pathogenic immune responses towards the bacterial flora of the gut (Shevach 2002).

In T cell-deficient mice and rats, colitis induced by CD4$^+$CD45RB^{high} T cells is prevented by co-transfer of CD4$^+$CD45RB^{low} T cells, cells which normally do not induce disease when transferred alone (Powrie et al. 1990, 1993). Recently it was shown that the protective capacity is enriched but not exclusively present in the CD25$^+$ subset of the CD4$^+$CD45RB^{low} T cell population (Annacker et al. 2001; Lehmann et al. 2002; Read et al. 2000). Annacker et al. (2001) observed that both the CD4$^+$CD25$^+$CD45RB^{low} and CD4$^+$CD25$^-$CD45RB^{low} purified cell populations were able to confer protection of colitis induced by CD45RB^{high} cells. In another study (Lehmann et al. 2002), subdivision of integrin $\alpha_E\beta_7^+$ (CD103) cells in CD4$^+$CD25$^-$ and CD4$^+$CD25$^+$ T cells revealed that both of the $\alpha_E\beta_7^+$ subsets can protect SCID mouse recipients from colitis. In agreement with these studies, observations from a model of *H. hepaticus*-induced colitis showed that the protective CD4$^+$ T cells are contained within both the CD25 positive and negative subsets of the CD45RB^{low} T cell fraction and that the CD25$^-$ T cells are the most effective inhibitors of inflammation (Kullberg et al. 2002). We have shown that development of colitis, induced by CD4$^+$ CD25$^-$ T cells, can be prevented both by co-transfer of CD4$^+$CD25$^+$ T cells or by co-transfer of unfractionated CD4$^+$ T cells derived from a 6-day co-culture with immature dendritic cells (DCs) (M. Gad et al. submitted). Finally, also other kinds of induced Treg cells such as IL-10-secreting Tr1 and TGF-β-secreting Tr3 Treg cells prevent T cell transfer-induced colitis (Groux et al. 1997; Neurath et al. 1996). However, the relationship between these phenotypically distinct subsets of Treg cells is not known.

Since even unfractionated CD4$^+$ T cells which include 10%–15% CD25$^+$ T cells have been reported to expand and induce colitis following transfer to SCID mice (Claesson et al. 1996), it has been suggested that the presence of *H hepaticus* in the animal facilities may play a role in the development of colitis (Annacker et al. 2000; Cahill et al. 1997; Claesson et al. 1999; Foltz et al. 1998). Thus, by transfer of unfractionated CD4$^+$ T cells to immunodeficient mice the surrounding environment, i.e., the presence or absence of *H. hepaticus*, may favor the expansion of pathogenic CD4$^+$ T cells or regulatory CD25$^+$ T cells, respectively, resulting in development of colitis or absence of disease.

6
Naturally Occurring Regulatory T Cells

Recently the focus has been largely on naturally occurring CD4$^+$ T cells constitutionally expressing the α chain of the IL-2 receptor (CD25); for a review see (Shevach 2002). Even though CD25$^-$ regulatory T cells exist (Apostolou et al. 2002; Lehmann et al. 2002), the CD25 marker has been used to define the properties of regulatory cells. The regulatory population was first identified as a subset of CD4$^+$ T cells able to prevent the development of organ-specific autoimmune disease in mice thymectomized on day 3 after birth (Asano et al. 1996; Sakaguchi et al. 1995). Subsequently, the regulatory T cells have been shown to inhibit many autoimmune diseases (Shevach 2000; von Herrath et al. 2003), transfer tolerance to alloantigens (Taylor et al. 2001), hinder anti-tumor immunity (Shimizu et al. 1999) and regulate the expansion of other peripheral CD4$^+$ T cells (Annacker et al. 2001). CD4$^+$CD25$^+$ regulatory T cells have also been isolated from the thymus and peripheral blood of humans and the cells have the same characteristics in mouse and man (Dieckmann et al. 2001; Jonuleit et al. 2001; Levings et al. 2001; Stephens et al. 2001). Naturally occurring regulatory CD4$^+$CD25$^+$ T cells are generated in the thymus (Thornton et al. 1998) and are therefore thought to recognize self-derived MHC-bound peptides. This raises the question of whether any self antigen in the thymus has the ability to generate regulatory cells. CD4$^+$CD25$^+$ T cells display a diverse TCR repertoire, suggesting that they undergo normal selection. Regulatory CD4$^+$CD25$^+$ T cells constitute around 10% of peripheral CD4$^+$ T cells (Sakaguchi et al. 1995) and are considered as resting antigen-experienced cells. Suppression mediated by the regulatory CD4$^+$CD25$^+$ T cells requires activation through their TCR (Dieckmann et al. 2001; Thornton et al. 1998). They are anergic in vitro as they do not proliferate or produce cytokines upon T cell receptor (TCR) stimulation. However, they regain responsiveness to TCR-mediated activation in the presence of exogenous IL-2 (Shevach 2002; Thornton et al. 1998). Although it is known that that CD4$^+$CD25$^+$ Treg cells suppress the transcription of the IL-2 gene in co-cultures with CD4$^+$CD25$^-$ responder cells (Shevach 2002), it has been suggested by Thornton and colleges (2004) that CD4$^+$CD25$^+$ Treg cells must respond to IL-2 before they can suppress proliferation of naïve responder cells. Somewhat unexpected from the in vitro data, recent evidence indicates that the regulatory T cells have a much more dynamic behavior than previously assumed. Thus regulatory T cells are capable of substantial antigen-induced expansion in vivo, accompanied by increased suppressive activity (Fisson et al. 2003; Klein et al. 2003; Walker et al. 2003; Yamazaki et al. 2003).

CD25 is not a very good marker for the regulatory T cells and a great effort has been made to define better markers. Numerous attempts to characterize and identify new markers revealed high expression of the negative regulator of T cell activation CTLA-4, the glucocorticoid-induced TNFR-related protein () (McHugh et al. 2002), and expression of membrane-bound tumor growth factor (TGF)-β1 after strong in vitro stimulation. Finally, the forkhead transcription factor FoxP3 which is expressed at high levels in murine regulatory CD4$^+$CD25$^+$ T cells, both in the thymus as in the periphery (Ramsdell 2003), but not or only weakly transcribed in naïve or recently activated CD25$^-$ T cells (Fontenot et al. 2003; Khattri et al. 2003; Ramsdell 2003) is an important marker. FoxP3-deficient mice develop massive autoimmune and inflammatory disease, whereas gene transfer of FoxP3 converts naïve CD4$^+$CD25$^-$ T cells into Treg cell (Fontenot et al. 2003; Khattri et al. 2003; Ramsdell 2003). However, as FoxP3 is found intracellular, it is not the best marker for functional studies.

Despite attempts to narrow the regulatory subset of cells, it was shown that $CD25^+$ cell-mediated in vitro regulation of a response to anti-CD3 was not altered much by further subdividing the cells into high and low expressers for CD62L, CD69, CD38, CD45RB (Thornton et al. 2000), or CD103 (McHugh et al. 2002). Nevertheless, in the SCID transfer model of colitis it was found that $CD4^+CD25^+$ T cells expressing $\alpha_E\beta_7$ had a higher regulatory capacity than the $\alpha_E\beta_7^-$ $CD4^+CD25^+$ T cell subset using a low regulator/target ratio, identified by a lower incidence of colitis, and lower clinical and histological colitis score in mice reconstituted with $CD4^+$ $CD45RB^{high}$ T cells and the $\alpha_E\beta_7^+$ $CD4^+CD25^+$ subset (Lehmann et al. 2002). The integrin $\alpha_E\beta_7$ is mainly expressed on intraepithelial lymphocytes residing in the gut wall and other epithelial compartments, such as skin and lung (Cerf-Bensussan et al. 1987), which suggest that $\alpha_E\beta_7$ may contribute to the regulatory function in the colitis model, e.g., by trafficking to inflamed tissues in the gut and acting directly at sites of inflammation. It should be mentioned that only $CD25^+$ $\alpha_E\beta_7^-$ cells are included among the natural Treg cells found in the thymus, whereas $CD25^+$ $\alpha_E\beta_7^+$ T cells may represent adaptive regulators which can be induced in the presence of, for example, TGF-β (Huehn et al. 2004). Thus, lately it has become clear that functionally distinct subsets of $CD4^+CD25^+$ Tregs with different phenotypes exist. It has been hypothesized by Blustone and Abbas (Bluestone et al. 2003) that there exist two subsets of $CD4^+$ Treg cells, natural and adaptive, that differ in terms of origin, specificity and mechanism of action. According to their model, natural self-antigen specific Treg develop during the normal process of T cell maturation in the thymus. In contrast, adaptive Tregs develop either from activation of natural $CD4^+CD25^+$ Treg cells or from naïve Th cells. Thus even the $CD4^+CD25^+$ Treg cells display a heterogeneous compartment of Treg cells.

7
Mechanisms of $CD4^+CD25^+$ Treg Cell-Mediated Immunosuppressive Functions

7.1
Cytokine Requirements for the Control of Colitis by $CD4^+CD25^+$ Treg

The mechanism by which regulatory T cells exert their function is currently a controversial issue. It has been demonstrated that that both TGF-β and IL-10 play important roles in regulatory T cell-induced protection of T cell-induced colitis (Asseman et al. 1999, 2003; Powrie et al. 1994; Read et al. 2000). Elevated levels of IL-10 and TGF-β mRNA were found in the $CD4^+CD25^+$ T cell subset ex vivo (Asano et al. 1996) as well as direct secretion of these cytokines by the CD4$^+$CD25$^+$ T cells when stimulated in an appropriate fashion (Nakamura et al. 2001). We know that IL-10 plays an important function in the intestinal homeostasis, revealed by the fact that IL-10-deficient mice (Rennick et al. 2000) or wild type mice treated with anti-IL-10R (Asseman et al. 2003) develop chronic inflammation in the intestine and IL-10 in general plays a role as a negative regulator of the immune response. In addition, administration of exogenous IL-10 inhibits the development of colitis in SCID mice reconstituted with CD4$^+$CD45RB^{high} T cells (Powrie et al. 1994) as well as in other models of IBD (Leach et al. 1999). Consistent with these studies, CD4$^+$CD45RB^{high} T cells isolated from transgenic mice, which expressed IL-10 under control of the IL-2 promoter, failed to induce colitis in SCID mice and were able to inhibit the disease when transferred with CD45RB^{high} CD4$^+$ T cells from normal mice. The importance of TGF-β in immune homeostasis is indicated by the fact that that TGF-β-deficient mice die within 3–5 weeks after birth due to a spontaneous autoimmune-like syndrome (Shull et al. 1992).

By adding antibodies that either block TGF-β (Powrie et al. 1996; Read et al. 2000) or the IL-10 receptor (IL-10R) (Asseman et al. 1999) to recipients of both pathogenic CD4$^+$CD45RB^{high} T cells and regulatory CD4$^+$CD45RB^{low} T cells, the protection against IBD is completely abrogated, suggesting that these cytokines are involved in the mechanisms of immune suppression. In addition, administration of anti-TGF-β to mice co-transferred with CD45RB^{high} and CD45RB^{low}CD25$^+$ T cells led to abrogation of suppression and induction of colitis in the recipients (Read et al. 2000). Very recently, it was stated that the CD4$^+$CD25$^+$ T cells produce the TGF-β1 themselves, as CD4$^+$CD25$^+$ T cells from TGF-β1$^{-/-}$ did not protect Rag-2$^{-/-}$ recipients of CD45RB^{high} T cells from developing colitis (Nakamura et al. 2004). Moreover, CD4$^+$CD45RB^{low} T cells isolated from IL10$^{-/-}$ mice failed to inhibit colitis when co-transferred with CD4$^+$CD45RB^{high} T cells (Asseman et al. 1999). However, the requirement for IL-10 in the suppression of IBD induced by transfer of naïve CD45RB^{high} T cells has until recently only been examined by using CD45RB^{low} cells as a source of Treg cells (Asseman et al. 1999). In light of these observations, stating the existence of colitis-inducing T cells within the CD45RB^{low} pool treated with anti- IL-10R Ab (Annacker et al. 2001; Asseman et al. 2003), it was suddenly very important to determine whether the regulation of naïve T cells by regulatory CD4$^+$CD25$^+$ T cells also requires IL-10. In a recent report, it was found that the CD4$^+$CD25$^+$ T cells isolated from IL-10$^{-/-}$ mice are still able to inhibit colitis induced by wild-type naïve CD4$^+$CD45RB^{high} T cells in the SCID model, which importantly states that CD4$^+$CD25$^+$ T cells themselves, in this system, do not have to produce IL-10 (Asseman et al. 2003). However, this is in conflict with an earlier report, using the RAG-2$^{-/-}$ model system of colitis, which states the opposite (Annacker et al. 2001). These discrepancies may simply be due to the use of immune-deficient recipients of different genetic backgrounds or different environmental conditions in the laboratories. In addition, the co-transfer of $CD4^+CD25^+$ T cells suppressed the development of colitis in SCID recipients by $CD4^+CD45RB^{high}$ cells, even in the presence of antiI-IL-10R, although a small but significant increase in the development of colitis was seen compared with control mice, indicating the control of colitis is partly dependent on IL-10 (Asseman et al. 2003).

In contrast to this, it was found that IL-10 is very necessary for the control of colitis induced by antigen-experienced cells (Asseman et al. 2003). Transfer of $CD4^+CD25^+$ T cells prevents the development of colitis induced by IL-$10^{-/-}$ $CD45RB^{low}CD25^-$ T cells and anti-IL-10R treatment induces colitis in recipients of unseparated $CD45RB^{low}$ cells. Although it was found that the control of antigen-experienced colitogenic T cells was highly dependent on IL-10, it was not investigated whether IL-10 secretion in this case was required by the $CD4^+CD25^+$ T cells themselves. Hence, the role of IL-10 in vivo seems very complex, as there are different requirements for IL-10 in the regulation of naïve and antigen experienced T cells, and the IL-10 requirements depend on the genetic lesion of the recipients, i.e., SCID vs $RAG^{-/-}$. In contrast, the role of TGF-β seems simpler. Thus in summery, TGF-β is sufficient to prevent colitis induced by naïve cells (Nakamura et al. 2004; Read et al. 2000), whereas IL-10 is required to control previously activated Th1 cells (Asseman et al. 2003). In support of this, TGF-β1 was shown to inhibit resting $CD4^+T$ cells in contrast to activated T cells, although addition of IL-10 restored TGF-β responsiveness on activated T cells (Cottrez et al. 2001), suggesting that IL-10 plays a role in potentiating the effects of TGF-β on differentiated effector T cells. Hence, both IL-10 and TGF-β seem to be involved in the function of regulatory T cells. In contrast, recombinant IL-4 had no positive effect on the health of mice injected with $CD45RB^{high}$ $CD4^+$ T cells (Powrie et al. 1994) and $IL-4^{-/-}CD45RB^{low}$ $CD4^+$ T cells were as efficient in protecting the recipient as their wild-type counterpart (Powrie et al. 1996).

It has been suggested that $CD4^+CD25^+$ Treg cells in addition to their direct inhibitory effect in vivo function indirectly by inducing the differentiation of naïve T cells into cytokine secreting Treg cells, a phenomenon termed infectious tolerance (Jonuleit et al. 2002). According to this view, the first step is a contact-dependent localized inhibitory effect, whereas the induced secondary Treg cells mediate a cell contact-independent widespread suppressive effect via cytokine secretion. This spreading of suppression from naturally occurring $CD4^+CD25^+$ cells to induced Treg cells may be a fundamental mechanism for the induction and maintenance of peripheral tolerance. Thus, the protective effect of IL-10 in some cases might depend on the ability

Table 2 Suppression of colitis by Treg cells in the SCID transfer model and the requirements of cytokines

Transfer of CD4+ T cells +cytokine addition	CD45RBlow	CD45RBlow IL-4-/-	CD45RBlow IL-10-/-	+Transfer of CD4+ Treg cells CD25+	CD25+ IL-10-/-	CD25+ TGF-β1-/-	Tr1+OVA	DC/CD4+ Treg
CD45RBhigh	No IBD	No IBD	IBD	No IBD	No IBD/IBD	IBD	No IBD	
CD45RBhigh + anti-IL-10R	IBD			No IBD/IBD			IBD	
CD45RBhigh + anti-TGF-β	IBD			IBD				
IL-10-/- CD45RBlow CD25-				No IBD				
CD25-								No IBD

The co-transfer of CD45RBlow T cells, CD25+ T cells, DC/CD4+ co-culture-induced Treg cells or Tr1 cells prevents induction of disease. However, the need for cytokines for control of colitis varies. See text for references.

of CD4$^+$CD25$^+$ Treg cells to induce other subsets of IL-10-producing Treg cells.

Table 2 shows an overview of the Treg cells used for suppression of colitis in the SCID transfer model and their requirements for cytokines to mediate suppression.

7.2
Cellular Requirements for the Regulation of Colitis by CD4$^+$CD25$^+$ Treg

It is well known that suppression mediated by the regulatory CD4$^+$CD25$^+$ T cells in vitro requires cell–cell interaction between the responder and regulatory populations and is independent of cytokines (Dieckmann et al. 2001; Jonuleit et al. 2001; Levings et al. 2001; Stephens et al. 2001; Takahashi et al. 2000; Thornton et al. 1998). A number of ligands and receptors have been suggested to be partially responsible for this inhibitory function and many of these are co-stimulatory molecules. It is widely accepted that T cell activation involves signals transduced by the TCR complex after recognition of antigen as well as from costimulatory molecules after encounter with their ligands present on APCs (Bretscher 1999). It is known that CD4$^+$CD25$^+$ T cells are present but in reduced numbers in both CD28$^{-/-}$ and B7$^{-/-}$ mice, suggesting that CD28-mediated co-stimulatory signals are involved in the homeostatic levels of this population in vivo (Salomon et al. 2000). In contrast to CD28, ligation of cytotoxic T-lymphocyte antigen (CTLA)-4 on the surface of activated T cells, by its ligands CD80/CD86 expressed on APCs, delivers a negative signal leading to inhibition of T cell activation (Chambers et al. 2001). Besides being expressed on activated T cells, an elevated CTLA-4 expression was found on regulatory T cells (Read et al. 2000; Takahashi et al. 2000), which suggests that the molecule might be functionally important. It has been suggested that Tregs expressing high levels of CTLA-4 may interact with APCs via B7 ligation and induce expression of the tryptophan-degrading enzyme indoleamine 2,3-dioxygenase (IDO). Expression of IDO by CD11c$^+$CD8α^+ DCs in mice and CD123$^+$DCs in humans allows these DCs to suppress T cell proliferation in vitro and suppress autoimmune disorders in vivo (Mellor et al. 2003), although its role in suppression of colitis has not been investigated yet. However, there is some disagreement about the importance of CTLA-4 for the inhibitory function of regulatory T cells. Takahashi et al. (2000) have shown that the addition of anti-CTLA-4 antibody or its Fab fragment reverse suppression in co-cultures of CD4$^+$CD25$^+$ T cells and CD4$^+$CD25$^-$ T cells. Similarly, Read et al. (2000) have shown that the treatment of recipients of co-transferred CD4$^+$CD45RB^{high} and CD4$^+$ CD45RB^{low}CD25$^+$ T cells with anti-CTLA-4 abrogated the suppression of colitis. Nevertheless, these studies have been difficult to reproduce by other groups, including our own group, which found that suppression in vitro is not abrogated by blockade of CTLA-4 (Gad et al. 2004; Jonuleit et al. 2001; Levings et al. 2001; McHugh et al. 2002; Thornton et al. 1998). As CTLA-4 is also expressed on activated $CD4^+CD25^-$ T cells, it has been suggested that the effect of anti-CTLA-4 Ab in vitro is the result of binding to the effector $CD4^+CD25^-$ T cells since anti-CTLA4 Ab may inhibit the normal down-regulatory effects of CTLA-4 on T cell activation and raise the threshold that is required for $CD4^+CD25^+$ T cells to mediate suppression (Shevach 2002).

The importance of another costimulatory molecule Ox40 (CD134) has also been investigated for its function on regulatory T cells. The Ox40 molecule is expressed transiently on activated $CD4^+$ T cells, whereas its ligand Ox40L (CD134L) has been reported to be present on dendritic cells after activation (Annacker et al. 2002; Ohshima et al. 1997). Administration of antibody against Ox40L has been shown to prevent T cell accumulation in the intestine of $CD4^+CD45RB^{high}$ T cell restored SCID mice and abrogate the development of colitis (Malmstrom et al. 2001), suggesting that that the Ox40 molecule may also play a role in the regulation of immune reactivity by regulatory T cells. However, although 30% of resting $CD4^+CD25^+$ T cells express Ox40, administration of antibody against Ox40 could not abrogate the ability of the $CD4^+CD25^+$ T to exert suppression in response to anti-CD3 in an in vitro system (McHugh et al. 2002). As mentioned above, a novel cell surface marker, glucocorticoid-induced TNF-receptor (GITR) has been identified on resting $CD4^+CD25^+$ T cells in the thymus and in the periphery (McHugh et al. 2002; Shimizu et al. 2002). GITR ligated with agonistic antibodies on $CD4^+CD25^+$ Treg cells results in loss of suppressive activity (Shimizu et al. 2002). It has been shown that $CD4^+GITR^+$ T cells regardless of their CD25 expression can prevent colitis development. Additionally, administration of anti-GITR mAb abrogates colitis suppression in mice restored with both $CD45RB^{high}$ and $CD45RB^{low}$ $CD4^+$ T cells (Uraushihara et al. 2003). Finally, it has been shown by Nakamura et al. that stimulated $CD4^+CD25^+$ T cells express high and persistent levels of TGF-β1 on the cell surface and that suppression mediated by these regulatory cells is abolished in the presence of anti-TGF-β Ab (Nakamura et al. 2001) or rLAP (Nakamura et al. 2004). This observation, together with the fact that the suppression in vitro requires cell–cell contact suggests that membrane-bound TGF-β1 could be involved in cell-mediated immune suppression. However, we and others have not been able to reverse suppression mediated by $CD4^+CD25^+$ T cells in vitro by administration of a soluble TGF-βRII-Fc complex or by mAb (Gad et al. 2004; Piccirillo et al. 2002; Read et al. 1998; Takahashi et al. 1998). The discrepancy may be due to the fact that $CD4^+CD25^+$ T cells only produce easily detectable amounts of TGF-β when maximally stimulated. Besides, Nakamura et al. (2001) found that only very high concentrations of anti-TGF-β mAb (50–100 µg/ml) can abrogate the suppression in vitro.

8
Other Subsets of Regulatory T Cells Involved in the Control of Colitis

Many studies suggest that SCID mice with colitis lack Treg cells. In addition to the naturally occurring regulatory $CD4^+CD25^+$ T cells, a number of different regulatory T cell populations, capable of inhibiting the response of other T cells, have been described (Cottrez et al. 2000; Gad et al. 2003; Neurath et al. 1996). Treg cells can be induced in vivo following oral exposure to antigen (Th3 cells) and in vitro after culture with antigen and IL-10 (Tr1 cells) or following co-culture of gut-derived $CD4^+$ T cells and immature DCs (Gad et al. 2003). All three subsets have been shown to prevent the development of colitis (Groux et al. 1997; Neurath et al. 1996; M. Gad et al. submitted).

The Tr1 cells are different from the classical Th1 and Th2 cells (Groux et al. 1997). They proliferate poorly, secrete neither IL-2 nor IL-4, but produce high levels of IL-10. They inhibit antigen-specific immune responses in vitro through the secretion of IL-10 and TGF-β. Besides mediating suppressing immune responses in vitro, Tr1 cells were shown to be immune suppressive in vivo. In the SCID transfer model of IBD co-transfer of OVA specific Tr1 cells and pathogenic $CD4^+CD45RB^{high}$ cells prevented the induction of Th1-mediated inflammation. The in vivo function of the Tr1 cells was antigen-dependent, as only mice receiving OVA were protected from disease (Groux et al. 1997). Therefore, it was suggested that these Tr1 cells can suppress immune responses to unknown antigens by an antigen-driven bystander suppression mechanism. Similar to the observations in in vitro experiments, it was observed that the Tr1-mediated suppression was completely abrogated when mice were treated with anti-IL-10R, confirming the importance of IL-10 for the function of Tr1 cells and as a general immunomodulator of immune responses (Foussat et al. 2003).

We have investigated the capacity of isolated $CD4^+$ T cells from the colonic LP of normal mice to suppress the extensive proliferation of enterobacteria-exposed Th1 cells from SCID mice with colitis (Gad et al. 2003). We found that freshly purified LP or MLN $CD4^+$ T cells do not inhibit proliferation, whereas LP or MLN $CD4^+$ T cells co-cultured with immature DCs for 2–6 days exert strong inhibitory activity. The majority of these DC-induced Treg cells display a nonactivated phenotype, and the suppression per se is enteroantigen-independent and mediated partly by soluble factors different from IL-10 and TGF-β. The CD4$^+$ T cells from the DC co-culture are a mixture of CD25$^+$ (10%–20%) and CD25$^-$ (80%–90%) T cells. However, in a recent report (M. Gad et al. submitted) it was revealed that all the suppressor activity both in vitro and in vivo resides in the CD25$^+$ T cell subset. The data show that the DC-induced CD25$^+$ Treg cells, in contrast to the prototype of CD25$^+$ Treg cells, display an immature phenotype and can function independently of cell activation and direct cellular contact. In addition, the DC-induced Treg cells mediate a stronger suppressive activity than the prototype CD25$^+$ regulatory T cells. Both unfractionated and CD25$^+$ DC-induced Treg cells were found to protect the recipients of CD4$^+$CD25$^-$ T cells in the SCID transfer model of colitis against development of colitis.

The Th3 cell is yet another type of regulatory T cell capable of inhibiting colitis induced by intraluminal exposure to TNBS (Neurath et al. 1996). Th3 cells induced during oral tolerance secrete TGFβ. However, the suppressive effect of Th3 cells is antigen nonspecific and is mediated as bystander suppression through secretion of TGF-β. It is known that Th2 conditions favor the induction of Th3 cells, whereas Th1 conditions inhibit this induction. Nevertheless, the exact cytokine milieu necessary for the induction of Th3 cells is not well understood.

9
Where Do the Treg Cells Localize and What Do They Target?

Although research has focused on the function or Treg cells in recent years, the exact mechanism by which CD4$^+$CD25$^+$ regulatory T cells exert their suppressive effects remain unknown. The anatomical locations in which the Treg cells act and how these cells migrate in vivo are important issues that have hardly been studied to date. Although it has been revealed that cell–cell contact but also suppressive cytokines are required for suppression, it is not known at which point in the inflammatory cascade that Treg cells work or whether they target the responder cells, the APCs or both. Neither, is it well defined whether the Treg cells inhibit the function of already activated effector cells.

It has been revealed that colitis is accompanied by an increase in the number of activated dendritic cells (DCs) in the mesenteric lymph nodes (MLN) (Malmstrom et al. 2001). As mentioned above, these DCs were found to express the costimulatory ligand CD134L and administration of anti-CD134L mAb inhibited the proliferation of T cells in the MLN and blocked the development of colitis (Malmstrom et al. 2001). Surprisingly, CD134L was found to be expressed by a proportion of DCs in the MLNs of unreconstituted SCID mice.

These activated DCs were present in a reduced number in SCID mice compared with mice restored with CD4$^+$CD45RB^{high} T cells but it was suggested that they may provide the initial costimulatory signals that drive the CD45RB^{high} cells into colitogenic Th1 cells. Importantly, mice protected from colitis by cotransfer of regulatory CD4$^+$CD25$^+$ T cells did not show an increase in activated CD134L$^+$ DCs in MLN, suggesting that modulation of DC function is one mechanism by which Treg cells may mediate their immune suppressive function. Whether the regulatory T cells inhibit the migration of DCs, their activation or life span still needs to be defined.

Suppression of colitis by Treg cells in vivo is characterized by a significant reduction in the number of activated Th1 cells that accumulate in the intestine (Annacker et al. 2001; Asseman et al. 1999; Mottet et al. 2003), which may be due to reduced expansion or migration of these cells. Recently, the influence of CD4$^+$CD25$^+$ T cells on local colitogenic T cell proliferation was examined using the CD4$^+$CD45RB^{high} T cell transfer model of colitis (Mottet et al. 2003). In colitic SCID mice, CD4$^+$CD45RB^{high} T cell proliferate vigorously in both MLN and LP 4 weeks after T cell transfer. It was found that CD4$^+$CD25$^+$ T cells transferred therapeutically at this time point proliferate vigorously in the MLN and in particular in the inflamed colonic LP a few weeks after transfer. However, the resolution of the inflammatory response, 10 weeks after the transfer of CD4$^+$CD25$^+$ T cells, correlates with a reduced number of proliferating pathogenic cells as well as of Treg cells. These results suggest that Treg cells control T cell effector responses not only in the lymph nodes but also in the inflamed tissue. Further, apparently the vigorous proliferation of Treg cells does not lead to loss of suppression as assessed by the resolution of inflammation (Mottet et al. 2003). Other studies agree with this assumption, as CD4$^+$CD25$^+$ T cells after expansion in vivo were found to be more potent suppressors in vitro (Gavin et al. 2002; Klein et al. 2003). Additionally, we have recently shown that in fully protected SCID mice co-injected with CD25$^-$ T cells and CD25$^+$ T cells, effector cells and Treg cells exist side by side. This was indicated by the fact that CD4$^+$ T cells recovered from both SCID mice with colitis and mice transplanted with CD25$^-$ T cells and Treg cells proliferate vigorously in response to enteroantigen ex vivo in contrast to unfractionated CD4$^+$ cells from normal BALB/c mice. Thus Treg cells cause neither effector cell depletion nor anergy. Finally, the regulatory CD4$^+$CD25$^+$ T cells were found to be in close contact with CD11c$^+$ DCs as well as pathogenic T cells in the colon and LP (Mottet et al. 2003). This location of Treg cells suggests that there is a direct physical contact between Tregs and CD11c$^+$ DCs, supporting a role for DC-Treg cell interaction.

The mechanisms for protection of colitis by Tr1 cells were also investigated (Foussat et al. 2003). CD4$^+$CD45RB^{high} T cell-reconstituted SCID mice

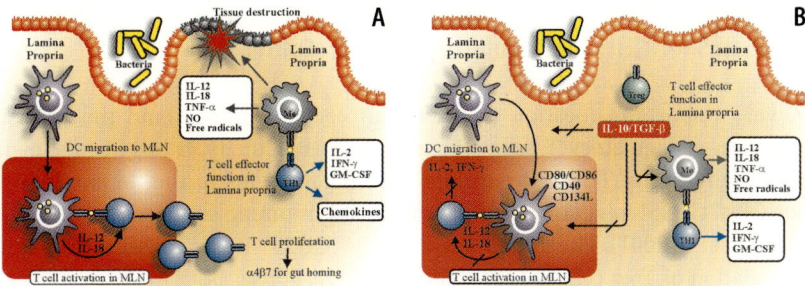

Fig. 1 A Development of intestinal inflammation. DCs sample antigens from bacterial flora, become activated and migrate to MLN. In the MLN, naïve T cells are activated in the presence of IL-12 and differentiate to Th1 cells expressing the gut-homing molecule $\alpha_4\beta_7$. The Th1 cells proliferate and enter LP, leading to recruitment of more inflammatory cells. **B** Inhibition of intestinal inflammation by regulatory T cells. It is suggested that Tregs may mediate their function at several sites. They may inhibit the migration of DCs to MLN. They may inhibit DC and T cell activation as well as T cell proliferation in the MLN by inhibiting co-stimulatory molecule expression. Finally, they may inhibit the T cell effector function in the LP by interfering with the homing capacity of activated T cells, or they may prevent the release of pro-inflammatory cytokines by macrophages, thereby inhibiting the progression of the inflammatory response. The inhibitory function of the Treg cells may be mediated either by direct cell–cell contact or by immune suppressive cytokines or both. One may hypothesize that $CD4^+CD25^+$ by infectious tolerance, via cell–cell contact, stimulates the differentiation of naïve T cell to become regulatory T cells (Tr1 or Tr3), which enhance and sustain the suppression by secretion of IL-10 and TGF-β. (Modified from Singh et al. 2001b)

co-transferred with Tr1 cells were treated with anti-IL-10R several weeks after cell transfer. The treatment completely reversed the protection of colitis up to 3 weeks after injection of Tr1 cells, which indicates that the protection of colitis is not due to a complete inhibition of the differentiation of the pro-inflammatory T cells in the colon. Indeed, some signs of inflammation were observed in the first weeks after co-transfer of pro-inflammatory $CD4^+CD45RB^{high}$ T cells and regulatory $CD4^+CD45RB^{low}$ T cells (Foussat et al. 2003), supporting the notion that Treg cells actively control inflammation.

Figure 1 shows a model for the development of intestinal inflammation and how Treg cells may regulate it at several sites.

10
Antigen Specificity for Regulatory T Cells in Colitis

A very important question to answer in order to understand the precise function of regulatory T cells is their antigen specificity. It has been shown that high-affinity TCR/self peptide–MHC interactions in the thymus select for $CD4^+CD25^+$ regulatory T cells displaying immune suppressive function (Jordan et al. 2001). The thymic derived $CD4^+CD25^+$ T cells constitute a major population of Treg cells able to inhibit T cell responses both in vitro (Read et al. 1998; Thornton et al. 1998) and in vivo (Read et al. 2000; Suri-Payer et al. 1998). The number of $CD4^+CD25^+$ T cells that are selected in the thymus has been shown to be proportional with the diversity of self-peptides presented in the context of MHC class II molecules on the thymic epithelium (Pacholczyk et al. 2002), suggesting that the Treg cells recognize self-antigens. As it was shown that the $CD4^+CD25^+$ T cells are a polyclonal population (Takahashi et al. 1998), it has been suggested that the Treg cells may react with a broad range of antigens.

We have demonstrated that $CD4^+CD25^+$ T cells derived from germfree mice have the ability to suppress the in vitro proliferation of $CD4^+CD25^-$ T cells stimulated with enteric bacteria (Gad et al. 2004). Consistent with our own results, $CD4^+CD45RB^{low}$ cells isolated from germfree mice can inhibit colitis (Annacker et al. 2000). We also found that the suppressive mechanism of Treg cells induced by DC/$CD4^+$ T cell co-culture is independent of exposure to the enteroantigen that stimulate the effector cells to proliferate in the absence of Treg cells (Gad et al. 2003). Thus apparently Treg cells in these model systems are not antigen experienced and in addition their specificity might not necessarily be the same as the effector cells. To date, there has been no evidence for a limited antigen repertoire of Treg cells, but most data point to the fact that $CD4^+CD25^+$ T cells require activation through their TCR in order to be suppressive, although once activated their suppressor function is completely nonspecific and does not require re-engagement of their TCR (Thornton et al. 1998, 2000). However, Treg cells might also function in an antigen specific way. Kullberg et al. (2002) used a modification of the SCID transfer model and found that Treg cells from *H. hepaticus*-infected but not from uninfected donor mice block colitis induced by *H. hepaticus*-specific effector T cells (Kullberg et al. 2002), suggesting antigen dependency. The antigen-specific protection was shown to be dependent on IL-10 both in vivo and in vitro (Kullberg et al. 2002) and the Treg cells thus resemble the IL-10 producing Ag-induced Tr1 cells more than the naturally occurring $CD25^+$ Treg cells.

11
Regulatory T Cells as a Therapeutic Agent for Inflammatory Bowel Disease

As described above, regulatory $CD4^+CD45RB^{low}$ T cells enriched within the $CD25^+$ subset as well as Tr1 cells and Treg cells from $DC/CD4^+$ T cell co-culture have been shown to prevent the development of colitis induced by transfer of $CD4^+CD45RB^{high}$ or $CD4^+CD25^-$ T cells to SCID mice (Foussat et al. 2003; Groux et al. 1997; Powrie et al. 1990, 1993; M. Gad et al. submitted). Recently, different groups have tried to cure already established colitis with regulatory T cells in the SCID transfer model (Foussat et al. 2003; Liu et al. 2003; Mottet et al. 2003). In a study by Mottet et al. (2003), immunodeficient SCID mice with clinical signs of colitis four weeks after transfer of $CD4^+CD45RB^{high}$ T cells were treated with $CD4^+CD25^+$ T cells. Histological changes, corresponding to an average colitis score of 3, confirmed the incidence of colitis at the time of treatment. In contrast to mice treated with $CD25^-$ T cell or control mice without a secondary transfer, the $CD4^+CD25^+$ T cells reduced the $CD4^+$ density in the colonic mucosa. Moreover, the transfer of the regulatory $CD4^+CD25^+$ T cells improved the clinical status, survival rate and intestinal pathology of mice with established colitis. Ten weeks after $CD4^+CD25^+$ T cell transfer, the recipient mice had almost completely recovered from colitis (Mottet et al. 2003). A second report investigated the therapeutic role of regulatory T cells in a model of colitis established by transfer of $CD4^+CD25^-$ T cells to SCID mice followed by infection of the protozoan parasite *Leishmania major* (Liu et al. 2003). Ten or 20 days after transfer of the pathogenic cells, mice were treated with freshly isolated, TGF-β-cultured or activated $CD4^+CD25^+$ T cells. In all cases, the colitis symptoms were reversed, and there were no differences in the pathology score among the mice treated with the different preparations of $CD4^+CD25^+$ T cells, indicating that it is possible to cure an established colitis. In addition, it was shown that the curative effect of the $CD4^+CD25^+$ T cell given day 21 was abolished by injecting the mice with anti-IL-10R, anti-TGF-β or anti-CTLA-4 Ab (Liu et al. 2003). These results demonstrate that the therapeutic effect of $CD4^+CD25^+$ T cell in this model is dependent on TGF-β, CTLA-4, which are in agreement with earlier prophylactic studies (Fuss et al. 2002; Read et al. 2000), and IL-10 (Annacker et al. 2001; Asseman et al. 2003). An explanation for the dependency of IL-10 in this model might be found in the authors' use of $CD4^+CD25^+$ donor T cells from both spleen and lymph nodes as $CD25^+$ T cells from MLN in the presence of anti-IL-10R may be colitogenic, as described by Asseman al. (2003). Finally, a recent study showed that Tr1 cells can also cure an ongoing colitis in the SCID transfer model even 6 weeks after transfer of the pathogenic $CD4^+CD45RB^{high}$ T cells

(Foussat et al. 2003). Treatment with Tr1 cells resulted in a very rapid remission of inflammation and mice were completely cured for colitis 3 weeks after treatment. Injection of mice with anti-IL-10R Ab abrogated the protective effect of the Tr1 cells. In contrast, Foussat et al. (2003) did not find any curative function of $CD4^+CD25^+$ T cells on colitis by looking at the colitis score 4–6 weeks after injection of the Treg cells. However, in the study by Mottet et al. (2003), the histological colonic abnormalities were not resolved before 10 weeks after $CD4^+CD25^+$ T cell transfer. Thus, $CD4^+CD25^+$ T cells seem to induce a slower remission of colitis as compared with Tr1 cells, a suggestion which supports the hypothesis of an indirect mechanism in the control of inflammation mediated by $CD4^+CD25^+$ T cells.

Taken together, the data show that adoptive transfer of regulatory T cell activity has the potential to reverse established inflammation leading to cure of colitis. However, the cured animals have not yet been observed over an extended time period and it is still unclear whether these mice can tolerate normal conventional environments including a higher risk for developing chronic infections and neoplastic diseases—issues that are of major importance for the practical use of adoptive regulatory T cell therapy in IBD.

12
Conclusion

The animal models of colitis have contributed to our understanding of the etiology, pathogenesis, immune pathology and the course of disease. Although the nature of antigens recognized by immune cells in IBD is still unknown, the triggering factors are most certainly of bacterial origin. Colitis in most experimental systems appears to be a result of a hyper-reactive Th1-mediated immune response due to lack of regulatory T cells. It is clear that Treg cells can inhibit colitis and even reverse established inflammation, leading to cure of disease. Treg cells perform multiple functions in the immune system, which altogether contribute to maintaining immune homeostasis. Recent observations open up the opportunity to use Treg cells in cellular therapy of patients with IBD. Results showing that regulatory $CD4^+CD25^+$ T cells maintain their ability to suppress after proliferation are important in the light of clinical use where induced expansion of autologous $CD4^+CD25^+$ T cells ex vivo or in vivo might be necessary. A better understanding of the physiology and pathology of regulatory T cells and the connection between its various subtypes will hopefully improve future therapies of the inflammatory diseases.

Acknowledgements Dr. Mogens H. Claesson is acknowledged for helpful discussions and critical reading of the manuscript. This work was supported by the Colitis Crohn Association, Physician SCE Friis and Wife's Fund, NovoNordic Fund, Kong Christian den tiendes Fund, Gerda and Aage Haensch's fund, Else and Mogens Wedellsborgs Fund and by The Danish Medical Research Agency.

References

Annacker O, Powrie F (2002) Homeostasis of intestinal immune regulation. Microbes Infect 4:567–574

Annacker O, Burlen-Defranoux O, Pimenta-Araujo R, Cumano A, Bandeira A (2000) Regulatory CD4 T cells control the size of the peripheral activated/memory CD4 T cell compartment. J Immunol 164:3573–3580

Annacker O, Pimenta-Araujo R, Burlen-Defranoux O, Barbosa TC, Cumano A, Bandeira A (2001) CD25+ CD4+ T cells regulate the expansion of peripheral CD4 T cells through the production of IL-10. J Immunol 166:3008–3018

Apostolou I, Sarukhan A, Klein L, von Boehmer H (2002) Origin of regulatory T cells with known specificity for antigen. Nat Immunol 3:756–763

Aranda R, Sydora BC, McAllister PL, Binder SW, Yang HY, Targan SR, Kronenberg M (1997) Analysis of intestinal lymphocytes in mouse colitis mediated by transfer of CD4+, CD45RBhigh T cells to SCID recipients. J Immunol 158:3464–3473

Asano M, Toda M, Sakaguchi N, Sakaguchi S (1996) Autoimmune disease as a consequence of developmental abnormality of a T cell subpopulation. J Exp Med 184:387–396

Asseman C, Mauze S, Leach MW, Coffman RL, Powrie F (1999) An essential role for interleukin 10 in the function of regulatory T cells that inhibit intestinal inflammation. J Exp Med 190:995–1004

Asseman C, Read S, Powrie F (2003) Colitogenic Th1 cells are present in the antigen-experienced T cell pool in normal mice: control by CD4+ regulatory T cells and IL-10. J Immunol 171:971–978

Bilsborough J, Viney JL (2002) Getting to the guts of immune regulation. Immunology 106:139–143

Bluestone JA, Abbas AK (2003) Natural versus adaptive regulatory T cells. Nat Rev Immunol 3:253–257

Borruel N, Carol M, Casellas F, Antolin M, de Lara F, Espin E, Naval J, Guarner F, Malagelada JR (2002) Increased mucosal tumour necrosis factor alpha production in Crohn's disease can be downregulated ex vivo by probiotic bacteria. Gut 51:659–664

Borruel N, Casellas F, Antolin M, Llopis M, Carol M, Espiin E, Naval J, Guarner F, Malagelada JR (2003) Effects of nonpathogenic bacteria on cytokine secretion by human intestinal mucosa. Am J Gastroenterol 98:865–870

Bregenholt S, Claesson MH (1998) Increased intracellular Th1 cytokines in SCID mice with inflammatory bowel disease. Eur J Immunol 28:379–389

Bregenholt S, Reimann J, Claesson MH (1998) Proliferation and apoptosis of lamina propria CD4+ T cells from SCID mice with inflammatory bowel disease. Eur J Immunol 28:3655–3663

Bretscher PA (1999) A two-step, two-signal model for the primary activation of precursor helper T cells. Proc Natl Acad Sci U S A 96:185–190

Brimnes J, Reimann J, Nissen M, Claesson M (2001) Enteric bacterial antigens activate CD4(+) T cells from SCID mice with inflammatory bowel disease. Eur J Immunol 31:23–31

Cahill RJ, Foltz CJ, Fox JG, Dangler CA, Powrie F, Schauer DB (1997) Inflammatory bowel disease: an immunity-mediated condition triggered by bacterial infection with Helicobacter hepaticus. Infect Immun 65:3126–3131

Campieri M, Gionchetti P (2001) Bacteria as the cause of ulcerative colitis. Gut 48:132–135

Cerf-Bensussan N, Jarry A, Brousse N, Lisowska-Grospierre B, Guy-Grand D, Griscelli C (1987) A monoclonal antibody (HML-1) defining a novel membrane molecule present on human intestinal lymphocytes. Eur J Immunol 17:1279–1285

Chambers CA, Kuhns MS, Egen JG, Allison JP (2001) CTLA-4-mediated inhibition in regulation of T cell responses: mechanisms and manipulation in tumor immunotherapy. Annu Rev Immunol 19:565–594

Chutkan RK (2001) Inflammatory bowel disease. Prim Care 28:539–56, vi

Claesson MH, Rudolphi A, Kofoed S, Poulsen SS, Reimann J (1996) CD4+ T lymphocytes injected into severe combined immunodeficient (SCID) mice lead to an inflammatory and lethal bowel disease. Clin Exp Immunol 104:491–500

Claesson MH, Bregenholt S, Bonhagen K, Thoma S, Moller P, Grusby MJ, Leithauser F, Nissen MH, Reimann J (1999) Colitis-inducing potency of CD4+ T cells in immunodeficient, adoptive hosts depends on their state of activation, IL-12 responsiveness, and CD45RB surface phenotype. J Immunol 162:3702–3710

Cottrez F, Groux H (2001) Regulation of TGF-beta response during T cell activation is modulated by IL-10. J Immunol 167:773–778

Cottrez F, Hurst SD, Coffman RL, Groux H (2000) T regulatory cells 1 inhibit a Th2-specific response in vivo. J Immunol 165:4848–4853

Darfeuille-Michaud A, Neut C, Barnich N, Lederman E, Di Martino P, Desreumaux P, Gambiez L, Joly B, Cortot A, Colombel JF (1998) Presence of adherent Escherichia coli strains in ileal mucosa of patients with Crohn's disease. Gastroenterology 115:1405–1413

Dieckmann D, Plottner H, Berchtold S, Berger T, Schuler G (2001) Ex vivo isolation and characterization of CD4(+)CD25(+) T cells with regulatory properties from human blood. J Exp Med 193:1303–1310

Duchmann R, May E, Heike M, Knolle P, Neurath M, Meyer zum Buschenfelde KH (1999) T cell specificity and cross reactivity towards enterobacteria, bacteroides, bifidobacterium, and antigens from resident intestinal flora in humans. Gut 44:812–818

Ehrhardt RO, Ludviksson BR, Gray B, Neurath M, Strober W (1997) Induction and prevention of colonic inflammation in IL-2-deficient mice. J Immunol 158:566–573

Fabia R, Ar'Rajab A, Johansson ML, Andersson R, Willen R, Jeppsson B, Molin G, Bengmark S (1993) Impairment of bacterial flora in human ulcerative colitis and experimental colitis in the rat. Digestion 54:248–255

Farrell RJ, Banerjee S, Peppercorn MA (2001) Recent advances in inflammatory bowel disease. Crit Rev Clin Lab Sci 38:33–108

Fisson S, Darrasse-Jeze G, Litvinova E, Septier F, Klatzmann D, Liblau R, Salomon BL (2003) Continuous activation of autoreactive CD4+ CD25+ regulatory T cells in the steady state. J Exp Med 198:737–746

Foltz CJ, Fox JG, Cahill R, Murphy JC, Yan L, Shames B, Schauer DB (1998) Spontaneous inflammatory bowel disease in multiple mutant mouse lines: association with colonization by Helicobacter hepaticus. Helicobacter 3:69–78

Fontenot JD, Gavin MA, Rudensky AY (2003) Foxp3 programs the development and function of CD4+CD25+ regulatory T cells. Nat Immunol 4:330–336

Foussat A, Cottrez F, Brun V, Fournier N, Breittmayer JP, Groux H (2003) A comparative study between T regulatory Type 1 and CD4+CD25+ T cells in the control of inflammation. J Immunol 171:5018–5026

Fuss IJ, Boirivant M, Lacy B, Strober W (2002) The interrelated roles of TGF-beta and IL-10 in the regulation of experimental colitis. J Immunol 168:900–908

Gad M, Brimnes J, Claesson MH (2003) CD4+ T regulatory cells from the colonic lamina propria of normal mice inhibit proliferation of enterobacteria-reactive, disease-inducing Th1-cells from SCID mice with colitis. Clin Exp Immunol 131:34–40

Gad M, Pedersen AE, Kristensen NN, Claesson MH (2004) Demonstration of strong enterobacterial reactivity of $CD4^+$ $CD25^-$ cells from conventional and germfree mice which is counter regulated by $CD4^+CD25^+$ T cells. Eur J Immunol 34:695–704

Gavin MA, Clarke SR, Negrou E, Gallegos A, Rudensky A (2002) Homeostasis and anergy of CD4(+)CD25(+) suppressor T cells in vivo. Nat Immunol 3:33–41

Gionchetti P, Rizzello F, Venturi A, Brigidi P, Matteuzzi D, Bazzocchi G, Poggioli G, Miglioli M, Campieri M (2000) Oral bacteriotherapy as maintenance treatment in patients with chronic pouchitis: a double-blind, placebo-controlled trial. Gastroenterology 119:305–309

Groux H, O'Garra A, Bigler M, Rouleau M, Antonenko S, de Vries JE, Roncarolo MG (1997) A CD4+ T-cell subset inhibits antigen-specific T-cell responses and prevents colitis. Nature 389:737–742

Hoffmann JC, Pawlowski NN, Kuhl AA, Hohne W, Zeitz M (2002) Animal models of inflammatory bowel disease: an overview. Pathobiology 70:121–130

Huehn J, Siegmund K, Lehmann JC, Siewert C, Haubold U, Feuerer M, Debes GF, Lauber J, Frey O, Przybylski GK, Niesner U, de la RM, Schmidt CA, Brauer R, Buer J, Scheffold A, Hamann A (2004) Developmental stage, phenotype, and migration distinguish naive- and effector/memory-like CD4+ regulatory T cells. J Exp Med 199:303–313

Jonuleit H, Schmitt E, Stassen M, Tuettenberg A, Knop J, Enk AH (2001) Identification and functional characterization of human CD4(+)CD25(+) T cells with regulatory properties isolated from peripheral blood. J Exp Med 193:1285–1294

Jonuleit H, Schmitt E, Kakirman H, Stassen M, Knop J, Enk AH (2002) Infectious tolerance: human CD25(+) regulatory T cells convey suppressor activity to conventional CD4(+) T helper cells. J Exp Med 196:255–260

Jordan MS, Boesteanu A, Reed AJ, Petrone AL, Holenbeck AE, Lerman MA, Naji A, Caton AJ (2001) Thymic selection of CD4+CD25+ regulatory T cells induced by an agonist self-peptide. Nat Immunol 2:301–306

Khattri R, Cox T, Yasayko SA, Ramsdell F (2003) An essential role for Scurfin in CD4+CD25+ T regulatory cells. Nat Immunol 4:337–342

Klein L, Khazaie K, von Boehmer H (2003) In vivo dynamics of antigen-specific regulatory T cells not predicted from behavior in vitro. Proc Natl Acad Sci U S A 100:8886–8891

Kullberg MC, Jankovic D, Gorelick PL, Caspar P, Letterio JJ, Cheever AW, Sher A (2002) Bacteria-triggered CD4(+) T regulatory cells suppress Helicobacter hepaticus-induced colitis. J Exp Med 196:505–515

Leach MW, Bean AG, Mauze S, Coffman RL, Powrie F (1996) Inflammatory bowel disease in C.B-17 SCID mice reconstituted with the CD45RBhigh subset of CD4+ T cells. Am J Pathol 148:1503–1515

Leach MW, Davidson NJ, Fort MM, Powrie F, Rennick DM (1999) The role of IL-10 in inflammatory bowel disease: "of mice and men". Toxicol Pathol 27:123–133

Lehmann J, Huehn J, de la Rosa M, Maszyna F, Kretschmer U, Krenn V, Brunner M, Scheffold A, Hamann A (2002) Expression of the integrin alpha Ebeta 7 identifies unique subsets of CD25+ as well as C25⁻ regulatory T cells. Proc Natl Acad Sci U S A 99:13031–13036

Levings MK, Sangregorio R, Roncarolo MG (2001) Human cd25(+)cd4(+) t regulatory cells suppress naive and memory T cell proliferation and can be expanded in vitro without loss of function. J Exp Med 193:1295–1302

Li X, Fox JG, Whary MT, Yan L, Shames B, Zhao Z (1998) SCID/NCr mice naturally infected with Helicobacter hepaticus develop progressive hepatitis, proliferative typhlitis, and colitis. Infect Immun 66:5477–5484

Liu H, Hu B, Xu D, Liew FY (2003) CD4+CD25+ regulatory T cells cure murine colitis: the role of IL-10, TGF-beta, and CTLA4. J Immunol 171:5012–5017

Madsen KL, Doyle JS, Jewell LD, Tavernini MM, Fedorak RN (1999) Lactobacillus species prevents colitis in interleukin 10 gene-deficient mice. Gastroenterology 116:1107–1114

Madsen KL, Doyle JS, Tavernini MM, Jewell LD, Rennie RP, Fedorak RN (2000) Antibiotic therapy attenuates colitis in interleukin 10 gene-deficient mice. Gastroenterology 118:1094–1105

Malmstrom V, Shipton D, Singh B, Al Shamkhani A, Puklavec MJ, Barclay AN, Powrie F (2001) CD134L expression on dendritic cells in the mesenteric lymph nodes drives colitis in T cell-restored SCID mice. J Immunol 166:6972–6981

Maloy KJ, Salaun L, Cahill R, Dougan G, Saunders NJ, Powrie F (2003) CD4+CD25+ T(R) cells suppress innate immune pathology through cytokine-dependent mechanisms. J Exp Med 197:111–119

McHugh RS, Whitters MJ, Piccirillo CA, Young DA, Shevach EM, Collins M, Byrne MC (2002) CD4(+)CD25(+) immunoregulatory T cells: gene expression analysis reveals a functional role for the glucocorticoid-induced TNF receptor. Immunity 16:311–323

Mellor AL, Munn DH (2003) Tryptophan catabolism and regulation of adaptive immunity. J Immunol 170:5809–5813

Mizoguchi A, Mizoguchi E, Chiba C, Bhan AK (1996) Role of appendix in the development of inflammatory bowel disease in TCR-alpha mutant mice. J Exp Med 184:707–715

Mombaerts P, Mizoguchi E, Grusby MJ, Glimcher LH, Bhan AK, Tonegawa S (1993) Spontaneous development of inflammatory bowel disease in T cell receptor mutant mice. Cell 75:274–282

Morrissey PJ, Charrier K, Braddy S, Liggitt D, Watson JD (1993) CD4+ T cells that express high levels of CD45RB induce wasting disease when transferred into congenic severe combined immunodeficient mice. Disease development is prevented by cotransfer of purified CD4+ T cells. J Exp Med 178:237–244

Mottet C, Uhlig HH, Powrie F (2003) Cutting edge: cure of colitis by CD4+CD25+ regulatory T cells. J Immunol 170:3939–3943

Nakamura K, Kitani A, Strober W (2001) Cell contact-dependent immunosuppression by CD4(+)CD25(+) regulatory T cells is mediated by cell surface-bound transforming growth factor beta. J Exp Med 194:629–644

Nakamura K, Kitani A, Fuss I, Pedersen A, Harada N, Nawata H, Strober W (2004) TGF-beta 1 plays an important role in the mechanism of CD4+CD25+ regulatory T cell activity in both humans and mice. J Immunol 172:834–842

Neurath MF, Fuss I, Kelsall BL, Presky DH, Waegell W, Strober W (1996) Experimental granulomatous colitis in mice is abrogated by induction of TGF-beta-mediated oral tolerance. J Exp Med 183:2605–2616

Ohshima Y, Tanaka Y, Tozawa H, Takahashi Y, Maliszewski C, Delespesse G (1997) Expression and function of OX40 ligand on human dendritic cells. J Immunol 159:3838–3848

Pacholczyk R, Kraj P, Ignatowicz L (2002) Peptide specificity of thymic selection of CD4+CD25+ T cells. J Immunol 168:613–620

Piccirillo CA, Letterio JJ, Thornton AM, McHugh RS, Mamura M, Mizuhara H, Shevach EM (2002) CD4(+)CD25(+) regulatory T cells can mediate suppressor function in the absence of transforming growth factor beta1 production and responsiveness. J Exp Med 196:237–246

Podolsky DK (2002) Inflammatory bowel disease. N Engl J Med 347:417–429

Powrie F, Mason D (1990) OX-22high CD4+ T cells induce wasting disease with multiple organ pathology: prevention by the OX-22low subset. J Exp Med 172:1701–1708

Powrie F, Leach MW, Mauze S, Caddle LB, Coffman RL (1993) Phenotypically distinct subsets of CD4+ T cells induce or protect from chronic intestinal inflammation in C. B-17 SCID mice. Int Immunol 5:1461–1471

Powrie F, Leach MW, Mauze S, Menon S, Caddle LB, Coffman RL (1994) Inhibition of Th1 responses prevents inflammatory bowel disease in SCID mice reconstituted with CD45RBhi CD4+ T cells. Immunity 1:553–562

Powrie F, Carlino J, Leach MW, Mauze S, Coffman RL (1996) A critical role for transforming growth factor-beta but not interleukin 4 in the suppression of T helper type 1-mediated colitis by CD45RB(low) CD4+ T cells. J Exp Med 183:2669–2674

Ramsdell F (2003) Foxp3 and natural regulatory T cells: key to a cell lineage? Immunity 19:165–168

Rath HC, Herfarth HH, Ikeda JS, Grenther WB, Hamm TE Jr, Balish E, Taurog JD, Hammer RE, Wilson KH, Sartor RB (1996) Normal luminal bacteria, especially Bacteroides species, mediate chronic colitis, gastritis, and arthritis in HLA-B27/human beta2 microglobulin transgenic rats. J Clin Invest 98:945–953

Read S, Mauze S, Asseman C, Bean A, Coffman R, Powrie F (1998) CD38+ CD45RB(low) CD4+ T cells: a population of T cells with immune regulatory activities in vitro. Eur J Immunol 28:3435–3447

Read S, Malmstrom V, Powrie F (2000) Cytotoxic T lymphocyte-associated antigen 4 plays an essential role in the function of CD25(+)CD4(+) regulatory cells that control intestinal inflammation. J Exp Med 192:295–302

Reimann J, Rudolphi A, Tscherning T, Claesson MH (1993) Selective engraftment of memory CD4+ T cells with an unusual recirculation pattern and a diverse T cell receptor-V beta repertoire into SCID mice. Eur J Immunol 23:350–356

Reimann J, Rudolphi A, Spiess S, Claesson MH (1995) A gut-homing, oligoclonal CD4+ T cell population in severe-combined immunodeficient mice expressing a rearranged, transgenic class I-restricted alpha beta T cell receptor. Eur J Immunol 25:1643–1653

Rembacken BJ, Snelling AM, Hawkey PM, Chalmers DM, Axon AT (1999) Non-pathogenic Escherichia coli versus mesalazine for the treatment of ulcerative colitis: a randomised trial. Lancet 354:635–639

Rennick DM, Fort MM (2000) Lessons from genetically engineered animal models. XII. IL-10-deficient (IL-10(-/-) mice and intestinal inflammation. Am J Physiol Gastrointest Liver Physiol 278:G829–G833

Rudolph U, Finegold MJ, Rich SS, Harriman GR, Srinivasan Y, Brabet P, Boulay G, Bradley A, Birnbaumer L (1995) Ulcerative colitis and adenocarcinoma of the colon in G alpha i2-deficient mice. Nat Genet 10:143–150

Rudolphi A, Boll G, Poulsen SS, Claesson MH, Reimann J (1994) Gut-homing CD4+ T cell receptor alpha beta+ T cells in the pathogenesis of murine inflammatory bowel disease. Eur J Immunol 24:2803–2812

Sakaguchi S, Sakaguchi N, Asano M, Itoh M, Toda M (1995) Immunologic self-tolerance maintained by activated T cells expressing IL-2 receptor alpha-chains (CD25). Breakdown of a single mechanism of self-tolerance causes various autoimmune diseases. J Immunol 155:1151–1164

Salomon B, Lenschow DJ, Rhee L, Ashourian N, Singh B, Sharpe A, Bluestone JA (2000) B7/CD28 costimulation is essential for the homeostasis of the CD4+CD25+ immunoregulatory T cells that control autoimmune diabetes. Immunity 12:431–440

Sanderson JD, Moss MT, Tizard ML, Hermon-Taylor J (1992) Mycobacterium paratuberculosis DNA in Crohn's disease tissue. Gut 33:890–896

Sartor RB (1997) The influence of normal microbial flora on the development of chronic mucosal inflammation. Res Immunol 148:567–576

Sartor RB, Rath H, Sellon R (1996) Microbial factors in chronic intestinal inflammation. Curr Opin Gastroenterol 12:327–333

Schultz M, Tonkonogy SL, Sellon RK, Veltkamp C, Godfrey VL, Kwon J, Grenther WB, Balish E, Horak I, Sartor RB (1999) IL-2-deficient mice raised under germfree conditions develop delayed mild focal intestinal inflammation. Am J Physiol 276:G1461–G1472

Sellon RK, Tonkonogy S, Schultz M, Dieleman LA, Grenther W, Balish E, Rennick DM, Sartor RB (1998) Resident enteric bacteria are necessary for development of spontaneous colitis and immune system activation in interleukin-10-deficient mice. Infect Immun 66:5224–5231

Shevach EM (2000) Regulatory T cells in autoimmmunity. Annu Rev Immunol 18:423–449

Shevach EM (2002) CD4+ CD25+ suppressor T cells: more questions than answers. Nat Rev Immunol 2:389–400

Shimizu J, Yamazaki S, Sakaguchi S (1999) Induction of tumor immunity by removing CD25+CD4+ T cells: a common basis between tumor immunity and autoimmunity. J Immunol 163:5211–5218

Shimizu J, Yamazaki S, Takahashi T, Ishida Y, Sakaguchi S (2002) Stimulation of CD25(+)CD4(+) regulatory T cells through GITR breaks immunological self-tolerance. Nat Immunol 3:135–142

Shull MM, Ormsby I, Kier AB, Pawlowski S, Diebold RJ, Yin M, Allen R, Sidman C, Proetzel G, Calvin D et al (1992) Targeted disruption of the mouse transforming growth factor-beta 1 gene results in multifocal inflammatory disease. Nature 359:693–699

Singh B, Powrie F, Mortensen NJ (2001a) Immune therapy in inflammatory bowel disease and models of colitis. Br J Surg 88:1558–1569

Singh B, Read S, Asseman C, Malmstrom V, Mottet C, Stephens LA, Stepankova R, Tlaskalova H, Powrie F (2001b) Control of intestinal inflammation by regulatory T cells. Immunol Rev 182:190–200

Spencer SD, Di Marco F, Hooley J, Pitts-Meek S, Bauer M, Ryan AM, Sordat B, Gibbs VC, Aguet M (1998) The orphan receptor CRF2-4 is an essential subunit of the interleukin 10 receptor. J Exp Med 187:571–578

Stephens LA, Mottet C, Mason D, Powrie F (2001) Human CD4(+)CD25(+) thymocytes and peripheral T cells have immune suppressive activity in vitro. Eur J Immunol 31:1247–1254

Strober W, Fuss IJ, Blumberg RS (2002) The immunology of mucosal models of inflammation. Annu Rev Immunol 20:495–549

Suri-Payer E, Amar AZ, Thornton AM, Shevach EM (1998) CD4+CD25+ T cells inhibit both the induction and effector function of autoreactive T cells and represent a unique lineage of immunoregulatory cells. J Immunol 160:1212–1218

Takahashi T, Kuniyasu Y, Toda M, Sakaguchi N, Itoh M, Iwata M, Shimizu J, Sakaguchi S (1998) Immunologic self-tolerance maintained by CD25+CD4+ naturally anergic and suppressive T cells: induction of autoimmune disease by breaking their anergic/suppressive state. Int Immunol 10:1969–1980

Takahashi T, Tagami T, Yamazaki S, Uede T, Shimizu J, Sakaguchi N, Mak TW, Sakaguchi S (2000) Immunologic self-tolerance maintained by CD25(+)CD4(+) regulatory T cells constitutively expressing cytotoxic T lymphocyte-associated antigen 4. J Exp Med 192:303–310

Taurog JD, Richardson JA, Croft JT, Simmons WA, Zhou M, Fernandez-Sueiro JL, Balish E, Hammer RE (1994) The germfree state prevents development of gut and joint inflammatory disease in HLA-B27 transgenic rats. J Exp Med 180:2359–2364

Taylor PA, Noelle RJ, Blazar BR (2001) CD4(+)CD25(+) immune regulatory cells are required for induction of tolerance to alloantigen via costimulatory blockade. J Exp Med 193:1311–1318

Thornton AM, Shevach EM (1998) CD4+CD25+ immunoregulatory T cells suppress polyclonal T cell activation in vitro by inhibiting interleukin 2 production. J Exp Med 188:287–296

Thornton AM, Shevach EM (2000) Suppressor effector function of CD4+CD25+ immunoregulatory T cells is antigen nonspecific. J Immunol 164:183–190

Thornton AM, Piccirillo CA, Shevach EM (2004) Activation requirements for the induction of CD4+CD25+ T cell suppressor function. Eur J Immunol 34:366–376

Uraushihara K, Kanai T, Ko K, Totsuka T, Makita S, Iiyama R, Nakamura T, Watanabe M (2003) Regulation of murine inflammatory bowel disease by CD25+ and CD25- CD4+ glucocorticoid-induced TNF receptor family-related gene+ regulatory T cells. J Immunol 171:708–716

Von Herrath MG, Harrison LC (2003) Antigen-induced regulatory T cells in autoimmunity. Nat Rev Immunol 3:223–232

Walker LS, Chodos A, Eggena M, Dooms H, Abbas AK (2003) Antigen-dependent proliferation of CD4+ CD25+ regulatory T cells in vivo. J Exp Med 198:249–258

Ward JM, Anver MR, Haines DC, Melhorn JM, Gorelick P, Yan L, Fox JG (1996) Inflammatory large bowel disease in immunodeficient mice naturally infected with Helicobacter hepaticus. Lab Anim Sci 46:15–20

Wittig BM, Zeitz M (2003) The gut as an organ of immunology. Int J Colorectal Dis 18:181–187

Yamazaki S, Iyoda T, Tarbell K, Olson K, Velinzon K, Inaba K, Steinman RM (2003) Direct expansion of functional CD25+ CD4+ regulatory T cells by antigen-processing dendritic cells. J Exp Med 198:235–247

Autoimmune Ovarian Disease in Day 3-Thymectomized Mice: The Neonatal Time Window, Antigen Specificity of Disease Suppression, and Genetic Control

K. S. K. Tung[1] (✉) · Y. Y. Setiady[1] · E. T. Samy[2] · J. Lewis[3] · C. Teuscher[4]

[1]Department of Pathology, Health Science Center, University of Virginia, P.O. Box 800214, Charlottesville, VA 22908, USA
kst7k@virginia.edu

[2]Department of Microbiology, University of Virginia, Charlottesville, VA 22908, USA

[3]Department of Medicine, University of Virginia, Charlottesville, VA 22908, USA

[4]Departments of Medicine and Pathology, University of Vermont, Burlington, VT 05405, USA

1	Introduction	211
2	Mechanism of Autoimmune Disease Induction in the Neonatal Mice	213
2.1	Deficiency of $CD4^+CD25^+$ Regulatory T Cells and d3tx Diseases	213
2.2	Induction of Neonatal Autoimmune Ovarian Disease and Tolerance to the Ovarian Zona Pellucida 3 autoAg and Other Self-Ags	215
2.2.1	Autoimmune Ovarian Disease Induction by Immunization with a ZP3 Peptide in Complete Freund's Adjuvant	215
2.2.2	Neonatal Exposure to Physiological Ovary-Derived Ag Induces Tolerance, and Neonatal Immunization with Self-peptide Results in Autoimmune Disease	215
2.2.3	An Environmental Factor Can Preferentially Co-stimulate Autoimmune Response and Disease in Neonatal Mice	216
2.2.4	Neonatal Immunization Induces Autoimmune Disease Besides Autoimmune Ovarian Disease	218
2.3	The Mechanism of Neonatal Autoimmune Ovarian Disease Induced by Maternal AutoAb to ZP3	219
2.3.1	Neonatal Autoimmune Ovarian Disease	219
2.3.2	Neonatal Autoimmune Ovarian Disease in the Euthymic Mice Is Mediated by De Novo Pathogenic T Cell Response	220
2.3.3	Why Are the Older Mice Resistant to nAOD?	220
2.3.4	Why Are Neonatal Mice (days 1–5) Susceptible to Neonatal Autoimmune Ovarian Disease?	222
2.3.5	Requirement of Neonatal NK Cells, Fcγ Receptor III (FcγRIII) Positive Cells and Proinflammatory Cytokines in Neonatal Autoimmune Ovarian Disease Induction	222

3	Endogenous Ag Specificity and Ag Requirement for Disease Suppression by CD4$^+$CD25$^+$ T Cells	224
3.1	The Location and Ag Dependency of Suppression	224
3.2	Suppression of Autoimmune Disease by Regulatory Cells from Donors with or Without the Relevant Self-Ag	225
4	Genetic Control of Susceptibility to D3tx-Induced Autoimmune Disease	227
4.1	Genetic Studies on Inbred Strains of Mice	227
4.2	Mapping Loci Controlling Susceptibility to D3Tx-Induced Autoimmune Disease	227
4.3	Positional-Candidate Genes for AOD and AIG QTL That Are Differentially Expressed by CD4$^+$CD25$^+$ Regulatory T Cells	231
4.3.1	Pdcd1 as a Candidate for Aod3	233
4.3.2	The Tumor Necrosis Factor Receptor Superfamily Genes	233
4.3.3	Tgfb1	234
4.3.4	H2	234
4.3.5	Il2	235
4.3.6	Positional-Candidate Genes for AOD and AIG QTL	236
4.3.7	The Autoantigen in d3tx-Induced Autoimmune Ovarian Disease	236

References 237

Abstract Discovery of the CD4$^+$CD25$^+$ T cells has stemmed from investigation of the AOD in the d3tx mice. Besides CD4$^+$CD25$^+$ T cell depletion, d3tx disease induction requires effector T cell activation prompted by lymphopenia. This is supported by other neonatal AOD models in which T cell-mediated injury has been found to be triggered by immune complex or Ag immunization. In addition, there is growing evidence that support a state of neonatal propensity to autoimmunity, which depends on concomitant endogenous antigenic stimulation, concomitant nematode infection, resistance to CD4$^+$CD25$^+$ T cell regulation, and participation of the neonatal innate system. The suppression of d3tx disease by polyclonal CD4$^+$CD25$^+$ T cells appears to be dependent on endogenous Ag and the persistence of regulatory T cells. Thus, suppression of AOD occurs in the ovarian LN, and AOD emerges upon ablation of the input regulatory T cells; and in AIP, the hormone-induced expression of prostate Ag in the CD4$^+$CD25$^+$ T cell donors rapidly enhances the capacity to suppress disease over Ag negative donors. Finally, genetic analysis of AOD and its component phenotypes has uncovered seven *Aod* loci. As the general themes that emerged, significant epistatic interactions among the loci play a role in controlling disease susceptibility, the majority of the *Aod* loci are linked to susceptibility loci of other autoimmune diseases, and the genetic intervals encompass candidate genes that are differentially expressed between CD4$^+$CD25$^+$ T cells and other T cells. The candidate genes include *Pdcd1*, TNFR superfamily genes, *H2*, *Il2*, *Tgfb*, *Nalp5* or *Mater*, an oocyte autoAg that reacts with autoantibody in sera of d3tx mice.

Abbreviations

Ab	Antibody
Ag	Antigen
AIG	Autoimmune gastritis
AOA	Antiovarian autoantibody
AOD	Autoimmune ovarian disease
AIP	Autoimmune prostatitis
APC	Antigen-presenting cell
AGM1	Asialo GM1
B6AF1	(C57BL/6xA/J)F1 mice
BC1	Backcross population
BTL	Binary trait loci
CFA	Complete Freund's adjuvant
CIM	Composite interval mapping
CP	Chimeric peptide
d3Tx	Thymectomy on day 3 of life
DC	Dendritic cell
FcγR	Fc γ receptor
IFA	Incomplete Freund's adjuvant
IFNγ	Interferon γ
LN	Lymph node
MHC	Major histocompatibility complex
nAOD	Neonatal AOD
NK	Natural killer
NOD	Nonobese diabetic
pZP3	Murine ZP3 peptide (330–342)
RIL	Recombinant inbred line
QTL	Quantitative trait loci
TCR	T cell receptor
TGFβ	Transforming growth factor β
TNFα	Tumor necrosis factor α
ZP	Zona pellucida

1
Introduction

To investigate T cell immunity in chemically induced murine mammary carcinoma, Nishizuka and Sakakura depleted T cells by neonatal thymectomy and were surprised to find that the mice did not develop mammary tumors (Y. Nishizuka, personal communication 1980). The finding was reported in 1969 as induction of ovarian dysgenesis in mice thymectomized on day 3 (d3tx) but not on days 0 or 7 after birth (Nishizuka and Sakakura 1969). Mammary tumors did not occur because of failure in mammary gland development due to ovarian failure. Although the ovarian abnormality was initially inter-

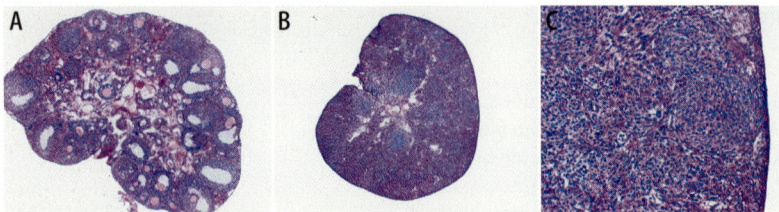

Fig. 1A–C The pathology of AOD of the d3tx mice. **A** Normal adult ovary with numerous ovarian follicles that contain growing and mature oocytes and is free of any inflammatory cells (this is also the appearance of ovaries from d3tx mice with disease suppression by half a million $CD4^+CD25^+$ T cells). **B** Ovarian atrophy in late stage of AOD, with disappearance of all oocytes and hypertrophy of interstitial gland cells. This appearance was initially called ovarian dysgenesis. Atrophy is preceded by oophoritis, or ovarian inflammation, shown in **C**. (H&E; **A** and **B**, ×50; **C**, ×200)

preted as evidence for hormonal interaction between the thymus and ovary, it was soon apparent that the ovarian change represented ovarian atrophy, the end stage of an autoimmune ovarian disease (AOD) (Fig. 1). Thus, the ovarian dysgenic changes were preceded by ovarian inflammation, the d3tx mice had autoantibody (autoAb) response to oocyte antigens (Ags) (Taguchi et al.1980; Alard et al. 2001), and AOD was adoptively transferable by spleen cells to young syngeneic recipients (Taguchi and Nishizuka 1980). Moreover, AOD was one of several autoimmune diseases attendant to d3tx in different mouse strains (Kojima and Prehn 1981). This phenomenon was subsequently confirmed by Penhale et al., who showed that adult thymectomy with fractional total body irradiation led to autoimmune disease of the thyroid and diabetes in the rats (Penhale et al. 1973 1990). Importantly, the diseases in d3tx mice and thymectomized rats were suppressed by transfer of normal adult $CD4^+$ spleen T cells (Penhale et al. 1976; Sakaguchi et al. 1982; Smith et al. 1991).

The d3tx model is a seminal milestone in autoimmunity research for at least three reasons:

1. It is a new paradigm of autoimmune disease pathogenesis—one due to perturbation of immunoregulation in normal individuals.
2. It defines suppression as an important mechanism of protection against spontaneous autoimmune disease.
3. The studies on d3tx mice, plus the data based on autoimmune disease in nu/nu mice that received $CD4^+CD5^{low}$ T cells (Sakaguchi et al. 1985; Smith et al. 1992), ultimately led to the discovery of the $CD4^+CD25^+$ T cells by Sakaguchi (1995) and Shevach (Suri-Payer et al. 1998).

For many years, the d3tx model and $CD4^+$ regulatory T cells were pursued by a handful of immunologists (Taguchi and Nishizuka 1987; Tung et al. 1987; Sakaguchi and Sakaguchi 1994; Gleeson et al. 1996; Suri-Payer et al. 1996), conducted independently of the highly-publicized but controversial $CD8^+$ suppressor T cell research initiated by Kondo and Gershon in 1970 (Gershon and Kondo 1970). The discovery of the $CD4^+CD25^+$ T cells has therefore stemmed directly from research on suppression of autoimmune diseases in the d3tx mice by normal $CD4^+$ T cells.

Since 1995, the $CD4^+CD25^+$ T cells have been defined as an important $CD4^+$ T cell functional subset, capable of regulating the innate and the adaptive immune responses, and have impact well beyond the context of autoimmunity. As described elsewhere in this monograph, many cellular, molecular, and functional properties of this regulatory T cell subset are being rapidly elucidated. In our laboratories, we have focused on the physiological function of $CD4^+CD25^+$ T cells in autoimmune disease prevention, as well as the mechanism and the genetic control of d3tx disease. We will discuss studies on the intriguing neonatal time window required for induction of AOD by d3tx and by other manipulations, summarize recent findings on the Ag specificity or Ag dependency of autoimmune disease prevention by $CD4^+CD25^+$ T cells in d3tx mice, and describe the genetic regulation of the d3tx disease.

2
Mechanism of Autoimmune Disease Induction in the Neonatal Mice

2.1
Deficiency of $CD4^+CD25^+$ Regulatory T Cells and d3tx Diseases

It has been proposed that autoimmune disease occurs in the d3tx mice because of depletion of the $CD4^+CD25^+$ T cells that have a late ontogeny (>day 5). However, the mechanism responsible for the d3tx disease is likely to be more complex because:

1. The evidence supporting this line of argument is not completely valid.
2. Disease induction is likely to depend on mechanisms besides $CD4^+CD25^+$ T cell depletion.
3. The neonatal mice have a propensity for autoimmunity for reasons besides $CD4^+CD25^+$ T cell deficiency.

It is argued that $CD4^+CD25^+$ T cell depletion is responsible for d3tx disease because autoimmune disease in the d3tx mice is suppressed by $CD4^+CD25^+$ T cells. Besides being a circular argument, it is possible that disease induction and disease suppression are phenomena that are not causally related.

For example, $CD4^+CD25^+$ T cells could inhibit disease by blocking innate inflammation rather than the Ag specific effector T cell response, as in the suppression of gastritis and colitis in *Helicobacter hepaticus*-infected mice devoid of T cells and B cells (Maloy et al. 2003). A similar argument of "two correct findings may not be related" can also be raised against the finding of $CD4^+CD25^+$ T cell suppression of disease in the athymic nu/nu mice induced by neonatal spleen T cells as evidence for neonatal deficiency of $CD4^+CD25^+$ T cells.

The $CD4^+CD25^-$ T cells are detected in the spleen of 3-day-old mice, whereas the $CD4^+CD25^+$ T cells emerge 2–3 days later, thus d3tx should enrich for effector T cells (Asano et al. 1996). This is true for the spleen; however, the lymph nodes (LNs) of normal day 3-day-old mice have the same fraction (~5%) of $CD4^+CD25^+$ cells as adult LNs (Suri-Payer et al. 1999). Neonatal LN $CD4^+CD25^+$ T cells suppress adult $CD4^+CD25^-$ T cells in vitro at a similar cell dose response as adult $CD4^+CD25^+$ T cells (Piccirillo et al. 2002; Samy and Tung, unpublished data); and recently, neonatal LN $CD4^+CD25^+$ T cells was found to suppress autoimmune disease in vivo (Samy and Tung, unpublished data). Although the $CD4^+CD25^+$ T cells transferred to adult mice are disseminated evenly in adult spleen and LNs, they preferentially home to the LNs in neonatal mice (A. Bayer and T. Malek, unpublished data). Thus differential homing of $CD4^+CD25^+$ T cells in neonatal mice may explain the different distribution of $CD4^+CD25^+$ T cells between the neonatal spleen and LNs. Because the initial T cell response in spontaneous organ specific autoimmune diseases occurs in regional LN, the cellular composition in the LN is most relevant in the regulation of the autoimmune response. Another argument in support of $CD4^+CD25^+$ T cell deficiency in d3tx mice is the finding that neonatal but not adult total spleen cells induce autoimmune disease when transferred to athymic nu/nu recipients (Smith et al. 1992; Asano et al. 1996). In retrospect, this might also be due to the selective $CD4^+CD25^+$ T cell deficiency in the spleen of neonatal cell donors.

On the other hand, autoimmune disease does not occur when the $CD4^+CD25^+$ T cells are depleted from normal mice unless accompanied by a second manipulation. For example, profound lymphopenia of d3tx mice allows expansion of pathogenic $CD4^+CD25^-$ T cells beyond the neonatal period (Min et al. 2003). Depletion of $CD25^+$ regulatory T cells from normal BALB/c adults did not cause autoimmune gastritis (AIG) unless they were injected with gastric autoAg H/K ATPase in incomplete Freund's adjuvant (IFA), which by itself is not pathogenic (for details, see the chapter by R.S. McHugh, this volume). Interestingly, $CD4^+$ T cells from the disease-free BALB/c mice with $CD4^+CD25^+$ T cell depletion were able to cause severe destructive AIG when transferred to lymphopenic nu/nu recipients (McHugh and Shevach 2002). In Sect. 2.3, we will show that immune complex created in neonatal mice also acts as a second stimulus. Together, these studies support the concept that autoimmune disease induction and prevention are determined by competition between the effector T cell response and the regulatory T cell response, and the balance of the two cell types determines the disease vs the non-disease state (Tung 1994).

Finally, as will be described below, other autoimmune disease models have documented a neonatal predisposition to autoimmune disease independent of $CD4^+CD25^+$ T cell deficiency. These findings will be summarized in Sect. 2.3, with emphasis on a new model of AOD that could only be induced in the neonate but not the adult and is caused by maternal Ab to an ovarian Ag.

2.2
Induction of Neonatal Autoimmune Ovarian Disease and Tolerance to the Ovarian Zona Pellucida 3 autoAg and Other Self-Ags

2.2.1
Autoimmune Ovarian Disease Induction by Immunization with a ZP3 Peptide in Complete Freund's Adjuvant

ZP3 is a major glycoprotein of the ZP that surrounds growing and mature oocytes, and is accessible to circulating Abs. The immunogen is the ZP3 (330–342) peptide (pZP3), which contains a well-defined pathogenic T cell autoepitope and a distinct B cell autoepitope that induces autoAb to native ZP3 (Lou and Tung 1993). The unique features of the AOD model include the opportunity to dissect autoimmune T cell and autoAb responses, the peptide being gender-specific, and the ability to manipulate the target organ (Tung et al. 1997). For example, the duration of expression of the physiological autoAg can be examined in mice with timed ovarian ablation, implanted ovarian grafts develop normally, remain viable and functional, and serve as an Ag source as well as a target for autoimmune effector cells in mice without ovaries.

2.2.2
Neonatal Exposure to Physiological Ovary-Derived Ag Induces Tolerance, and Neonatal Immunization with Self-peptide Results in Autoimmune Disease

Neonatal mice are traditionally considered as immunologically immature, prone to development of tolerance. This is true when the tolerogen is tissue-derived. In the study on AOD induced by pZP3, adult male mice mounted a stronger T cell response than adult female mice against the female-specific Ag, and male mice developed more frequent and severe AOD in ovarian grafts. However, the differences were eliminated by ablation of endogenous

Ag (Garza et al. 2000). In a "gain of function" experiment, when male mice were engrafted with neonatal ovaries as neonates, their response to pZP3 as adults was reduced to the level of female mice (Pramoonjago et al., unpublished data). In contrast, in studies involving neonatal injection of Ag (usually of foreign origin), the neonates develop a Th2-biased response rather than tolerance (Singh et al. 1996; Garza et al. 1997; Adkins 2000). On the other hand, we have found that neonatal response to the self-peptide frequently led to autoimmune response and autoimmune disease. Indeed, neonatal mice mounted autoimmune responses and elicited autoimmune memory in situations where adult mice would be resistant (Tung et al. 2001). Thus, the nature of neonatal immune response can vary greatly depending on the nature of the antigenic stimulus.

In AOD, injection of pZP3 in IFA in neonatal female mice elicited a pathogenic autoimmune response rather than tolerance (Garza et al. 1997). AOD and ZP autoAbs were evident by 5 weeks, and subsequent challenge with pZP3 led to memory response and severe AOD. In contrast, injection of pZP3 in IFA in neonatal male mice resulted in a nonpathogenic Th2 response without AOD. Interestingly, a similar Th2 response was found in female mice whose endogenous ovarian ZP3 Ag had been surgically removed on day 2 or day 5 of life. However, Th2 deviation did not occur when the ovarian Ag was depleted at day 7 or day 14. Therefore, the neonatal immune system perceives and responds to ovarian autoAg stimulation, and the neonatal Ag exposure supports the generation of a pathogenic rather than a nonpathogenic autoimmune response. In these studies, an ovarian graft was used to monitor AOD.

2.2.3
An Environmental Factor Can Preferentially Co-stimulate Autoimmune Response and Disease in Neonatal Mice

The neonatal but not adult response to self-Ags is also uniquely modified by the environmental pinworm infection (Agersborg et al. 2001). Without pinworm infection, neonatal injection of pZP3 in water did not elicit an immune response. However, when infected with the rodent pinworm *Syphacia obvelata*, neonatal mice injected with self-pZP3 in water developed strong ZP3-specific Th2 responses and severe eosinophilic AOD, followed by a strong pathogenic Th2 memory when challenged with pZP3 in CFA. In contrast, pinworm-infected adults mounted a pathogenic Th1 response when immunized with pZP3 in CFA. Therefore, pinworm infection dramatically promotes a strong autoimmune Th2 pathogenic response; however, the effect only impacts neonatal mice.

Pinworm infection also influences the neonatal response to a peptide of the lupus Ag, Ro60 (Fig. 2). Neonatal but not adult mice, infected with rodent pinworm, produced a strong and diversified autoAb response when injected with the human Ro60 (316–335) peptide. Although adult SJL mice immunized with the Ro60 peptide (316–335) in CFA produced Abs indicative of intramolecular and intermolecular spreading (Deshmukh et al. 1999), this was not observed in adult BALB/c mice (Fig. 2D). However, as shown in Fig. 2A–C, a single injection of the Ro60 (316–335) peptide in water, in pinworm-infected neonatal BALB/c mice, induced Ab against both human and murine Ro60. In addi-

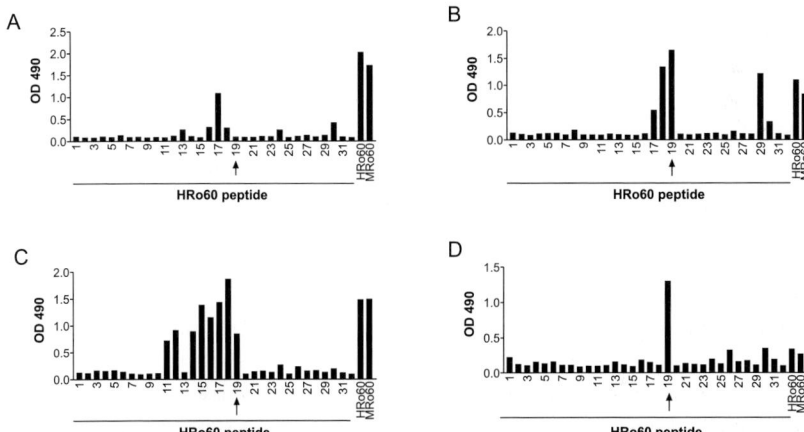

Fig. 2A–D The influence of pinworm infection on the murine antibody response to the human lupus autoantigen Ro60. Mice with pinworm infection were injected with human Ro60 peptide 316–335 (or peptide 19, *arrows*) in water. The human and murine Ro60 peptides 316–335 differ from each other by three amino acid residues. The overlapping Ro60 peptides were 20–25 amino acids long overlapped by five to ten amino acids and spanned the human Ro60. All samples used in the ELISA were diluted 1:100. **A** Reaction of serum antibody pooled from BALB/c mice 4 weeks after injection of Ro60 peptide 316–335 in water at age 2 days. The only antibody response is directed to Ro60 peptide 296–315 (peptide 17), distinct from the immunizing peptide. **B** shows the antibody response of another pinworm-infected BALB/c mouse to neonatal injection of Ro60 peptide in water, but was studied at 10 weeks. **C** The reaction of serum antibody pooled from four BALB/c mice 10 weeks following a single neonatal injection of the human Ro60 peptide 316–335 in water. **D** The response of BALB/c mice 4 weeks following a single Ro60 peptide 316–335 immunization in CFA administered in adulthood. Note that the antisera shown in **A**, **B**, and **C** also react with the recombinant Ro60 antigens; the ELISA reaction to the murine Ro60 protein was confirmed by immunoprecipitation using Ro60-associated mYRNAs derived from a radiolabeled murine cell line (data not shown)

tion, when the mice were studied at 4 weeks, they produced Ab to the Ro60 (296–315) peptide, an epitope distinct from the immunizing Ro60 (316–335) peptide (Fig. 2A). Over time, the Ab response was further diversified to additional Ro60 epitopes, indicative of intramolecular epitope spreading (Fig. 2B, 2C). The diversified Ab response occurred only in pinworm-infected neonatal mice, and this was not observed in pinworm-infected BALB/c adults and uninfected neonates (Fig. 2D). Both the pathogenic Th2 response to pZP3 and the diversified Ab response to the Ro60 peptide instantly stopped when pinworm infection was eliminated, and they resurfaced when mice were re-infected with pinworm.

These two studies document pinworm as a strong environmental factor that impacts exclusively on neonatal autoimmune response and autoimmune disease. Pinworm infection does not cause autoimmune disease per se but modulates or co-stimulates the neonatal response to self-peptide presented in a nonimmunogenic form. Moreover, in the setting of the nematode infection, pZP3 imprints a strong pathogenic Th2 memory response and stimulates a diversified B cell response. This study therefore supports the thesis of neonatal propensity to autoimmune responsiveness.

2.2.4
Neonatal Immunization Induces Autoimmune Disease Besides Autoimmune Ovarian Disease

AIG develops in neonatal rats that are injected with the gastric parietal cell H^+K^+ ATPase Ag in water (Claeys et al. 1997). Lupus autoAbs and nephritis develop in mice injected neonatally with a peptide that mimics double-stranded DNA in IFA (Singh et al. 1996). In double transgenic mice expressing influenza virus hemagglutinin and its cognate T cell receptor (TCR), a state of tolerance of the transgenic $CD8^+$ T cells is preceded by transient neonatal autoimmune response (Morgan et al. 1999). In addition, tolerance to the allogeneic lymphocytes is preceded by an early and transient graft-versus-host response to the donor MHC class II alloAg (Schurmans et al. 1991), and by a transient lupus-like disease that becomes fatal in mice with bcl-2 overexpressing B cells (Lopez-Hoyos et al. 1996).

The studies on murine AOD and other autoimmune models indicate that neonatal mice are more sensitive than adults to disease induction, and this is in turn influenced by factors including endogenous Ag expression, resistance to apoptosis, and environmental factors. We next describe the response of neonatal mice to ZP3 immune complex that results in a new intergenerational autoimmune disease known as neonatal AOD (nAOD). The nAOD model has permitted more precise dissection of the underlying mechanisms; because of this and the relevance of the model to autoimmunity of the d3tx mice, it will be described in more detail.

2.3
The Mechanism of Neonatal Autoimmune Ovarian Disease Induced by Maternal AutoAb to ZP3

2.3.1
Neonatal Autoimmune Ovarian Disease

To investigate autoAb without concomitant T cell response, we studied a chimeric peptide (CP) that contains the foreign T cell epitope of bovine ribonuclease (94–104) and the ZP3 (335–342) native B cell epitope. The peptide (CP2) elicited strong epitope-specific Abs that bound to the ovarian ZP in vivo. Despite this, the adult ovaries were free of pathology (Lou et al. 1995). The only observable effect in adult mice was the retargeting the location of ZP3-specific Th1 or Th2-mediated tissue destruction from the ovarian interstitium to the ovarian follicles (Lou et al. 2000).

Unexpectedly, over 80% of the progenies from the ZP3-positive dams developed severe nAOD at 2 weeks of age, and 40% of those with nAOD developed ovarian atrophy, premature ovarian failure and infertility (Setiady et al. 2003) (Fig. 3). Severe nAOD was induced by serum or purified serum IgG from adult female or male mice immunized with CP2 in CFA, or by transfer of a mouse monoclonal Ab to ZP3 (335–342). Therefore, autoAb to the ZP3 (335–342) B cell epitope is sufficient to trigger severe and frequent nAOD, a process independent of maternal lymphocytes or pregnancy-associated factors.

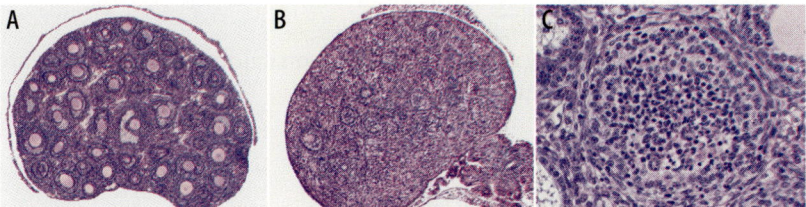

Fig. 3A–C The pathology of nAOD. **A** Normal ovary of a 2-week-old mouse, with numerous growing ovarian follicles. **B** Atrophic ovary in severe nAOD shows loss of all oocytes. **C** Ovarian inflammation has replaced the oocyte of an ovarian follicle in nAOD. (H&E; **A**, ×50; **B**, ×75; **C**, ×400)

2.3.2
Neonatal Autoimmune Ovarian Disease in the Euthymic Mice Is Mediated by De Novo Pathogenic T Cell Response

In nAOD, a 7-day interval existed between ovarian immune complex deposition and ovarian inflammation, and the inflammation was enriched in T cells and activated antigen-presenting cells (APCs) (Fig. 3, data not shown). Strikingly, when both CD4 and CD8 T cells of the neonates were depleted, the neonates did not develop nAOD. More importantly, $CD4^+$ T cells from mice with nAOD transferred severe nAOD to naive neonatal mice. Thus, maternal ZP3 autoAbs form immune complex with the endogenous Ag, and this can trigger de novo pathogenic T cell response to ovarian Ag in the neonatal mice (Setiady et al. 2003).

When neonates from untreated dams were fostered-fed milk from CP2-immunized dams, they developed high incidences and severity of nAOD when feeding commenced on day 3 or day 5 of life. However, pups fed CP2 Ab-positive milk from day 7 or day 9 did not develop nAOD. Thus frequent and severe nAOD develops only when neonatal mice are exposed to CP2 Ab within the first 5 days of life. This neonatal propensity is not due a differential rate of maternal Ab transfer in the neonatal period or to a propensity of neonatal ovaries to immune injury. When neonatal and adult ovaries were implanted under the kidney capsule of postpartum females with CP2 Ab, all the ovarian grafts contained immune complexes but they were free of AOD. In contrast, pups fostered-fed milk from the same dams developed severe nAOD. Therefore, neonatal ovaries are not uniquely prone to AOD; instead, the unique neonatal environment of days 1–5 predisposes to nAOD.

To further elucidate the unusual propensity of neonatal mice to autoimmune disease, we studied the mechanism of nAOD with respect to $CD4^+CD25^+$ T cell function and the state of innate immunity, by addressing three questions:

1. Why are older mice (>day 5) resistant to autoimmunity?
2. Why are mice more susceptible to autoimmunity during the first 5 days of life?
3. What are the cells and molecules of the neonatal innate system that are required for nAOD induction?

2.3.3
Why Are the Older Mice Resistant to nAOD?

To address whether the emergence of $CD4^+CD25^+$ regulatory T cell function could explain the resistance of the older mice to nAOD, we studied the effect of in vivo $CD25^+$ T cell depletion. Indeed, when neonatal mice were treated with CD25 Ab and fed CP2 Ab-positive milk from postnatal day 9, 90% of them developed severe nAOD (Fig. 4A). In contrast, day 9 mice that received CD25 Ab alone were free of nAOD. Therefore, the presence of $CD4^+CD25^+$ regulatory T cell function can explain the resistance to nAOD in mice older than 7 days. As mentioned earlier (Sect. 2.1), depletion of $CD25^+$ regulatory T cells in normal mice at this age does not elicit autoimmune disease unless it is accompanied by a second event which, in this case, is autologous immune complex.

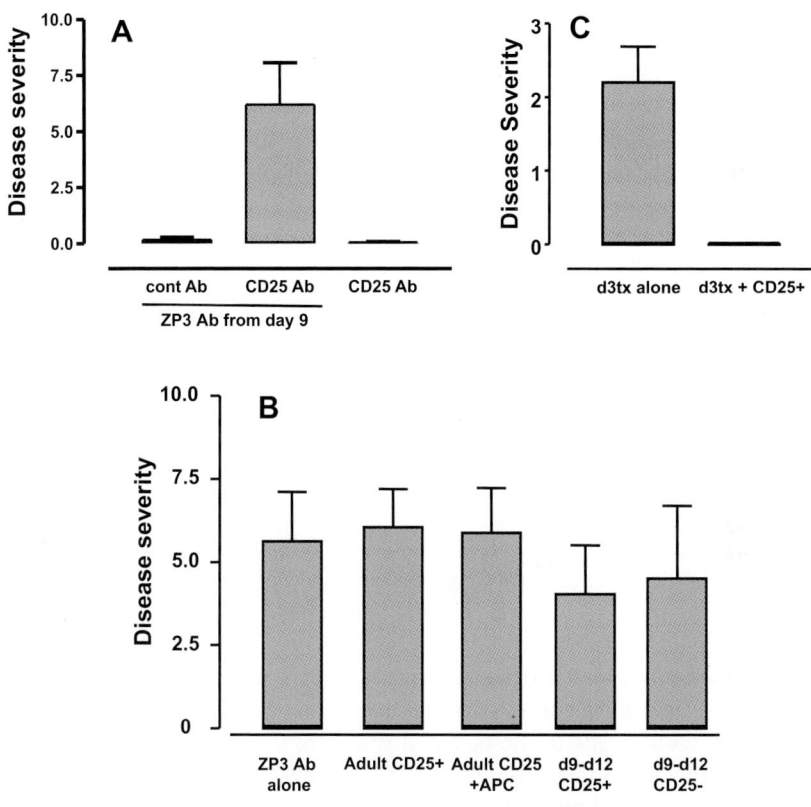

Fig. 4A–C The influence of in vivo depletion or infusion of $CD4^+CD25^+$ on nAOD development. **A** The exposure of neonatal mice to Ab to pZP3 from day 9 did not induce nAOD unless the mice were treated with Ab to CD25 (PC61); whereas CD25 Ab treatment alone did not induce nAOD. **B** The infusion of adult or d9–12 $CD4^+CD25^+$ T cells into neonatal mice did not affect disease development. The co-transfer of adult $CD4^+CD25^+$ T cells with adult APC also had no effect. **C** As control, the adult $CD4^+CD25^+$ T cells that did not affect nAOD completely inhibited AOD in the d3tx mice

2.3.4
Why Are Neonatal Mice (days 1–5) Susceptible to Neonatal Autoimmune Ovarian Disease?

If the neonatal time window of disease susceptibility is due to immaturity or preferential deficiency of $CD4^+CD25^+$ T cells, transfer of adult $CD25^+$ regulatory T cells may close the window. However, despite many attempts to prevent nAOD by infusion of $CD4^+CD25^+$ T cells from 9-day-old or adult mice, with or without co-transfer of adult APCs, we did not change the course of nAOD (Fig. 4B). These negative results suggest that the neonatal mice are resistant to suppression by $CD4^+CD25^+$ T cells. Because cells of the innate immune system [including natural killer (NK) cells, macrophages, and dendritic cells (DCs)] are known to influence adaptive immune response but also inhibit the regulatory function of $CD4^+CD25^+$ T cells (Pasare and Medzhitov 2003), we investigate the neonatal innate system in nAOD, specifically NK cells.

2.3.5
Requirement of Neonatal NK Cells, Fcγ Receptor III (FcγRIII) Positive Cells and Proinflammatory Cytokines in Neonatal Autoimmune Ovarian Disease Induction

Current knowledge on the ontogeny, phenotype, and function of neonatal NK cells is limited. In vitro studies suggest that neonatal mice have few NK cells and they are immature. Purified neonatal NK cells are barely cytotoxic against the classical NK cell targets, and do not reach adult activity until 2–3 weeks of age (Dussault and Miller 1995; Hackett, Jr. et al. 1986). The progenitors of neonatal NK cells are noted to divide more rapidly than adult NK cells (Jamieson et al. 2004). Expression of receptors for the MHC class I or class I-like molecule on neonatal NK cells is more restricted; they express predominantly CD94/NKG2A (Sivakumar et al. 1999; Kubota et al. 1999), and the Ly49 receptors are not detected before 1 week (Ortaldo et al. 2000).

We were therefore surprised to readily detect $NK1.1^+$ TCRVβ (but not $NK1.1^+$ TCRVβ^+) cells in the neonatal spleen of (C56BL/6xA/J)F1 (B6AF1) mice. The average ratio of NK cell to $\alpha\beta TCR^+$ T cells in 3-day-old mice was 0.6, which declined to 0.2 by day 9 as the T cell numbers increased. The neonatal NK cells were functional in vivo: their asialo GM1 (AGM1) positive cells, in response to lipopolysaccharide, produced as much interferon γ (IFNγ) as adult mice. Most importantly, when $NK1.1^+$ or $AGM1^+$ NK cells were depleted, the neonatal mice did not develop nAOD (Setiady et al. 2004). Neonatal NK cells are operative in both the induction and the effector phase of nAOD. Thus in adoptive transfer of nAOD, the recipient disease was ameliorated when either the donor or the recipient NK cells were depleted.

Adult NK cells can induce maturation and cytokine production by DCs, which in turn can activate naïve neonatal T cells (Ferlazzo et al. 2002; Piccioli et al. 2002; Gerosa et al. 2002; Mocikat et al. 2003; Mailliard et al. 2003). In nAOD, neonatal NK cells may function by modifying the APC function of neonatal DCs, or by stimulating T cells directly through engagement of 2B4 with CD48 on T cells (Assarsson et al. 2004). NK cell/DC interaction is bi-directional, thus both DC and T cells, when activated, can induce proliferation, activation, and cytokine production of NK cells (Fernandez et al. 1999; Ferlazzo et al. 2002; Piccioli et al. 2002; Gerosa et al. 2002; Ferlazzo et al. 2003). They may communicate by cell contact or via proinflammatory cytokines such as IFNγ and tumor necrosis factor α (TNFα) (Fernandez et al. 1999; Ferlazzo et al. 2002; Piccioli et al. 2002; Gerosa et al. 2002). Indeed, the ovaries with nAOD expressed high levels of IFNγ and TNFα that correlated with disease severity. In vivo, nAOD was inhibited by anti-IFNγ or anti-TNFα Ab. Interestingly, when cell donors were treated with IFNγ Ab, adoptively transfer of nAOD was also inhibited, thus IFNγ is likely operative during T cell induction, and NK cells a probable source of IFNγ (Setiady et al. 2004).

nAOD development is strongly influenced by the FcγR expressed on the innate cells because blockade of FcγRIIB and FcγRIII (by 2.4G2 monoclonal Ab) completely inhibited nAOD (Setiady et al. 2004). In addition, nAOD can be modulated by the stimulatory FcγRIII and the inhibitory FcγRIIb, thus the disease was ameliorated in mice deficient in FcγRIII but was greatly enhanced in FcγRIIB-deficient mice. In nAOD, the ZP3 immune complex may engage the FcγR on the NK cells, the DCs, or both. Since NK cells express predominantly FcγRIII, this may explain a dominant effect of FcγRIII deficiency in nAOD development. On the other hand, FcγRIIB and FcγRIII are co-expressed on DCs and they can potentially modulate the response of the neonatal T cells to DCs as an APC. Finally, FcγR expressed in granulocytes, monocytes, and macrophages may also contribute to nAOD through cytophilic anti-ZP3 Ab.

Many in vitro studies describe that murine neonatal T cell, neonatal NK cells, and neonatal APCs are deficient in number and function (Lu and Unanue 1982; Adkins 1999; Muthukkumar et al. 2000; Dakic et al. 2004). In contrast, the in vivo neonatal T cell and B cell responses to viral infections and vaccines are often comparable to adults (Forsthuber et al. 1996; Ridge et al. 1996; Sarzotti et al. 1996). Studies on nAOD indicate that the neonatal lymphoid compartment is far more responsive to autoantigenic stimulation than one might anticipate from the in vitro studies. Perhaps some of the discrepancies between the in vitro and in vivo findings are reconciled if the neonatal innate cells are included in the equation. In nAOD, the innate immune system including neonatal NK cells are documented to have an important role in promoting neonatal autoimmunity by enhancing neonatal APC function in other types of immune responses. It will be important to determine whether the neonatal innate response affects CD4$^+$CD25$^+$ T cell function and provides another piece of the puzzle in the pathogenesis of d3tx autoimmunity.

3
Endogenous Ag Specificity and Ag Requirement for Disease Suppression by CD4$^+$CD25$^+$ T Cells

3.1
The Location and Ag Dependency of Suppression

To understand the physiological function of the CD4$^+$CD25$^+$ T cell, it is important to elucidate whether disease suppression in vivo is Ag specific. Ag specificity can have several interpretations. First, it defines the range and Ag specificity of the target cells being regulated. Does it differ in suppression of T cell subsets vs B cell and cells of the innate system (NK cells, DCs)? For example, do CD4$^+$CD25$^+$ T cells regulate only the T cells with shared Ag specificity, or can they cross-regulate other T cells when both cognate epitopes are presented? Second, there is the repertoire issue: how biased are the CD4$^+$CD25$^+$ T cells directed to self epitopes? Third, it can be the specificity of the antigenic stimulus required to expand and maintain the regulatory capacity of CD4$^+$CD25$^+$ T cells in the periphery, an issue important for the CD4$^+$CD25$^+$ T cells to maintain self-tolerance. Fourth, specificity can also imply the Ag dependency and Ag specificity during the process of regulation; and this in turn addresses the location of regulation, the source of antigenic stimulus, and the persistence of regulatory T cell action. Our recent studies have addressed the last two topics on the Ag specificity of CD4$^+$CD25$^+$ T cell function.

In several systems, the target organ has been found to be a site of suppression where CD4$^+$CD25$^+$ T cells are often co-localized with CD4$^+$CD25$^-$ T cells (Mottet et al. 2003; Suvas et al. 2004). On the other hand, we recently identified the regional LN as a unique site of suppression of AOD in the d3tx mice (Samy et al., unpublished data). Although the infused CD4$^+$CD25$^+$ T cells were widely disseminated, the ovarian draining LN was the only lymphoid organ where recipient CD4$^+$ T cell response was completely inhibited. This finding implies that suppression of AOD by polyclonal CD4$^+$CD25$^+$ T cells depends on stimulation of the regulatory T cells by endogenous Ags. This is also supported by an earlier study that documented the critical requirement of endogenous ovarian Ag for maintenance of the physiological tolerance state. As mentioned earlier (Sect. 2.2.2), the supremacy of male over female response to the female specific self-Ag pZP3 indicates female mice are tolerant to ZP3 and this was terminated by ovarian ablation (Garza et al. 2000). In addition, continuous Ag stimulation was found to be required to maintain tolerance, which was terminated within 1 week after ovarian ablation. In our recent study on suppression of AOD in d3tx mice, depletion of the input $CD4^+CD25^+$ T cells also promptly led to emergence of severe AOD (Samy et al., unpublished data). Similar reversibility of suppression has been reported in experimental autoimmune encephalomyelitis (EAE) induced by T cells with transgenic TCR to myelin basic protein (Hori et al. 2002). The requirement of persistence of $CD4^+CD25^+$ T cells in suppression of autoimmunity argues against the importance of clonal elimination of effector T cells or induction of infectious tolerance.

3.2
Suppression of Autoimmune Disease by Regulatory Cells from Donors with or Without the Relevant Self-Ag

Earlier studies reported that AOD in the d3tx mice was suppressed by thymic graft or spleen cells from female mice, whereas male thymic cells and male spleen cells either do not suppress AOD or only in excess cell numbers (Nishizuka and Sakakura 1969; Sakaguchi et al. 1982). Our attempt to reproduce this finding was not successful (Smith et al. 1991). More recently, we have confirmed that our result was correct by showing that $CD4^+CD25^+$ T cells from male and female donors suppressed AOD equally, with identical cell dose responses (Setiady et al., preliminary data).

In view of differential suppression of autoimmune prostatitis (AIP) and autoimmune thyroiditis by T cells from Ag-positive vs Ag-negative cell donors (described below), how do we explain their equal suppression of AOD? Our interpretation is that even if the regulatory capacities of male and female $CD4^+CD25^+$ T cells for AOD suppression are different, they are equalized when the cells encounter the endogenous ovarian Ag in the young d3tx host. Indeed, we have shown that ovarian Ags (mater and ZP3) are expressed from birth and have the capacity to stimulate T cells on day 3 (Alard et al. 2001). This is also exemplified by the process of diversified autoAb response that depends on de novo B cell response to endogenous ovarian Ag. Immunized female mice with a ZP3 peptide that contains T but not native B epitope (in CFA) elicited Ab response to a distant native ZP3 B cell epitope within 7 days, 2 days after detectable response to the ZP3 T cell epitope (Lou et al. 1996). Other examples of endogenous ovarian antigenic stimulation, mentioned in Sect. 2.2.2, are:

1. The endogenous Ag requirement (in days 1–5) in promoting pathogenic Th1 response attendant to neonatal stimulation by pZP3 in IFA.
2. The rapid termination of female tolerance to pZP3 within 1 week of ovarian ablation.

Because of the highly accessible ovarian Ags, the AOD model may not be suitable for differentiating the regulatory capacity of $CD4^+CD25^+$ T cells from Ag-positive vs Ag-negative donors. Indeed, more clear-cut results have come from studies on autoimmune thyroiditis and AIP.

Seddon and Mason (1999) studied total $CD4^+$ T cells in suppression of autoimmune thyroiditis in nu/nu rats induced by the $CD4^+CD46RC^{high}$ effector T cells. Using a single cell dose, suppression was evident only when the $CD4^+$ T cells came from euthyroid donors, whereas autoimmune diabetes was suppressed by cells from both euthyroid and athyroid donors.

In murine autoimmune prostatitis, in which prostate Ags are expressed at the age of 2 weeks, it was found that total male spleen cells suppressed better than female cells (Taguchi and Nishizuka 1987). The male supremacy was lost when the cell donors were neonatally orchiectomized to prevent prostate development, but it was restored when prostate development was subsequently induced by dihydrotestosterone. We have confirmed this interesting finding by showing that $CD4^+CD25^+$ T cells from male donors also suppressed more efficiently than cells from female donors (Setiady et al., unpublished data). Importantly, exposure of cell donors to endogenous Ag for only 10 days was sufficient to enhance the regulatory capacity of $CD4^+CD25^+$ T cells of Ag-negative donors to that of Ag-positive donors. This finding is relevant to AOD suppression. For example, for the inexperienced male cells to rapidly gain regulatory capacity through encounter with the ovarian Ag in the d3tx recipients, it may need to occur before effector T cell activation at 2–3 weeks (Alard et al. 2001). On the other hand, this would not be possible in AIP suppression because of the late ontogeny of prostate Ag expression.

Taken together, the in vivo studies in d3tx mice support Ag-specific suppression of autoimmune diseases by $CD4^+CD25^+$ T cells, though the findings do not rule out additional suppression by nonspecific means. Our study on Ag specificity further emphasizes the dynamic nature of immune suppression by the $CD4^+CD25^+$ T cells:

1. The regulatory T cell function is critically dependent on their persistent stimulation by endogenous Ag.
2. Effective disease suppression (or tolerance) is critically dependent on the persistence of the $CD4^+CD25^+$ T cells in the host.

These important findings will influence the design of immunotherapy based on $CD4^+CD25^+$ T cells.

4
Genetic Control of Susceptibility to D3tx-Induced Autoimmune Disease

4.1
Genetic Studies on Inbred Strains of Mice

Kojima and Prehn's study (1981) examining susceptibility to d3Tx-induced autoimmune disease in 21 different inbred and congenic strains of mice found strain variation in organ involvement, incidence, and severity of disease; they also found that AIP was the only disease with a clear *H2* association. However, *H2*-linkage has subsequently been extended to include susceptibility to both AOD and AIG (Silveira et al. 2001; Roper et al. 2002). Additional studies were carried out to address the inheritance of d3tx-induced autoimmune disease. The results obtained using reciprocal F1 hybrid, backcross, and F2 intercross populations are consistent with oligogenic control by a limited number of interacting loci. Importantly, however, they revealed that susceptibility to AOD exhibits a maternal parent-of-origin effect in that the incidence of disease observed in F1 hybrid mice is significantly greater when the dam is the susceptible parental strain (Kojima and Prehn 1981). Preliminary attempts to map the genes controlling susceptibility to AOD, AIG, and AIP utilizing recombinant inbred lines (RIL) derived from BALB/cByJ and C57BL/6ByJ mice suggested a possible association of AIG with the minor histocompatibility locus *H27*, whose map location is unknown, and again, AIP with *H2*.

4.2
Mapping Loci Controlling Susceptibility to D3Tx-Induced Autoimmune Disease

There is little doubt that transgenic and gene knockout technologies provide insight into identifying genes involved in various aspects of immune processes (Yeung et al. 1993; Fischer and Malissen 1998). However, less is known about the function of a particular molecule as it pertains to its larger ecologically relevant and evolutionarily selected role in the immune system. Such information can only be obtained by identifying and characterizing the naturally occurring, evolutionarily selected alleles giving rise to phenotypic variation.

AOD and AIG are amenable to forward genetic analysis based on disease incidence (Kojima and Prehn 1981; Tung et al. 1987; Silveira et al. 1999). Approximately 90% of d3Tx female A/J and B6AF1 hybrid mice develop AOD and 80% of BALB/cCrSlc mice develop AIG with C57BL/6 J mice exhibiting less than 10% disease. Genome scans and linkage analyses carried out using mapping populations segregating susceptibility to AOD, AIG, and their component phenotypes are consistent with genetic control by a limited number of disease genes rather than polygenic inheritance. A summary of the binary trait loci (BTL) and quantitative trait loci (QTL) controlling susceptibility to AOD and AIG and their component phenotypes is presented in Table 1.

Genetic analysis of AOD utilizing a (C57BL/6 J × A/J) × C57BL/6 J backcross population (BC1) initially indicated that susceptibility was controlled by a single dominant locus (*Aod1*) with the results of the initial genome scan placing *Aod1* on central chromosome 16 (Wardell et al. 1995). Subsequently, *Aod2*, a second locus associated with susceptibility to ovarian atrophy was mapped to chromosome 3 (Teuscher et al. 1996). These studies, however, focused on susceptibility to AOD as a binary trait (affected vs. unaffected).

Composite interval mapping (CIM) -based QTL analysis (Zeng 1993, 1994), utilizing semi-quantitative histopathological lesion scores for oophoritis and atrophy as well as anti-ovarian autoantibody (AOA) titers, verified *Aod1* and *Aod2*; and identified three new QTL involved in AOD; *Aod3* (Chr. 1), *Aod4* (Chr. 2) and *Aod5* (Chr. 7) (Roper et al. 2002). CIM-QTL analysis using the A × B and B × A RILs also verified *Aod3* and detected linkage to *H2*. Importantly, statistical genetic-based interaction analysis (Wendell and Gorski 1997; Roper et al. 1999) also predicted the existence of epistasis between *Aod1–5*, *Gasa2*, a QTL controlling d3Tx-induced AIG (Silveira et al. 1999, 2001), and with *H2* (Table 2). For example, *Aod3* was predicted to interact with *Gasa2*. Similar results were observed for AOD with *Aod3* and *Aod5*, *Aod3* and *H2*, and *Aod1* and *Aod4* and together explained 35.8% of the AOD trait variance (Roper et al. 2002).

As the first step toward positionally cloning *Aod1*, we generated a panel of interval-specific bidirectional recombinant congenic lines encompassing the genetic interval on chromosome 16 (Roper et al. 2003). The results of these studies indicated that *Aod1* does control AOD but rather than being a single locus, *Aod1* is comprised of two linked QTL with opposing allelic effects. *Aod1a* resides between *D16Mit211* (23.3 cM) and *D16Mit51* (66.75 cM) on chromosome 16, whereas *Aod1b* maps proximal of *Aod1a* between *D16Mit89* (20.9 cM) and *D16Mit211* (23.3 cM).

A similar genetic analysis for AIG was carried out using a (BALB/cCrSlc × C57BL/6) F2 intercross population (Silveira et al. 1999). Two linked QTL on telomeric chromosome 4, *Gasa1* at ~60–70 cM and *Gasa2* at ~78–82 cM, were implicated in the genetic control of susceptibility to AIG, as assessed by the existence of histopathological lesions and H^+/K^+ ATPase-specific autoAb titers. A subsequent study utilizing partitioned Chi-square analysis revealed the existence of two additional QTL controlling susceptibility to AIG: *Gasa3* on chromosome 6 at ~42–49 cM and *Gasa4 (H2)* (Silveira et al. 2001). Potential epistatic interactions between the QTL controlling susceptibility to AIG were also implicated in susceptibility to AIG, i.e., *Gasa2* × *Gasa4* (*H2*).

The detection of epistasis among and between the QTL controlling AOD and AIG as well as with *H2* (Table 2) suggest that the QTL controlling d3Tx-

Table 1 Summary of QTL controlling d3Tx-induced autoimmune diseases identified to date

Disease	Locus	Cross	Chr.	Marker(s)	cM	Phenotype	Reference
AOD	Aod1	BC1	16	D16Mit58–D16Mit59	23–28	Oophoritis	Wardell et al. 1995; Roper et al. 2002
	Aod1a	Congenic	16	D16Mit211–D16Mit51	23.3–66.8	Oophoritis	Roper et al. 2003
	Aod1b	Congenic	16	D16Mit89–D16Mit211	20.9–23.3	Oophoritis	Roper et al. 2003
	Aod2	BC1	3	D16Mit21–D16Mit94	19–22	Atrophy	Teuscher et al. 1996; Roper et al. 2002
	Aod3	BC1	1	D1Mit417	63	Oophoritis	Roper et al. 2002
		BC1	1	D1Mit45	58	Atrophy	Roper et al. 2002
		RIL	1	D1Mit128	37	Oophoritis	Roper et al. 2002
	Aod4	BC1	2	D2Mit452	79	Atrophy	Roper et al. 2002
	Aod5	BC1	7	D7Mit340–D7Mit77	1–7	Auto-Ab	Roper et al. 2002
	Aod6 (H2)	RIL	17	D17Mit62	17.4	Oophoritis	Roper et al. 2002
AIG	Gasa1	F2	4	D4Mit203–D4Mit284	60–70	Gastritis	Silveira et al. 1999
	Gasa2	F2	4	D4Mit127–D4Mit344	78–82	Gastritis, auto-Ab	Silveira et al. 1999
	Gasa3	F2	6	D6Mit67–D6Mit287	42–49	Gastritis	Silveira et al. 2001
	Gasa4 (H2)	Congenic	17		19	Gastritis	Silveira et al. 2001

Table 2 Interaction of QTL among AOD and AG phenotypes

Phenotype	Trait-specific QTL[a]	Interacting QTL[b]	% Variance[c]	F	P value
Oophoritis			35.8	6.2	<0.0001
	Aod1	Aod3 × Gasa2			
	Aod3	Aod3 × Aod5			
		Aod3 × Aod6 (H2)			
		Aod1 × Aod4			
Atrophy			43.6	9.3	<0.0001
	Aod2	Aod1 × Aod4			
	Aod3	Aod2 × Aod6 (H2)			
	Aod4				
AOA			13.9	3.6	0.0180
	Aod5	Aod2 × Aod4			
Gastritis					
	Gasa1	Gasa2 × Gasa4 (H2)	ND[d]	ND	ND
	Gasa2				
	Gasa3				
	Gasa4				

[a] Independent variables in linear regression model represented by loci identified by CIM.
[b] Independent variables that represent significant interactions as found by stepwise selection.
[c] Variance, F and P values are for entire model with all terms included in the linear regression model.
[d] Not determined.

induced autoimmunity may be both organ-specific and more generalized in their effects with respect to the genesis and activity of the immunoregulatory mechanisms maintaining peripheral tolerance. The non-MHC-linked "shared" autoimmune disease gene hypothesis, first proposed by Teuscher in 1985 (Teuscher 1985; Sudweeks et al. 1993; Meeker et al. 1995), was recently validated by our identification of *Bphs* as *Hrh1*, a "shared" gene in EAE and autoimmune orchitis (Ma et al. 2002). Additionally, given the role of $CD4^+CD25^+$ regulatory T cells in d3Tx-induced diseases, it is likely that one or more of the QTL controlling d3Tx-induced autoimmune disease play a role in the genesis and maintenance of these cells or in controlling their effector functions.

4.3
Positional-Candidate Genes for AOD and AIG QTL That Are Differentially Expressed by CD4$^+$CD25$^+$ Regulatory T Cells

The pathway to gene discovery using the positional-candidate gene approach involves genetic mapping of trait loci; physically delineating a support interval for each locus by congenic mapping; gene identification using expression or structural polymorphisms to guide the selection from a list of candidate genes within the interval; and tests for expression of that gene in relevant cells, the mechanism of its action, and the way that natural alleles of the gene shape its behavior, all in the context of environmental influences. In this scheme, candidate gene selection is primarily based on phenotype-genotype relationships delineated by congenic mapping. However, additional criteria can be used to aid in considering a particular gene, or set of genes, as potential candidates when congenic mapping-based genotype–phenotype relationships are unavailable (Abiola et al. 2003). For example, genes residing within the AOD and AIG BTL and QTL intervals that exhibit differential expression in CD4$^+$CD25$^+$ regulatory T cells are promising candidates for initial evaluation.

Comparative microarray analyses between CD4$^+$CD25$^+$ T cells and other T cells in several different models resulted in the identification of a limited set of differentially expressed genes (Bystry et al. 2001; Lechner et al. 2001; Gavin et al. 2002; McHugh et al. 2002; Graca et al. 2002; Zelenika et al. 2002). To identify which of these genes map within the genetic intervals encompassing the AOD and AIG disease susceptibility loci we determined their map locations by searching the MGI and NCBI linkage maps. The locations for the unmapped genes were determined by locating their sequence within the mouse genome using the ENSEMBL or UCSC genome browsers and identifying the closest linked gene or marker whose map location was known. The list of genes that was identified in this way is presented in Table 3. Surprisingly, a number of the differentially expressed genes mapped within the genetic intervals encompassing the AOD and AIG susceptibility loci. Importantly, there were no differentially expressed loci that mapped within the *Aod1a*, *Aod1b* and *Gasa1* intervals, suggesting that the detected occurrences are not simply random events. Additionally, it is worth nothing that several of the associations co-localize with QTL involved in other autoimmune diseases (http://www.informatics.jax.org/) in which CD4$^+$CD25$^+$ regulatory T cells have been implicated (multiple reviews in Parham 2001). Thus, structural- or expression-level polymorphism in these genes could underlie "shared" autoimmune disease susceptibility loci.

Of the genes exhibiting differential expression in CD4$^+$CD25$^+$ regulatory T cells several were identified in more than one study (Table 3, highlighted in bold type). These include *Pdcd1* (programmed cell death-1); *Tnfrsf1b*

Table 3 Summary of positional-candidate genes that are differentially expressed by CD4$^+$CD25$^+$ T-cells mapping within the genetic intervals encompassing QTL controlling AOD and AG

QTL	Differentially expressed positional candidate genes			
	Chr.[a]	cM[a]	Gene designation[b]	Process/functional category[c]
Aod2	3	19	*Il2*	Cell proliferation, cellular defense response, IL-2 receptor activity
Aod3	1	54–59	**Pdcd1**	Apoptosis
Aod4	2	81	*Tde1*	Induction of apoptosis
Aod3×Gasa2, Gasa1,	4	76	*Tnfrsf1b*	Cell proliferation, cell surface receptor linked signal transduction
Gasa2, Gasa2 × Gasa4 (H2)		76	*Tnfrsf9*	Defense response
		79	*Tnfrsf4*	Cellular defense response
		79	*Tnfrsf18*	Receptor activity
Aod5	7	3	*Pira1*	Unknown
		4	*Apoe*	Lipid transport, lipoprotein metabolism
		7	**Tgfb1**	Cell growth, cell proliferation
Aod6, Gasa4 (H2)	17	16	*Pim1*	Cell growth and/or maintenance, protein amino acid phosphorylation
		19	**Psmb9**	Protein metabolism, proteasome complex
		19	**Psmb8**	Immune response, ubiquitin-dependent protein catabolism, endopeptidase
		19	**Lta**	Cell growth and/or maintenance, cell proliferation
		19	**Ltb**	Lymph gland development
		20	*H2-M3*	Defense response

[a] Locations are based on the MGI linkage map (http://www.informatics.jax.org/). Map locations for unmapped EST were determined by BLAST analysis and placed according to the closest linked, mapped marker or gene.
[b] Enboldened genes are those that appeared in two or more comparisons (Bystry et al., 2001; Lechner et al., 2001; Gavin et al., 2002; McHugh et al., 2002; Graca et al., 2002; Zelenika et al., 2002).
[c] Process and functional classifications are according to MGI (http://www.informatics.jax.org/).

(tumor necrosis factor receptor superfamily, member 1b); *Tnfrsf9* (tumor necrosis factor receptor superfamily, member 9); *Tnfrsf4* (tumor necrosis factor receptor superfamily, member 4); *Tnfrsf18* (tumor necrosis factor receptor superfamily, member 18); *Tgfb1* (transforming growth factor, beta 1); *Psmb9* (proteosome subunit, beta type 9); *Lta* (lymphotoxin A); and *Ltb* (lymphotoxin B).

4.3.1
Pdcd1 as a Candidate for Aod3

Pdcd1, an inhibitory co-stimulatory receptor induced on activated T, B, and myeloid cells, plays a role in the regulation of peripheral tolerance in that Pdcd1 signaling in T cells induces anergy (Okazaki et al. 2002; Leibson 2004). Disruption of *Pdcd1* also leads to strain-specific autoimmune phenomena, i.e., C57BL/6 *Pdcd1$^{-/-}$* mice develop spontaneous lupus-like disease, whereas BALB/c *Pdcd1$^{-/-}$* mice exhibit autoAb-mediated dilated cardiomyopathy (Nishimura et al. 1999, 2001; Okazaki et al. 2003). In addition, *Pdcd1* has been implicated in the regulation of both autoimmune diabetes (Ansari et al. 2003) and EAE (Salama et al. 2003). The role of *Pdcd1* in the genesis and/or function of CD4$^+$CD25$^+$ regulatory T cells is unclear but it was recently shown to be upregulated on CD4$^+$CD25$^+$ regulatory T cells generated by exposure of CD4$^+$CD25- T cells to TGFβ (Park et al. 2004). It has also been shown to play a role in thymocyte development (Nishimura et al. 2000). Most importantly, with respect to *Pdcd1* as a candidate for *Aod3*, polymorphism in *Pdcd1* has been reported to be associated with susceptibility to systemic lupus erythematosus (Prokunina et al. 2002), type I diabetes (Nielsen et al. 2003), and rheumatoid arthritis (Prokunina et al. 2004).

4.3.2
The Tumor Necrosis Factor Receptor Superfamily Genes

Of the tumor necrosis factor receptor superfamily genes that are candidates for *Gasa1*, *Gasa2*, *Aod3* (based on the interaction between *Aod3* and *Gasa2*) (Roper et al. 2002), and the interaction between *Gasa2* and *Gasa4* (*H2*) (Silveira et al. 2001), *Tnfrsf18/Gitr* is of particular note. Depletion of Tnfrsf18$^+$ cells or stimulation of Tnfrsf18 was shown to abrogate CD4$^+$CD25$^+$ regulatory T cell activity resulting in the development of autoimmune disease (Shimizu et al. 2002; McHugh et al. 2002).

4.3.3
Tgfb1

Tgfb1 is a pleiotropic factor that plays a central function in maintenance of immune homeostasis (reviewed in Letterio and Roberts 1998) and several studies suggest a possible link between *Tgfb1* and regulatory T cells (Nakamura et al. 2001; Yamagiwa et al. 2001). It has been suggested that TCR activation in the presence of Tgfb1 converts naïve mouse $CD4^+CD25^-$ T cells into $CD4^+CD25^+$ regulatory T cells through the induction of Foxp3 (Chen et al. 2003; Schramm et al. 2004), a gene that has been proposed to be a master switch for $CD4^+CD25^+$ regulatory T cell development and function (Hori et al. 2003; Fontenot et al. 2003; Khattri et al. 2003; reviewed in Fehervari and Sakaguchi 2004). Interestingly, it was recently reported that Tgfb1 co-stimulation of $CD4^+CD25^-$ T cells leads to an increase in the level of Pdcd1 expression upon conversion to $CD4^+CD25^+$ regulatory T cells (Park et al. 2004). The existence of this amplification loop may reflect the epistatic interaction observed between *Aod3* and *Aod5* in the genetic control of oophoritis (Table 2).

4.3.4
H2

Genetic linkage of autoimmune disease susceptibility to the MHC is believed to reflect class I- and class II-based genetic restriction of autoantigenic peptide presentation to T cells (Rhodes and Trowsdale 1999; Sonderstrup and McDevitt 2001; Fourneau et al. 2004). However, the existence of other MHC-linked genes functioning in susceptibility to autoimmune and infectious diseases is becoming increasingly evident (Hattori et al. 1999; Morel et al. 1999; Boulard et al. 2002a; Teuscher et al. 2004). *Psmb9*, *Lta* and *Ltb*, the three *H2*-linked genes differentially expressed in $CD4^+CD25^+$ regulatory T cells have all received considerable attention as candidates for MHC-linked autoimmune disease susceptibility genes. *Psmb9* is known to have three structural alleles, $Psmb9^d$, $Psmb9^b$, and $Psmb9^q$ that correlate with the *H2* haplotypes of various inbred strains of mice (Zhou et al. 1993). The $Psmb9^d$ (A/J and BALB/cCrSlc allele) and $Psmb9^b$ (C57BL/6 J) alleles are segregating in both the AOD and AIG BC1 populations. Ltb has been shown to affect the function of *aire* (Chin et al. 2003). The mutation of *aire* alone has been shown to result in human autoimmune polyglandular syndromes type I (APECED) (Ruan and She 2004), and mice with targeted deletion of *aire* develop autoimmune disease of the stomach, ovary, and eye (Anderson et al. 2002), the typical autoimmune diseases that develop in d3tx mice.

4.3.5
Il2

Of the genes exhibiting differential expression in CD4$^+$CD25$^+$ regulatory T cells, *Il2* is a particularly strong candidate for a "shared" autoimmune disease susceptibility gene. *Il2* was originally identified as a candidate for *Aod2*, and based on its co-localization with *Idd3*, the strongest QTL associated with resistance to IDDM in the NOD mouse (Lyons et al. 2000; Podolin et al. 2000; Ikegami et al. 2002; Ikegami et al. 2003), we hypothesized that a structural polymorphism in *Il2* (Chesnut et al. 1993) may reflect a "shared" autoimmune disease susceptibility gene underlying the two QTL (Teuscher et al. 1996). Subsequent studies also implicated *Il2* as a candidate for *eae3/20* (Butterfield et al. 1998; Encinas et al. 1999) and *Ssial2*, controlling autoimmune sialoadenitis in NOD mice (Boulard et al. 2002b). Importantly, recombinant IL2 allelic proteins have been reported to differentially influence IL2 regulated responses (Matesanz and Alcina 1996, 1998; Choi et al. 2002). IL2 expression at the mRNA level also differs between EAE-susceptible SJL/J and EAE-resistant B10.S/DvTe CD4$^+$ T cells following stimulation with anti-CD3/CD28 monoclonal Ab (unpublished data). Thus, IL2 is a candidate gene based on the existence of both a structural- and expression-level polymorphism. Interestingly, a sequence polymorphism in the human *Il2* promoter (G/T and T/T) at −330 (−384 from the ATG), influencing IL2 synthesis, has been reported to be associated with susceptibility to multiple sclerosis (Matesanz et al. 2001, 2004).

Support for *Il2* as a candidate gene in the genesis, maturation, and maintenance of CD4$^+$CD25$^+$ regulatory T cells is based on the differential expression of IL2 and IL2ra between CD4$^+$CD25$^+$ and CD4$^+$CD25$^-$ T cells after stimulation with anti-CD3 and IL2 (McHugh et al. 2002); *Il2*-knockout (*Il2*KO), *Il2ra*KO (CD25), and *Il2rb*KO mice all develop autoimmune phenomenon (Sadlack et al. 1993; Willerford et al. 1995; Suzuki et al. 1995), with 25%–50% of *Il2*KO and *Il2ra*KO mice dying from severe hemolytic anemia and the remaining mice developing wasting disease (Sadlack et al. 1993; Willerford et al. 1995); *Il2ra*KO mice lack functional CD4$^+$CD25$^+$ regulatory T cells (Furtado et al. 2002); adoptive transfer of normal CD4$^+$CD25$^+$ T cells into neonatal *Il2rb*KO mice prevents autoimmunity (Malek et al. 2002); autoimmunity seen in *Il2rb*KO mice can be prevented by selectively expressing *Il2rb* in the thymus (Malek et al. 2000); CD4$^+$CD25$^+$ regulatory T cells "de-anergized" by stimulation with high levels of IL2 lose their capacity to suppress disease (Takahashi et al. 1998); and CD4$^+$CD25$^+$ regulatory T cells constitutively express CD25 (Sakaguchi et al. 1995). These observations suggest that IL2–IL2r signaling plays an essential role in the genesis, maturation, and maintenance of CD4$^+$CD25$^+$ regulatory T cells mediating peripheral tolerance (Malek 2003;

Nelson 2004) and underscores the concept that the *Il2* polymorphisms may have selectively unique ontogenic effects within the thymus during the genesis and selection of these cells and in the periphery during their maturation and maintenance of regulatory activity.

4.3.6
Positional-Candidate Genes for AOD and AIG QTL

Immunologically relevant positional-candidate genes for *Gasa3* on chromosome 6 have yet to be identified within the linkage interval (http://www.informatics.jax.org/). Similarly, given the current size of the interval encompassing *Aod1a*, identification of potential candidates is highly speculative. However, *Il10rb* (interleukin-10 receptor β) at 61 cM is an intriguing candidate since IL10 has been implicated in the establishment and maintenance of $CD4^+CD25^+$ T cells (Annacker et al. 2001). *Trfr* (transferrin receptor or Cd71) at 21.2 cM is a potential candidate for *Aod1b*. Trfr is downregulated during adult T cell development as well as in ontogeny prior to the appearance of the α/β TCR and therefore serves as a marker of immature, proliferating T cells (Brekelmans et al. 1994). *Stfa1*, *Stfa2*, *Stfa3* (stefin A1, A2 and A3) at 22.85 cM are inhibitors of cysteine endo- and exopeptidases (Bode and Huber 2000) such as cathepsin L and S involved in Ag processing (Pluger et al. 2002; Hsieh et al. 2002). Most importantly, cathepsin S inhibitors were shown to prevent autoAg presentation in vitro, and in vivo treatment with cathepsin inhibitors blocks lymphocytic infiltration into the salivary and lacrimal glands, abrogates autoAb production, and promotes the recovery from autoimmune disease in these organs in d3tx NFS/sld mice (Saegusa et al. 2002). These polymorphisms have the potential of functioning at both the selection phase of $CD4^+CD25^+$ T cells during thymopoiesis and their maturation and maintenance within the periphery (Parham 2001; Fehervari and Sakaguchi 2004), and at the effector or inflammatory phase of the disease mediated by $CD4^+CD25^-$ effector T cells. However, to date, the polymorphic residues of *Stfa1* and *Stfa2* have not been modeled with respect to their functionality as inhibitors of cathepsin activity.

4.3.7
The Autoantigen in d3tx-Induced Autoimmune Ovarian Disease

A potential candidate gene within the *Aod5* interval is *Nalp5* (NACHT, leucine-rich repeat and PYD containing 5; also known as *Mater*, *Op1*, and PAN11). *Nalp5* is an ovarian specific autoAg identified by its reactivity with autoAb present in the sera of d3tx mice (Tong and Nelson 1999). We sequenced

Nalp5 and identified it as a structurally polymorphic candidate gene for *Aod5* (Roper et al. 2003). Importantly, sequencing results from other strains of mice that exhibit differential susceptibility to AOD also express the same polymorphic splice variants (unpublished data). The polymorphic peptides arising from the A/J and C57BL/6 J Nalp5 alleles may affect the genesis, maturation, and maintenance of $CD4^+CD25^-$ effector T cells, $CD4^+CD25^+$ regulatory T cells or both, and thereby directly impact disease susceptibility. $CD4^+CD25^+$ regulatory T cells appear to be selected from a cellular pool with different affinities compared to regulatory T cells that are CD25 negative (Suto et al. 2002); and our studies described in Sect. 3 on the requirement for self-Ags in the generation and maintenance of $CD4^+CD25^+$ T cells is consistent with this possibility. Moreover, any polymorphism in the ontogeny of autoAg expression during the first few days of life may also strongly influence disease susceptibility in d3tx mice.

References

Abiola O, Angel JM, Avner P, Bachmanov AA, Belknap JK, Bennett B, Blankenhorn EP, Blizard DA, Bolivar V, Brockmann GA, Buck KJ, Bureau JF, Casley WL, Chesler EJ, Cheverud JM, Churchill GA, Cook M, Crabbe JC, Crusio WE, Darvasi A, de Haan G, Dermant P, Doerge RW, Elliot RW, Farber CR, Flaherty L, Flint J, Gershenfeld H, Gibson JP, Gu J, Gu W, Himmelbauer H, Hitzemann R, Hsu HC, Hunter K, Iraqi FF, Jansen RC, Johnson TE, Jones BC, Kempermann G, Lammert F, Lu L, Manly KF, Matthews DB, Medrano JF, Mehrabian M, Mittlemann G, Mock BA, Mogil JS, Montagutelli X, Morahan G, Mountz JD, Nagase H, Nowakowski RS, O'Hara BF, Osadchuk AV, Paigen B, Palmer AA, Peirce JL, Pomp D, Rosemann M, Rosen GD, Schalkwyk LC, Seltzer Z, Settle S, Shimomura K, Shou S, Sikela JM, Siracusa LD, Spearow JL, Teuscher C, Threadgill DW, Toth LA, Toye AA, Vadasz C, Van Zant G, Wakeland E, Williams RW, Zhang HG, Zou F (2003) The nature and identification of quantitative trait loci: a community's view. Nat Rev Genet 4:911–916

Adkins B (1999) T-cell function in newborn mice and humans. Immunol Today 20:330–335

Adkins B (2000) Development of neonatal Th1/Th2 function. Int Rev Immunol 19:157–171

Agersborg SS, Garza KM, Tung KS (2001) Intestinal parasitism terminates self tolerance and enhances neonatal induction of autoimmune disease and memory. Eur J Immunol 31:851–859

Alard P, Thompson C, Agersborg SS, Thatte J, Setiady Y, Samy E, Tung KS (2001) Endogenous oocyte antigens are required for rapid induction and progression of autoimmune ovarian disease following day-3 thymectomy. J Immunol 166:4363–4369

Anderson MS, Venanzi ES, Klein L, Chen Z, Berzins SP, Turley SJ, von Boehmer H, Bronson R, Dierich A, Benoist C, Mathis D (2002) Projection of an immunological self shadow within the thymus by the aire protein. Science 298:1395–1401

Annacker O, Pimenta-Araujo R, Burlen-Defranoux O, Barbosa TC, Cumano A, Bandeira A (2001) CD25+ CD4+ T cells regulate the expansion of peripheral CD4 T cells through the production of IL-10. J Immunol 166:3008–3018

Ansari MJ, Salama AD, Chitnis T, Smith RN, Yagita H, Akiba H, Yamazaki T, Azuma M, Iwai H, Khoury SJ, Auchincloss H Jr, Sayegh MH (2003) The programmed death-1 (PD-1) pathway regulates autoimmune diabetes in nonobese diabetic (NOD) mice. J Exp Med 198:63–69

Asano M, Toda M, Sakaguchi N, Sakaguchi S (1996) Autoimmune disease as a consequence of developmental abnormality of a T cell subpopulation. J Exp Medicine 184:387–396

Assarsson E, Kambayashi T, Schatzle JD, Cramer SO, von Bonin A, Jensen PE, Ljunggren HG, Chambers BJ (2004) NK cells stimulate proliferation of T and NK cells through 2B4/CD48 interactions. J Immunol 173:174–180

Bode W, Huber R (2000) Structural basis of the endoproteinase-protein inhibitor interaction. Biochim Biophys Acta 1477:241–252

Boulard O, Damotte D, Deruytter N, Fluteau G, Carnaud C, Garchon HJ (2002a) An interval tightly linked to but distinct from the H2 complex controls both overt diabetes (Idd16) and chronic experimental autoimmune thyroiditis (Ceat1) in nonobese diabetic mice. Diabetes 51:2141–2147

Boulard O, Fluteau G, Eloy L, Damotte D, Bedossa P, Garchon HJ (2002b) Genetic analysis of autoimmune sialadenitis in nonobese diabetic mice: a major susceptibility region on chromosome 1. J Immunol 168:4192–4201

Brekelmans P, van Soest P, Voerman J, Platenburg PP, Leenen PJ, van Ewijk W (1994) Transferrin receptor expression as a marker of immature cycling thymocytes in the mouse. Cell Immunol 159:331–339

Butterfield RJ, Sudweeks JD, Blankenhorn EP, Korngold R, Marini JC, Todd JA, Roper RJ, Teuscher C (1998) New genetic loci that control susceptibility and symptoms of experimental allergic encephalomyelitis in inbred mice. J Immunol 161:1860–1867

Bystry RS, Aluvihare V, Welch KA, Kallikourdis M, Betz AG (2001) B cells and professional APCs recruit regulatory T cells via CCL4. Nat Immunol 2:1126–1132

Canto E, Vidal S, Rodriguez-Sanchez JL (2003) HK-ATPase expression in the susceptible BALB/c and the resistant DBA/2 strains of mice to autoimmune gastritis. Autoimmunity 36:275–283

Chen W, Jin W, Hardegen N, Lei KJ, Li L, Marinos N, McGrady G, Wahl SM (2003) Conversion of peripheral CD4+. J Exp Med 198:1875–1886

Chesnut K, She JX, Cheng I, Muralidharan K, Wakeland EK (1993) Characterizations of candidate genes for IDD susceptibility from the diabetes-prone NOD mouse strain. Mamm. Genome 4:549–554

Chin RK, Lo JC, Kim O, Blink SE, Christiansen PA, Peterson P, Wang Y, Ware C, Fu YX (2003) Lymphotoxin pathway directs thymic Aire expression. Nat Immunol 4:1121–1127

Choi Y, Simon-Stoos K, Puck JM (2002) Hypo-active variant of IL-2 and associated decreased T cell activation contribute to impaired apoptosis in autoimmune prone MRL mice. Eur J Immunol 32:677–685

Claeys D, Saraga E, Rossier BC, Kraehenbuhl JP (1997) Neonatal injection of native proton pump antigens induces autoimmune gastritis in mice. Gastroenterology 113:1136–1145

Dakic A, Shao QX, D'Amico A, O'Keeffe M, Chen WF, Shortman K, Wu L (2004) Development of the dendritic cell system during mouse ontogeny. J Immunol 172:1018–1027

Deshmukh US, Lewis JE, Gaskin F, Kannapell CC, Waters ST, Lou YH, Tung KS, Fu SM (1999) Immune responses to Ro60 and its peptides in mice. I. The nature of the immunogen and endogenous autoantigen determine the specificities of the induced autoantibodies. J Exp Med 189:531–540

Dussault I, Miller SC (1995) Suppression of natural killer cell activity in infant mice occurs after target cell binding. Nat Immun 14:35–43

Encinas JA, Wicker LS, Peterson LB, Mukasa A, Teuscher C, Sobel R, Weiner HL, Seidman CE, Seidman JG, Kuchroo VK (1999) QTL influencing autoimmune diabetes and encephalomyelitis map to a 0.15-cM region containing Il2. Nat Genet 21:158–160

Fehervari Z, Sakaguchi S (2004) Development and function of CD25+CD4+ regulatory T cells. Curr Opin Immunol 16:203–208

Ferlazzo G, Morandi B, D'Agostino A, Meazza R, Melioli G, Moretta A, Moretta L (2003) The interaction between NK cells and dendritic cells in bacterial infections results in rapid induction of NK cell activation and in the lysis of uninfected dendritic cells. Eur J Immunol 33:306–313

Ferlazzo G, Tsang ML, Moretta L, Melioli G, Steinman RM, Munz C (2002) Human dendritic cells activate resting natural killer (NK) cells and are recognized via the NKp30 receptor by activated NK cells. J Exp Med 195:343–351

Fernandez NC, Lozier A, Flament C, Ricciardi-Castagnoli P, Bellet D, Suter M, Perricaudet M, Tursz T, Maraskovsky E, Zitvogel L (1999) Dendritic cells directly trigger NK cell functions: cross-talk relevant in innate anti-tumor immune responses in vivo. Nat Med 5:405–411

Fischer A, Malissen B (1998) Natural and engineered disorders of lymphocyte development. Science 280:237–243

Fontenot JD, Gavin MA, Rudensky AY (2003) Foxp3 programs the development and function of CD4+CD25+ regulatory T cells. Nat Immunol 4:330–336

Forsthuber T, Yip HC, Lehmann PV (1996) Induction of TH1 and TH2 immunity in neonatal mice. Science 271:1728–1730

Fourneau JM, Bach JM, van Endert PM, Bach JF (2004) The elusive case for a role of mimicry in autoimmune diseases. Mol Immunol 40:1095–1102

Furtado GC, Curotto de Lafaille MA, Kutchukhidze N, Lafaille JJ (2002) Interleukin 2 signaling is required for CD4(+) regulatory T cell function. J Exp Med 196:851–857

Garza KM, Agersborg SS, Baker E, Tung KS (2000) Persistence of physiological self antigen is required for the regulation of self tolerance. J Immunol 164:3982–3989

Garza KM, Griggs ND, Tung KS (1997) Neonatal injection of an ovarian peptide induces autoimmune ovarian disease in female mice: requirement of endogenous neonatal ovaries. Immunity 6:89–96

Gavin MA, Clarke SR, Negrou E, Gallegos A, Rudensky A (2002) Homeostasis and anergy of CD4(+)CD25(+) suppressor T cells in vivo. Nat Immunol 3:33–41

Gerosa F, Baldani-Guerra B, Nisii C, Marchesini V, Carra G, Trinchieri G (2002) Reciprocal activating interaction between natural killer cells and dendritic cells. J Exp Med 195:327–333

Gershon RK, Kondo K (1970) Cell interactions in the induction of tolerance: the role of thymic lymphocytes. Immunology 18:723–737

Gleeson PA, Toh BH, van Driel IR (1996) Organ-specific autoimmunity induced by lymphopenia. Immunol Rev 149:97–125

Graca L, Thompson S, Lin CY, Adams E, Cobbold SP, Waldmann H (2002) Both CD4(+)CD25(+) and CD4(+)CD25(-) regulatory cells mediate dominant transplantation tolerance. J Immunol 168:5558–5565

Hackett J Jr, Tutt M, Lipscomb M, Bennett M, Koo G, Kumar V (1986) Origin and differentiation of natural killer cells. II. Functional and morphologic studies of purified NK-1.1+ cells. J Immunol 136:3124–3131

Hattori M, Yamato E, Itoh N, Senpuku H, Fujisawa T, Yoshino M, Fukuda M, Matsumoto E, Toyonaga T, Nakagawa I, Petruzzelli M, McMurray A, Weiner H, Sagai T, Moriwaki K, Shiroishi T, Maron R, Lund T (1999) Cutting edge: homologous recombination of the MHC class I K region defines new MHC-linked diabetogenic susceptibility gene(s) in nonobese diabetic mice. J Immunol 163:1721–1724

Hori S, Haury M, Lafaille JJ, Demengeot J, Coutinho A (2002) Peripheral expansion of thymus-derived regulatory cells in anti-myelin basic protein T cell receptor transgenic mice. Eur J Immunol 32:3729–3735

Hori S, Nomura T, Sakaguchi S (2003) Control of regulatory T cell development by the transcription factor Foxp3. Science 299:1057–1061

Hsieh CS, deRoos P, Honey K, Beers C, Rudensky AY (2002) A role for cathepsin L and cathepsin S in peptide generation for MHC class II presentation. J Immunol 168:2618–2625

Ikegami H, Fujisawa T, Makino S, Ogihara T (2002) Genetic dissection of type 1 diabetes susceptibility gene, Idd3, by ancestral haplotype congenic mapping. Ann N Y Acad Sci 958:325–328

Ikegami H, Fujisawa T, Makino S, Ogihara T (2003) Congenic mapping and candidate sequencing of susceptibility genes for Type 1 diabetes in the NOD mouse. Ann N Y Acad Sci 1005:196–204

Jamieson AM, Isnard P, Dorfman JR, Coles MC, Raulet DH (2004) Turnover and proliferation of NK cells in steady state and lymphopenic conditions. J Immunol 172:864–870

Khattri R, Cox T, Yasayko SA, Ramsdell F (2003) An essential role for Scurfin in CD4+CD25+ T regulatory cells. Nat Immunol 4:337–342

Kojima A, Prehn RT (1981) Genetic susceptibility to post-thymectomy autoimmune diseases in mice. Immunogenetics 14:15–27

Kubota A, Kubota S, Lohwasser S, Mager DL, Takei F (1999) Diversity of NK cell receptor repertoire in adult and neonatal mice. J Immunol 163:212–216

Lechner O, Lauber J, Franzke A, Sarukhan A, von Boehmer H, Buer J (2001) Fingerprints of anergic T cells. Curr Biol 11:587–595

Leibson PJ (2004) The regulation of lymphocyte activation by inhibitory receptors. Curr Opin Immunol 16:328–336

Letterio JJ, Roberts AB (1998) Regulation of immune responses by TGF-beta. Annu Rev Immunol 16:137–161

Lopez-Hoyos M, Carrio R, Merino R, Buelta L, Izui S, Nunez G, Merino J (1996) Constitutive expression of bcl-2 in B cells causes a lethal form of lupus-like autoimmune disease after induction of neonatal tolerance to H-2b alloantigens. J Exp Med 183:2523–2531

Lou Y, Ang J, Thai H, McElveen F, Tung KS (1995) A zona pellucida 3 peptide vaccine induces antibodies and reversible infertility without ovarian pathology. J Immunol 155:2715–2720

Lou Y, Tung KS (1993) T cell peptide of a self-protein elicits autoantibody to the protein antigen. Implications for specificity and pathogenetic role of antibody in autoimmunity. J Immunol 151:5790–5799

Lou YH, McElveen MF, Garza KM, Tung KS (1996) Rapid induction of autoantibodies by endogenous ovarian antigens and activated T cells: implication in autoimmune disease pathogenesis and B cell tolerance. J Immunol 156:3535–3540

Lou YH, Park KK, Agersborg S, Alard P, Tung KS (2000) Retargeting T cell-mediated inflammation: a new perspective on autoantibody action. J Immunol 164:5251–5257

Lu CY, Unanue ER (1982) Ontogeny of murine macrophages: functions related to antigen presentation. Infect Immun 36:169–175

Lyons PA, Armitage N, Argentina F, Denny P, Hill NJ, Lord CJ, Wilusz MB, Peterson LB, Wicker LS, Todd JA (2000) Congenic mapping of the type 1 diabetes locus, Idd3, to a 780-kb region of mouse chromosome 3: identification of a candidate segment of ancestral DNA by haplotype mapping. Genome Res 10:446–453

Ma RZ, Gao J, Meeker ND, Fillmore PD, Tung KS, Watanabe T, Zachary JF, Offner H, Blankenhorn EP, Teuscher C (2002) Identification of Bphs, an autoimmune disease locus, as histamine receptor H1. Science 297:620–623

Mailliard RB, Son YI, Redlinger R, Coates PT, Giermasz A, Morel PA, Storkus WJ, Kalinski P (2003) Dendritic cells mediate NK cell help for Th1 and CTL responses: two-signal requirement for the induction of NK cell helper function. J Immunol 171:2366–2373

Malek TR (2003) The main function of IL-2 is to promote the development of T regulatory cells. J Leukoc Biol 74:961–965

Malek TR, Porter BO, Codias EK, Scibelli P, Yu A (2000) Normal lymphoid homeostasis and lack of lethal autoimmunity in mice containing mature T cells with severely impaired IL-2 receptors. J Immunol 164:2905–2914

Malek TR, Yu A, Vincek V, Scibelli P, Kong L (2002) CD4 regulatory T cells prevent lethal autoimmunity in IL-2Rbeta-deficient mice. Implications for the nonredundant function of IL-2. Immunity 17:167–178

Maloy KJ, Salaun L, Cahill R, Dougan G, Saunders NJ, Powrie F (2003) CD4+CD25+ T(R) cells suppress innate immune pathology through cytokine-dependent mechanisms. J Exp Med 197:111–119

Matesanz F, Alcina A (1996) Glutamine and tetrapeptide repeat variations affect the biological activity of different mouse interleukin-2 alleles. Eur J Immunol 26:1675–1682

Matesanz F, Alcina A (1998) High expression in bacteria and purification of polymorphic mouse interleukin 2 molecules. Cytokine 10:249–253

Matesanz F, Fedetz M, Collado-Romero M, Fernandez O, Guerrero M, Delgado C, Alcina A (2001) Allelic expression and interleukin-2 polymorphisms in multiple sclerosis. J Neuroimmunol 119:101–105

Matesanz F, Fedetz M, Leyva L, Delgado C, Fernandez O, Alcina A (2004) Effects of the multiple sclerosis associated −330 promoter polymorphism in IL2 allelic expression. J Neuroimmunol 148:212–217

McHugh RS, Shevach EM (2002) Cutting edge: depletion of CD4+CD25+ regulatory T cells is necessary, but not sufficient, for induction of organ-specific autoimmune disease. J Immunol 168:5979–5983

McHugh RS, Whitters MJ, Piccirillo CA, Young DA, Shevach EM, Collins M, Byrne MC (2002) CD4(+)CD25(+) immunoregulatory T cells: gene expression analysis reveals a functional role for the glucocorticoid-induced TNF receptor. Immunity 16:311–323

Meeker ND, Hickey WF, Korngold R, Hansen WK, Sudweeks JD, Wardell BB, Griffith JS, Teuscher C (1995) Multiple loci govern the bone marrow-derived immunoregulatory mechanism controlling dominant resistance to autoimmune orchitis. Proc Natl Acad. Sci U S A 92:5684–5688

Min B, McHugh R, Sempowski GD, Mackall C, Foucras G, Paul WE (2003) Neonates support lymphopenia-induced proliferation. Immunity 18:131–140

Mocikat R, Braumuller H, Gumy A, Egeter O, Ziegler H, Reusch U, Bubeck A, Louis J, Mailhammer R, Riethmuller G, Koszinowski U, Rocken M (2003) Natural killer cells activated by MHC class I(low) targets prime dendritic cells to induce protective CD8 T cell responses. Immunity 19:561–569

Morel L, Tian XH, Croker BP, Wakeland EK (1999) Epistatic modifiers of autoimmunity in a murine model of lupus nephritis. Immunity 11:131–139

Morgan DJ, Kurts C, Kreuwel HT, Holst KL, Heath WR, Sherman LA (1999) Ontogeny of T cell tolerance to peripherally expressed antigens. Proc Natl Acad Sci U S A 96:3854–3858

Mottet C, Uhlig HH, Powrie F (2003) Cutting edge: cure of colitis by CD4+CD25+ regulatory T cells. J Immunol 170:3939–3943

Muthukkumar S, Goldstein J, Stein KE (2000) The ability of B cells and dendritic cells to present antigen increases during ontogeny. J Immunol 165:4803–4813

Nakamura K, Kitani A, Strober W (2001) Cell contact-dependent immunosuppression by CD4(+)CD25(+) regulatory T cells is mediated by cell surface-bound transforming growth factor beta. J Exp Med 194:629–644

Nelson BH (2004) IL-2, regulatory T cells, and tolerance. J Immunol 172:3983–3988

Nielsen C, Hansen D, Husby S, Jacobsen BB, Lillevang ST (2003) Association of a putative regulatory polymorphism in the PD-1 gene with susceptibility to type 1 diabetes. Tissue Antigens 62:492–497

Nishimura H, Honjo T, Minato N (2000) Facilitation of beta selection and modification of positive selection in the thymus of PD-1-deficient mice. J Exp Med 191:891–898

Nishimura H, Nose M, Hiai H, Minato N, Honjo T (1999) Development of lupus-like autoimmune diseases by disruption of the PD-1 gene encoding an ITIM motif-carrying immunoreceptor. Immunity 11:141–151

Nishimura H, Okazaki T, Tanaka Y, Nakatani K, Hara M, Matsumori A, Sasayama S, Mizoguchi A, Hiai H, Minato N, Honjo T (2001) Autoimmune dilated cardiomyopathy in PD-1 receptor-deficient mice. Science 291:319–322

Nishizuka Y, Sakakura T (1969) Thymus and reproduction: sex-linked dysgenesia of the gonad after neonatal thymectomy in mice. Science 166:753–755

Okazaki T, Iwai Y, Honjo T (2002) New regulatory co-receptors: inducible co-stimulator and PD-1. Curr Opin Immunol 14:779–782

Okazaki T, Tanaka Y, Nishio R, Mitsuiye T, Mizoguchi A, Wang J, Ishida M, Hiai H, Matsumori A, Minato N, Honjo T (2003) Autoantibodies against cardiac troponin I are responsible for dilated cardiomyopathy in PD-1-deficient mice. Nat Med 9:1477–1483

Ortaldo JR, Winkler-Pickett R, Wiegand G (2000) Activating Ly-49D NK receptors: expression and function in relation to ontogeny and Ly-49 inhibitor receptors. J Leukoc Biol 68:748–756

Parham P (ed) (2001) Regulatory T cells. Immunol Rev 182

Park HB, Paik DJ, Jang E, Hong S, Youn J (2004) Acquisition of anergic and suppressive activities in transforming growth factor-beta-costimulated CD4+. Int Immunol 16:1203–1213

Pasare C, Medzhitov R (2003) Toll pathway-dependent blockade of CD4+CD25+ T cell-mediated suppression by dendritic cells. Science 299:1033–1036

Penhale WJ, Farmer A, McKenna RP, Irvine WJ (1973) Spontaneous thyroiditis in thymectomized and irradiated Wistar rats. Clin Exp Immunol 15:225–236

Penhale WJ, Irvine WJ, Inglis JR, Farmer A (1976) Thyroiditis in T cell-depleted rats: suppression of the autoallergic response by reconstitution with normal lymphoid cells. Clin Exp Immunol 25:6–16

Penhale WJ, Stumbles PA, Huxtable CR, Sutherland RJ, Pethick DW (1990) Induction of diabetes in PVG/c strain rats by manipulation of the immune system. Autoimmunity 7:169–179

Piccioli D, Sbrana S, Melandri E, Valiante NM (2002) Contact-dependent stimulation and inhibition of dendritic cells by natural killer cells. J Exp Med 195:335–341

Piccirillo CA, Letterio JJ, Thornton AM, McHugh RS, Mamura M, Mizuhara H, Shevach EM (2002) CD4(+)CD25(+) Regulatory T cells can mediate suppressor function in the absence of transforming growth factor beta1 production and responsiveness. J Exp Med 196:237–246

Pluger EB, Boes M, Alfonso C, Schroter CJ, Kalbacher H, Ploegh HL, Driessen C (2002) Specific role for cathepsin S in the generation of antigenic peptides in vivo. Eur J Immunol 32:467–476

Podolin PL, Wilusz MB, Cubbon RM, Pajvani U, Lord CJ, Todd JA, Peterson LB, Wicker LS, Lyons PA (2000) Differential glycosylation of interleukin 2, the molecular basis for the NOD Idd3 type 1 diabetes gene? Cytokine 12:477–482

Prokunina L, Castillejo-Lopez C, Oberg F, Gunnarsson I, Berg L, Magnusson V, Brookes AJ, Tentler D, Kristjansdottir H, Grondal G, Bolstad AI, Svenungsson E, Lundberg I, Sturfelt G, Jonssen A, Truedsson L, Lima G, Alcocer-Varela J, Jonsson R, Gyllensten UB, Harley JB, Alarcon-Segovia D, Steinsson K, Alarcon-Riquelme ME (2002) A regulatory polymorphism in PDCD1 is associated with susceptibility to systemic lupus erythematosus in humans. Nat Genet 32:666–669

Prokunina L, Padyukov L, Bennet A, de Faire U, Wiman B, Prince J, Alfredsson L, Klareskog L, Alarcon-Riquelme M (2004) Association of the PD-1.3A allele of the PDCD1 gene in patients with rheumatoid arthritis negative for rheumatoid factor and the shared epitope. Arthritis Rheum 50:1770–1773

Rhodes DA, Trowsdale J (1999) Genetics and molecular genetics of the MHC. Rev Immunogenet 1:21–31

Ridge JP, Fuchs EJ, Matzinger P (1996) Neonatal tolerance revisited: turning on newborn T cells with dendritic cells. Science 271:1723–1726

Roper RJ, Griffith JS, Lyttle CR, Doerge RW, McNabb AW, Broadbent RE, Teuscher C (1999) Interacting quantitative trait loci control phenotypic variation in murine estradiol-regulated responses. Endocrinology 140:556–561

Roper RJ, Ma RZ, Biggins JE, Butterfield RJ, Michael SD, Tung KS, Doerge RW, Teuscher C (2002) Interacting quantitative trait loci control loss of peripheral tolerance and susceptibility to autoimmune ovarian dysgenesis after day 3 thymectomy in mice. J Immunol 169:1640–1646

Roper RJ, McAllister RD, Biggins JE, Michael SD, Min SH, Tung KS, Call SB, Gao J, Teuscher C (2003) Aod1 controlling day 3 thymectomy-induced autoimmune ovarian dysgenesis in mice encompasses two linked quantitative trait loci with opposing allelic effects on disease susceptibility. J Immunol 170:5886–5891

Ruan QG, She JX (2004) Autoimmune polyglandular syndrome type 1 and the autoimmune regulator. Clin Lab Med 24:305–317

Sadlack B, Merz H, Schorle H, Schimpl A, Feller AC, Horak I (1993) Ulcerative colitis-like disease in mice with a disrupted interleukin-2 gene. Cell 75:253–261

Saegusa K, Ishimaru N, Yanagi K, Arakaki R, Ogawa K, Saito I, Katunuma N, Hayashi Y (2002) Cathepsin S inhibitor prevents autoantigen presentation and autoimmunity. J Clin Invest 110:361–369

Sakaguchi S, Fukuma K, Kuribayashi K, Masuda T (1985) Organ-specific autoimmune diseases induced in mice by elimination of T cell subset. I. Evidence for the active participation of T cells in natural self-tolerance; deficit of a T cell subset as a possible cause of autoimmune disease. J Exp Med 161:72–87

Sakaguchi S, Sakaguchi N (1994) Thymus, T cells, and autoimmunity: various causes but a common mechanism of autoimmune disease. In Coutinho A, Kazatchine M (eds) Autoimmunity: physiology and disease. New York: Wiley-Liss, pp 203–227

Sakaguchi S, Sakaguchi N, Asano M, Itoh M, Toda M (1995) Immunologic self-tolerance maintained by activated T cells expressing IL-2 receptor alpha-chains (CD25). Breakdown of a single mechanism of self-tolerance causes various autoimmune diseases. J Immunol 155:1151–1164

Sakaguchi S, Takahashi T, Nishizuka Y (1982) Study on cellular events in post-thymectomy autoimmune oophoritis in mice. II. Requirement of Lyt-1 cells in normal female mice for the prevention of oophoritis. J Exp Med 156:1577–1586

Salama AD, Chitnis T, Imitola J, Ansari MJ, Akiba H, Tushima F, Azuma M, Yagita H, Sayegh MH, Khoury SJ (2003) Critical role of the programmed death-1 (PD-1) pathway in regulation of experimental autoimmune encephalomyelitis. J Exp Med 198:71–78

Sarzotti M, Robbins DS, Hoffman PM (1996) Induction of protective CTL responses in newborn mice by a murine retrovirus. Science 271:1726–1728

Schramm C, Huber S, Protschka M, Czochra P, Burg J, Schmitt E, Lohse AW, Galle PR, Blessing M (2004) TGF(beta) regulates the CD4+CD25+ T-cell pool and the expression of Foxp3 in vivo. Int Immunol 16:1241–1249

Schurmans S, Brighouse G, Kramer G, Wen L, Izui S, Merino J, Lambert PH (1991) Transient T and B cell activation after neonatal induction of tolerance to MHC class II or Mls alloantigens. J Immunol 146:2152–2160

Seddon B, Mason D (1999) Peripheral autoantigen induces regulatory T cells that prevent autoimmunity. J Exp Med 189:877–882

Setiady YY, Pramoonjago P, Tung KS (2004) Requirements of NK cells and proinflammatory cytokines in T cell-dependent neonatal autoimmune ovarian disease triggered by immune complex. J Immunol 173:1051–1058

Setiady YY, Samy ET, Tung KS (2003) Maternal autoantibody triggers de novo T cell-mediated neonatal autoimmune disease. J Immunol 170:4656–4664

Shimizu J, Yamazaki S, Takahashi T, Ishida Y, Sakaguchi S (2002) Stimulation of CD25(+)CD4(+) regulatory T cells through GITR breaks immunological self-tolerance. Nat Immunol 3:135–142

Silveira PA, Baxter AG, Cain WE, van Driel IR (1999) A major linkage region on distal chromosome 4 confers susceptibility to mouse autoimmune gastritis. J Immunol 162:5106–5111

Silveira PA, Wilson WE, Esteban LM, Jordan MA, Hawke CG, van Driel IR, Baxter AG (2001) Identification of the Gasa3 and Gasa4 autoimmune gastritis susceptibility genes using congenic mice and partitioned, segregative and interaction analyses. Immunogenetics 53:741–750

Singh RR, Hahn BH, Sercarz EE (1996) Neonatal peptide exposure can prime T cells and, upon subsequent immunization, induce their immune deviation: implications for antibody vs. T cell-mediated autoimmunity. J Exp Med 183:1613–1621

Sivakumar PV, Gunturi A, Salcedo M, Schatzle JD, Lai WC, Kurepa Z, Pitcher L, Seaman MS, Lemonnier FA, Bennett M, Forman J, Kumar V (1999) Cutting edge: expression of functional CD94/NKG2A inhibitory receptors on fetal NK1.1+Ly-49- cells: a possible mechanism of tolerance during NK cell development. J Immunol 162:6976–6980

Smith H, Lou YH, Lacy P, Tung KS (1992) Tolerance mechanism in experimental ovarian and gastric autoimmune diseases. J Immunol 149:2212–2218

Smith H, Sakamoto Y, Kasai K, Tung KS (1991) Effector and regulatory cells in autoimmune oophoritis elicited by neonatal thymectomy. J Immunol 147:2928–2933

Sonderstrup G, McDevitt HO (2001) DR, DQ, and you: MHC alleles and autoimmunity. J Clin Invest 107:795–796

Sudweeks JD, Todd JA, Blankenhorn EP, Wardell BB, Woodward SR, Meeker ND, Estes SS, Teuscher C (1993) Locus controlling Bordetella pertussis-induced histamine sensitization (Bphs), an autoimmune disease-susceptibility gene, maps distal to T-cell receptor beta-chain gene on mouse chromosome 6. Proc Natl Acad Sci U S A 90:3700–3704

Suri-Payer E, Amar AZ, McHugh R, Natarajan K, Margulies DH, Shevach EM (1999) Post-thymectomy autoimmune gastritis: fine specificity and pathogenicity of anti-H/K ATPase-reactive T cells. Eur J Immunol 29:669–677

Suri-Payer E, Amar AZ, Thornton AM, Shevach EM (1998) CD4+CD25+ T cells inhibit both the induction and effector function of autoreactive T cells and represent a unique lineage of immunoregulatory cells. J Immunol 160:1212–1218

Suri-Payer E, Kehn PJ, Cheever AW, Shevach EM (1996) Pathogenesis of post-thymectomy autoimmune gastritis. Identification of anti-H/K adenosine triphosphatase-reactive T cells. J Immunol 157:1799–1805

Suto A, Nakajima H, Ikeda K, Kubo S, Nakayama T, Taniguchi M, Saito Y, Iwamoto I (2002) CD4(+)CD25(+) T-cell development is regulated by at least 2 distinct mechanisms. Blood 99:555–560

Suvas S, Azkur AK, Kim BS, Kumaraguru U, Rouse BT (2004) CD4(+)CD25(+) regulatory T cells control the severity of viral immunoinflammatory lesions. J Immunol 172:4123–4132

Suzuki H, Kundig TM, Furlonger C, Wakeham A, Timms E, Matsuyama T, Schmits R, Simard JJ, Ohashi PS, Griesser H (1995) Deregulated T cell activation and autoimmunity in mice lacking interleukin-2 receptor beta. Science 268:1472–1476

Taguchi O, Nishizuka Y (1980) Autoimmune oophoritis in thymectomized mice: T cell requirement in adoptive cell transfer. Clin Exp Immunol 42:324–331

Taguchi O, Nishizuka Y (1987) Self tolerance and localized autoimmunity. Mouse models of autoimmune disease that suggest tissue-specific suppressor T cells are involved in self tolerance. J Exp Med 165:146–156

Taguchi O, Nishizuka Y, Sakakura T, Kojima A (1980) Autoimmune oophoritis in thymectomized mice: detection of circulating antibodies against oocytes. Clin Exp Immunol 40:540–553

Takahashi T, Kuniyasu Y, Toda M, Sakaguchi N, Itoh M, Iwata M, Shimizu J, Sakaguchi S (1998) Immunologic self-tolerance maintained by CD25(+)CD4(+) naturally anergic and suppressive T cells: induction of autoimmune disease by breaking their anergic/suppressive state. Int Immunol 10:1969–1980

Teuscher C (1985) Experimental allergic orchitis in mice. II. Association of disease susceptibility with the locus controlling Bordetella pertussis-induced sensitivity to histamine. Immunogenetics 22:417–425

Teuscher C, Bunn JY, Fillmore PD, Butterfield RJ, Zachary JF, Blankenhorn EP (2004) Gender, age and season at immunization uniquely influence the genetic control of susceptibility to histopathological lesions and clinical signs of experimental allergic encephalomyelitis: implications for the genetic of multiple sclerosis. Am J Pathol 16:1593–1602

Teuscher C, Wardell BB, Lunceford JK, Michael SD, Tung KS (1996) Aod2, the locus controlling development of atrophy in neonatal thymectomy-induced autoimmune ovarian dysgenesis, co-localizes with Il2, Fgfb, and Idd3. J Exp Med 183:631–637

Thorstenson KM, Khoruts A (2001) Generation of anergic and potentially immunoregulatory CD25+CD4 T cells in vivo after induction of peripheral tolerance with intravenous or oral antigen. J Immunol 167:188–195

Tong ZB, Nelson LM (1999) A mouse gene encoding an oocyte antigen associated with autoimmune premature ovarian failure. Endocrinology 140:3720–3726

Tung KS (1994) Mechanism of self-tolerance and events leading to autoimmune disease and autoantibody response. Clin Immunol Immunopathol 73:275–282

Tung KS, Agersborg SS, Alard P, Garza KM, Lou YH (2001) Regulatory T-cell, endogenous antigen and neonatal environment in the prevention and induction of autoimmune disease. Immunol Rev 182:135–148

Tung KS, Lou YH, Garza KM, Teuscher C (1997) Autoimmune ovarian disease: mechanism of disease induction and prevention. Curr Opin Immunol 9:839–845

Tung KS, Smith S, Teuscher C, Cook C, Anderson RE (1987) Murine autoimmune oophoritis, epididymoorchitis, and gastritis induced by day 3 thymectomy. Immunopathology. Am J Pathol 126:293–302

Wardell BB, Michael SD, Tung KS, Todd JA, Blankenhorn EP, McEntee K, Sudweeks JD, Hansen WK, Meeker ND, Griffith JS (1995) Aod1, the immunoregulatory locus controlling abrogation of tolerance in neonatal thymectomy-induced autoimmune ovarian dysgenesis, maps to mouse chromosome 16. Proc Natl Acad Sci U S A 92:4758–4762

Wendell DL, Gorski J (1997) Quantitative trait loci for estrogen-dependent pituitary tumor growth in the rat. Mamm Genome 8:823–829

Willerford DM, Chen J, Ferry JA, Davidson L, Ma A, Alt FW (1995) Interleukin-2 receptor alpha chain regulates the size and content of the peripheral lymphoid compartment. Immunity 3:521–530

Yamagiwa S, Gray JD, Hashimoto S, Horwitz DA (2001) A role for TGF-beta in the generation and expansion of CD4+CD25+ regulatory T cells from human peripheral blood. J Immunol 166:7282–7289

Yeung RS, Penninger J, Mak TW (1993) Genetically modified animals and immunodeficiency. Curr Opin Immunol 5:585–594

Zelenika D, Adams E, Humm S, Graca L, Thompson S, Cobbold SP, Waldmann H (2002) Regulatory T cells overexpress a subset of Th2 gene transcripts. J Immunol 168:1069–1079

Zeng ZB (1993) Theoretical basis for separation of multiple linked gene effects in mapping quantitative trait loci. Proc Natl Acad Sci U S A 90:10972–10976

Zeng ZB (1994) Precision mapping of quantitative trait loci. Genetics 136:1457–1468

Zhou P, Cao H, Smart M, David C (1993) Molecular basis of genetic polymorphism in major histocompatibility complex-linked proteasome gene (Lmp-2) Proc Natl Acad Sci U S A 90:2681–2684

Regulatory T Cells in Transplantation Tolerance

H. Waldmann (✉) · L. Graca · E. Adams · P. Fairchild · S. Cobbold

Sir William Dunn School of Pathology, South Parks Road, Oxford OX1 3RE, UK
herman.waldmann@path.ox.ac.uk

1	Aim	250
2	Introduction	250
2.1	Overview	250
2.2	Rejuvenation of Research into Regulatory T Cells in Transplantation	251
3	Dominant Tolerance Can Be Associated with Linked Suppression	251
4	How Does Co-receptor Blockade Set up the Regulatory Pathway?	252
5	The Controversial Issue of the Phenotype of Regulatory T Cells That Mediate Transplantation Tolerance	253
5.1	Regulatory T Cells Within the Tolerated Grafts	254
6	How Might Persistent Exposure to Donor Antigens Promote Infectious Tolerance?	257
7	At What Stage Do Regulatory T Cells Block Graft Rejection In Vivo?	259
8	What Are Regulatory T Cells Doing in the Tissues?	260
9	Conclusions	261
	References	261

Abstract Our ability to harness tolerance mechanisms will have a major impact in organ transplantation if it becomes possible to minimize drug maintenance, or even wean off immunosuppressive drugs. An improved understanding of the biology of regulatory T cells will make it possible to replace current induction regimens with those favouring the vaccination and selection of T cells that prevent graft rejection. Once tolerance is established, the continuous supply of graft antigens should sustain T cell mediated regulation as the dominant mechanism preventing graft rejection.

1
Aim

In this chapter we aim to summarize what we think we know about mechanisms underlying *regulation* and *infectious tolerance* in transplantation. More important, we will attempt to highlight uncertainties in our knowledge. We hope that this chapter will be one of many that will bury the unhealthy scepticism that has surrounded this field over the past 15 years.

2
Introduction

2.1
Overview

Currently the successful transplantation of organs is critically dependent on the long-term use of combinations of immunosuppressive drugs. These drugs not only penalize the whole immune system, but also inflict a wide range of unwanted side effects, some of which limit the life of the transplanted organ and indeed the patient. One of the major goals in improving immunosuppressive therapy is to be able to harness tolerance processes so as to minimize the number, dose and frequency of maintenance drugs. Full tolerance would be the ideal, but this might be hard to achieve as a routine procedure.

Following Medawar's classical description of acquired tolerance in the neonatal mouse (Billingham et al. 1953), it has long been recognized that one route to tolerance would be to establish a state of mixed (host + donor) chimerism using a source of donor stem cells as the tolerizing inoculum. This strategy is based on the notion that one would need to delete or inactivate all host alloreactive T cells. This may be difficult to achieve without aggressive manipulation of the blood and immune systems (Waldmann and Cobbold 2004). The alternative, but not mutually exclusive, strategy derives from the discovery in rodent models that regulatory T cells can be harnessed to prevent allograft rejection, even in the presence of potential effector cells within the host. This necessitates the generation of regulatory T cells sufficient in both numbers and potency to dominate over effector T cells (Waldmann 2002; Zheng et al. 2003). To do this, we need to understand the biology of regulatory T cells, how they are affected by immunosuppressive drugs, and how they might be amplified by selective vaccination for therapeutic purposes. Future immunosuppressive therapies should be directed to maximizing the function of these T cells in synergy with selected immunosuppressive and anti-inflammatory drugs.

2.2
Rejuvenation of Research into Regulatory T Cells in Transplantation

Historically, there has been much confusion about the phenotype of regulatory T cells, much of the early work implicating $CD8^+$ T cells in suppressive function (Gershon and Kondo 1971; Gershon 1975). These early claims preceded the development of monoclonal antibodies, and were very dependent on the limitations of the, then available, alloantisera that lacked reagents which could distinguish $CD4^+$ T cells. The first indication that $CD4^+$ T cells might mediate suppression in transplantation came from adoptive transfer studies showing that splenic $CD4^+$ T cells from rats, holding long-term grafts after treatment with cyclosporin A, could suppress rejection by naive lymphocytes (Hall et al. 1985). This was followed by the finding that mice rendered tolerant to skin grafts by co-receptor (anti-CD4 + anti-CD8) blockade, contained within them $CD4^+$ T cells that could prevent rejection by freshly infused naive T cells (Qin et al. 1993). $CD4^+$ T cells from tolerant animals could suppress rejection by naive splenocytes, or indeed separately purified $CD4^+$ or $CD8^+$ T cells on adoptive transfer (Qin et al. 1993; Davies et al. 1996b; Marshall et al. 1996). Using genetically marked T cells, it could be shown that naive T cells introduced into tolerant animals themselves became tolerant, and over time, they too showed suppressive function in preventing rejection by a further cohort of newly introduced naive T cells (Qin et al. 1993). As tolerance and suppression could be passed on from one population of T cells to naive T cells, we termed this phenomenon infectious tolerance. This was a different usage of the term to that first coined by Gershon (Gershon and Kondo 1971), where he simply used it as an alternative to "suppression". Since that time, infectious tolerance has been demonstrated in models of skin (Qin et al. 1993), marrow (Bemelman et al. 1998), and heart transplantation (Chen et al. 1996), and not only across multiple minor, but also across MHC, incompatibilities. The same outcome could also be elicited by so-called co-stimulation blockade with CD40L antibodies (Honey et al. 1999; Graca et al. 2000).

3
Dominant Tolerance Can Be Associated with Linked Suppression

Animals rendered tolerant to skin grafts through co-receptor, co-stimulation or combined blockade of both, demonstrate an impaired capacity to reject grafts that carry third-party antigens combined with the tolerated set (Chen et al. 1996; Davies et al. 1996a; Bemelman et al. 1998; Honey et al. 1999; Graca et al. 2002b). In other words, A-strain animals tolerant of B-type grafts become able to accept $(BxC)F_1$ grafts, and can in time, become tolerant of C-type antigens without further immunosuppressive treatment. Linked suppression was shown to be mediated by CD4$^+$ T cells.

In transplantation, the immune system is confronted with two sets of antigens, those which are presented directly on graft derived cells (direct presentation), and those that are reprocessed by host dendritic cells (indirect presentation). In vivo studies have clearly demonstrated that T cells that mediate linked suppression can make use of donor alloantigens processed through the indirect pathway (Wise et al. 1998).

When tolerant T cells are removed from the graft-bearing host and parked in T cell deficient animals, they lose their tolerant state unless the tolerizing antigen is restored (Scully et al. 1994; Cobbold et al. 1996). Removal of antigen also appears to reduce the "memory" state for regulation (Onodera et al. 1998). This may mean that the regulatory T cells require antigen to stay alive or need antigen to stay activated and suppressive.

These findings suggest that host dendritic cells, even in a quiescent state, are continuously involved in maintaining dominant regulation, with the implication that the signalling needs of regulatory T cells might be less stringent than those of T cells destined to reject the graft (Waldmann et al. 2004). We will return to this issue when we discuss the form of antigen needed to drive regulation.

4
How Does Co-receptor Blockade Set up the Regulatory Pathway?

Although co-receptor blockade can be used to elicit tolerance to allografts, T cells taken from the treated animal, early on in the induction period, still remain competent to reject [when adoptively transferred to T cell depleted hosts (Scully et al. 1994)]. This suggests that co-receptor blockade has two operational functions: namely to restrain T cells from mounting aggressive responses in the first instance, and following that, to create the conditions that selectively promote regulation.

Recent work using TCR transgenic mice has given us some insights into mechanisms that underlie these events. Female A1.RAG1$^{-/-}$ TCR transgenic mice contain a monoclonal T cell population bearing a single TCR that recognizes the male DBY peptide (Zelenika et al. 1998; Scott et al. 2000). Female mice reject male grafts, but can be easily tolerized by co-receptor blockade with a nondepleting CD4 antibody. Animals tolerized in this way maintain their male grafts even after a challenge infusion of naive T cells, indicating that resistance and dominant tolerance have been established (Cobbold et al. 2004). CD4$^+$CD25$^+$ and foxP3-expressing regulatory T cells can be demonstrated in both the tolerated grafts and in the spleen. As these mice normally have no such T cells in their thymus or in their periphery, they must have been induced as a result of the treatment. Quite remarkably, however, tolerance induction could be prevented by antibody neutralization of TGFβ during the induction phase (Cobbold et al. 2004).

In-vitro analysis of the process has shown that what we think of as co-receptor blockade is profoundly dependent on the presence of TGFβ. TGFβ neutralization has a major impact on the extent to which proliferation to antigen is inhibited (Cobbold et al. 2004). This hitherto unpredicted role of TGFβ is consistent with the finding that TGFβ may be involved in raising the TCR-signalling threshold (Bommireddy et al. 2003), a role that is amplified or exposed in the presence of co-receptor blockade. Furthermore, TGFβ is able to induce expression of foxP3 mRNA, and to induce both anergy and the capacity to regulate naive TCR transgenic T cells whose TCR are exposed to antigen (Chen et al. 2003; Cobbold et al. 2004).

These findings lead us to conclude that co-receptor blockade in conjunction with an internal source of TGFβ (whose cell source is, as yet, unspecified) is responsible for containing rejection responses, while regulatory T cells (including those which are foxP3$^+$) are induced and expanded in the periphery of the treated animals. In conventional mice that already possess a cohort of natural $CD4^+CD25^+$ regulators, we suggest that the induced regulators probably act in concert with these natural regulators in restraining the rejection process. Graft antigens continuously released from the tolerated tissue, and indirectly processed by host dendritic cells, would be expected to constantly recruit and sustain regulatory T cells, so maintaining dominant tolerance.

5
The Controversial Issue of the Phenotype of Regulatory T Cells That Mediate Transplantation Tolerance

Traditionally, the phenotype of T cells responsible for a known function has been determined by negative and positive selection of such cells, followed by functional testing in adoptive transfer studies. Transfers into T cell replete mice have shown transferrable suppression is mediated by $CD4^+$ T cells from donors tolerized by co-receptor blockade (Chen et al. 1996; Bemelman et al. 1998). This type of analysis does, however, necessitate large numbers of T cells. In order to examine which subpopulations of $CD4^+$ T cells are involved, in-vivo readout systems were developed which would allow the analysis of relatively small numbers of T cells (Graca et al. 2002b; Kingsley et al. 2002; Zheng et al. 2003; Graca et al. 2004). These systems have largely focused on use of lymphocyte-deprived recipients (e.g. nude, T cell-depleted, lightly irradiated, RAG$^{-/-}$ or SCID mice).

Although established in good faith, these readouts may have an inherent defect that would confound the interpretation of results. Recent studies have demonstrated enhanced effector properties of small numbers of naive T cells introduced into lymphopenic mice, through a process termed homeostatic expansion (Barthlott et al. 2003; Stockinger et al. 2004). CD4$^+$CD25$^+$ T cells from tolerant animals are nearly always suppressive in transfers using lymphopenic hosts, but so too are CD4$^+$CD25$^+$ T cells from naive animals (Graca et al. 2004). Although some researchers have claimed alloantigen-specificity of regulatory T cells in such models (Kingsley et al. 2002; Zheng et al. 2003), none have performed criss-cross studies, and where these have been conducted, no clear alloantigen specificity has been demonstrated (Graca et al. 2004). For CD4$^+$CD25$^+$ T cells, this apparent lack of alloantigen specificity might arise as an artefact of homeostatic expansion and/or because the repertoire of the natural CD4$^+$CD25$^+$ population is itself dominated by self-reactivity (Hsieh et al. 2004). If so, then it is quite likely that any alloreactive specificity acquired by induced regulators would be obscured.

CD4$^+$CD25$^+$ T cells are not the only T cells capable of regulation in dominant transplantation tolerance. CD4$^+$CD25$^-$ T cells are also able to act in this way, although they appear be much less efficient (Graca et al. 2002b). However, as CD4$^+$CD25$^-$ T cells contribute more than 90% of the CD4 population, they would be expected to make a very significant contribution to the process. One study has provided some preliminary evidence that CD4$^+$CD25$^+$ and CD4$^+$CD25$^-$ T cells from tolerant donors may indeed synergize, as the regulatory potency of each population when separated was less that when they were together (Graca et al. 2002b). Criss-cross experiments have not been possible with CD4$^+$CD25$^-$ T cells given their propensity to reject the third-party grafts. Therefore the issue of alloantigen specificity in these T cells is also unclear. This can only be resolved if one could isolate the subset of CD4$^+$CD25$^-$ T cells that suppresses, to further analyse their alloantigen specificity.

5.1
Regulatory T Cells Within the Tolerated Grafts

Tolerated grafts are known to harbour regulatory T cells (Graca et al. 2002a). The transfer of such grafts onto lymphocyte-depleted hosts allows these hosts to be re-colonized with T cells that prevent rejection by naive T cells. This suggests that we may gain knowledge of the diversity of regulatory T cells by examining the T cells that reside in the tolerated graft (Cobbold et al. 2003a, 2003b, 2004)

Other types of T cells capable of regulating immune responses have been implicated from a range of in vitro and in vivo studies. One type, characterized through its singular secretion of the cytokine IL-10, has been loosely referred to as a Tr1 cell (Groux et al. 1997; Roncarolo et al. 2003). Tr1-like cells have been shown capable of preventing GVHD (Roncarolo et al. 2003) and graft rejection (Zelenika et al. 2001). The question arises as to whether these T cells also participate in dominant and infectious tolerance.

Since Tr1-like cells lack a unique surface marker to identify them, it is hard to answer this question. Gene expression studies using T cell clones from the transgenic mouse cited above indicate that Tr1-like cells are related to Th2 T cells, differing only in that certain genes are under-expressed (e.g. GATA-3), while other genes are over-expressed but not unique (Zelenika et al. 2002; Cobbold et al. 2003b). However, Tr1-like clones can be grown from the skin of tolerated grafts, suggesting that they are indeed present. Other studies indicating that anti-IL10R antibodies may also block suppression are consistent with a role for IL-10 (Kingsley et al. 2002). Given the potential promiscuous origins of IL-10 in such systems, it has been difficult to establish whether or not Tr1 T cells are relevant. The identification of ROG (repressor of GATA) as a potential marker of Tr1-like cells may prove helpful in this context (Cobbold et al. 2003a, 2003b).

In summary, there is evidence that $CD4^+CD25^+foxP3^+$ T cells (both natural and induced) participate in dominant transplantation tolerance and that Tr1-like cells are also capable of suppressing graft rejection. Our current synthesis of how co-stimulation blockade may induce these regulatory T cells in transplantation tolerance is depicted in Fig. 1. There is, however, compelling evidence that other regulatory T cell populations may also be involved, depending on the circumstances and microenvironments of antigen exposure. Figure 2 summarizes the four main types of regulatory T cells that have been defined so far and some of their known mechanisms of action. The "natural" regulatory T cells originally recognized by their constitutive expression of CD4 and CD25 are further defined by expression of the transcription factor foxP3 and surface CD152 (Hori et al. 2003). Their generation and some of their suppressive activity is dependent on TGFβ and it has been shown that they can induce IDO in appropriate DCs by CD152-mediated ligation of CD80/86 (Mellor et al. 2004). TGFβ-producing Th3 cells (Weiner 2001) may also be related to this population. Anergic $CD4^+$ T cells generated by antigen stimulation in the absence of co-stimulation seem to be characterized by an intrinsic raising of their threshold for antigen stimulation, which may be maintained by expression of E3 ubiquitin ligases such as GRAIL, c-cbl and Itch (Mueller 2004). Anergic cells can act as regulatory T cells by competing at the sites of antigen presentation and adsorbing out stimulatory cytokines

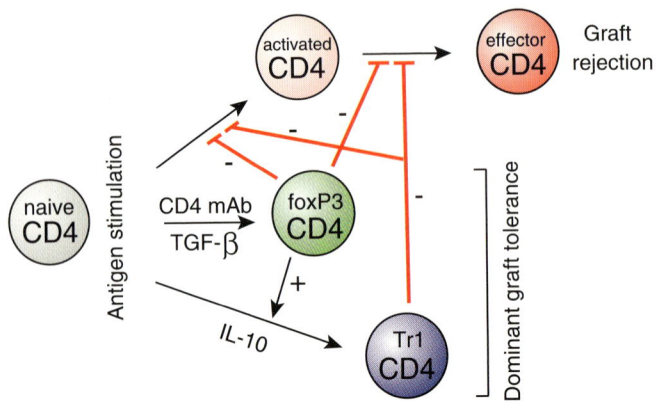

Fig. 1 Induction of tolerance and regulatory T cells by CD4 blockade. Effective antigen stimulation of CD4⁺ T cells would normally lead to activation, proliferation and eventual differentiation into effector T cells, which would lead to graft rejection. It has now been clearly demonstrated that in the presence of antigen and CD4 mAb blockade, the naïve T cells are able to acquire expression of the transcription factor foxP3, which is known to be sufficient to induce regulatory T cell activity. This induction of foxP3 is a TGFβ-dependent process, although the source of TGFβ is not yet defined. Skin graft tolerance is initially dependent on the presence of TGFβ and the generation of these foxP3⁺ CD25⁺ regulatory T cells, but there is accumulating evidence that robust transplantation tolerance may further involve the presence of IL-10-dependent, foxP3⁻ Tr1-like cells. It remains to be determined whether foxP3⁺ T cells directly recruit Tr1-like cells or act by allowing Tr-1 cells to develop as a result of longer graft survival. It can be demonstrated that either Tr1 or foxP3⁺ T cells are able to suppress graft rejection and that both populations are able to act on both the inductive (activation/proliferation) and differentiated (IFN-γ and cytotoxicity) functions of effector T cells

and chemokines (Lombardi et al. 1994; Taams and Wauben 2000; James et al. 2003). Tr1 cells represent an induced subset of CD4⁺ helper T cells that are dependent on IL-10 for their differentiation and for some of their regulatory properties (Groux et al. 1997). They do not express foxP3 but may express markers associated with Th2 cells and repressor of GATA (ROG) (Zelenika et al. 2002). Like natural Tregs, they express high levels of surface CD152 and can induce IDO and trypophan catabolism in appropriate DCs (Mellor et al. 2004). CD8⁺CD28⁻ suppressor T (Ts) cells were first characterized in humans, but have recently also been demonstrated in rodents. Like Tr1 cells, they are induced in the presence of IL-10, and IL-10 may be involved in the downregulation of dendritic cell co-stimulation and the upregulation of ILT-3 and ILT-4 (in human dendritic cells) that seem to play an important role in presenting antigen to tolerize further cohorts of T cells (Manavalan et al. 2004).

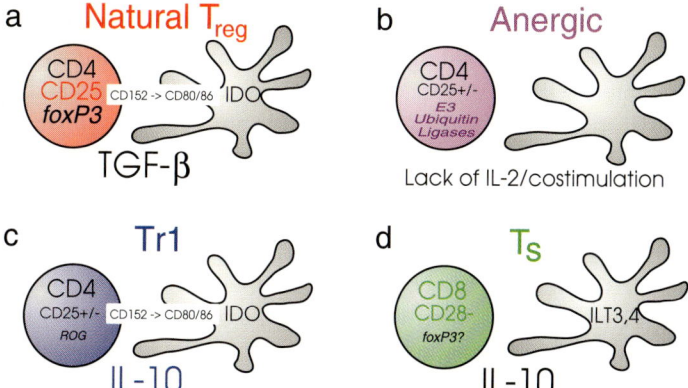

Fig. 2A–D Mechanisms of action of the different regulatory T cell subsets. Four of the major regulatory T cell subsets that have been described are depicted in the left of each panel (**A–D**) together with their appropriate antigen presenting cells on the right. **A** The "natural" $CD4^+DC25^+foxP3^+$ regulatory T cells. **B** Anergic $CD4^+$ T cells competing for antigen presentation. **C** Tr1 cells representing an induced subset of $CD4^+$ helper T cells that are dependent on IL-10. **D** $CD8^+CD28^-$ suppressor T (T_s) cells that induce ILT3 and ILT4 in dendritic cells

6
How Might Persistent Exposure to Donor Antigens Promote Infectious Tolerance?

In considering how infectious tolerance might arise, we need to remind ourselves that once the graft is healed, it remains a permanent source of antigen, which will be constitutively processed by dendritic cells in the local lymphoid tissue and, indeed, in the graft itself. As these dendritic cells would have no source of inflammatory (or danger) signals to activate them, they should be providing a constant source of low immunogenicity antigen to T cells without the co-stimulatory signals needed to activate T cell aggression. We have proposed that persistent exposure of T cells to antigens that cannot signal fully may result in T cells being driven towards anergy, and some of these may be polarized towards becoming regulatory T cells (Waldmann et al. 2004).

We tested this hypothesis by deriving an altered peptide ligand (APL) of the DBY male peptide. This ligand was a poor stimulator of T cells in vitro. However, multiple doses of APL given in vivo to female A1.RAG-$1^{-/-}$ mice resulted in these mice becoming tolerant to male skin grafts, such tolerance showing dominant features reflected through resistance to rejection by naive T cells, and with evidence of newly induced $foxP3^+CD4^+CD25^+$ T cells in the tolerated graft and spleen (Chen et al. 2004b).

In another related model, female TCR$^+$ T cells injected into male RAG-1$^{-/-}$ hosts became remarkably anergic to in vitro stimulation by male peptide, and were potently suppressive in vitro (Chen et al. 2004a). We could find no foxp3 mRNA nor CD25$^+$ T cells in the spleen, nor could the splenic T cells produce IL-10 in vitro. This suggests that regulatory T cells can be generated by persistent stimulation by antigen, and that such T cells need not be the conventional foxP3$^+$CD25$^+$ nor Tr1-like cells. Here is an example of a T cell population that is profoundly anergic but that can also be powerfully suppressive through an as yet undetermined mechanism. Such T cells behave as "civil servants", where anergic T cells compete for effector T cells in the model for T cell regulation that we proposed over a decade ago (Waldmann et al. 1992). We were then trying to explain results where we had used co-receptor blockade to establish low-level donor chimerism, where tolerant animals could be shown to have (Mls) antigen-specific anergic T cells in the periphery, evidence of resistance to breakdown of tolerance by naive T cells, and to boosting by further challenge with immunogen (Qin et al. 1989).

Our overall interpretation of these data is that when T cells perceive antigen in circumstances where they cannot be fully stimulated, and when that stimulation is persistent, it is likely that a proportion of these T cells will develop into regulatory T cells. We propose that the local micro-environment of cytokines will determine the type of regulatory T cells which emerges. The presence of TGFβ may encourage polarization towards foxP3$^+$CD25$^+$ T cells, and of IL-10 the development of Tr1-like cells. There may yet be other routes of polarization that have not yet been recognized.

This hypothesis provides some symmetry between the initial induction phase of tolerization and the maintenance phase. We propose that in the induction phase, drugs and antibodies that can induce tolerance do so by partially blocking signalling. If, in that induction period, the exposure to antigen has resulted in some potentially aggressive clones being deleted, others anergized, and yet others polarized to become regulatory T cells, then the balance of regulation to effector function could be permanently reset in favour of tolerance. Processed antigens from the healed graft would continue to recruit new naive T cells into regulatory activity, so ensuring that regulation would continue to stay dominant through infectious tolerance. This model would predict many different drug regimens capable of generating dominant tolerance. However, tolerance once established would be maintained by a distinct set of mechanisms wholly determined by the nature of donor antigen exposure to the immune system in its constitutive resting mode. The model would also argue that linked suppression and infectious tolerance are facets of the same biological processes (Fig. 3).

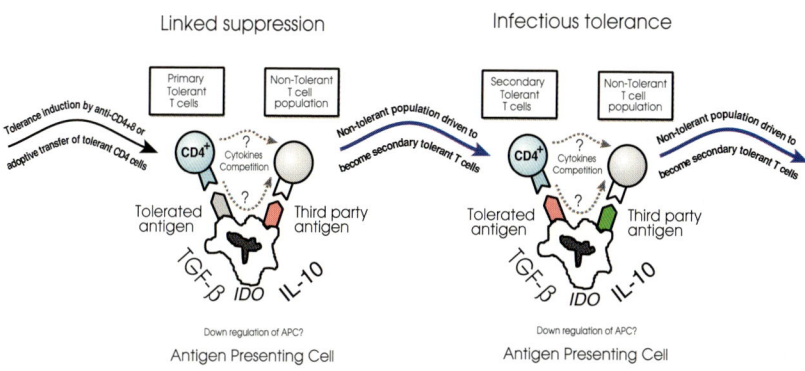

Fig. 3 Linked suppression and infectious tolerance. Tolerance can be induced either by exposing T cells to antigen under the cover of nondepleting CD4 and CD8 monoclonal antibodies (co-receptor blockade) or by the adoptive transfer of an excess of tolerant/regulatory CD4$^+$ T cells. These primary tolerant T cells are able suppress the response of nontolerant T cells that are recognizing third-party antigens expressed on the same antigen-presenting cells. This suppression may be dependent on a number of factors, including the production of modulatory cytokines by the tolerant T cells, competition for antigen presentation, and the state of the local microenvironment that includes factors such as the presence of TGFβ, IL-10 or the utilization of tryptophan by indoleamine dioxygenase (*IDO*) expressed by modulated antigen-presenting cells. The result of suppression is the generation of a fresh cohort of CD4$^+$ regulatory T cells that can continue to act sequentially on further cohorts of naïve T cell populations in a similar fashion during the process known as infectious tolerance

Drugs that totally block T cell signalling might themselves interfere with the development of tolerance and regulation. We suggest that all currently available and future immunosuppressive drugs should be monitored for their ability to antagonize as well synergize in the induction of regulatory T cells.

7
At What Stage Do Regulatory T Cells Block Graft Rejection In Vivo?

CD4$^+$CD25$^+$ regulatory T cells, whether natural (Sakaguchi et al. 1995) or induced, have the ability to block T cell proliferation in vitro (Piccirillo and Shevach 2004), as indeed do Tr1-like cells (Roncarolo et al. 2003). This has led to the widespread assumption that proliferation blockade is the mechanism of suppression in vivo. Indeed there are some data tracking TCR transgenic cells in vivo consistent with that idea (Lee et al. 2004).

However, we observed this not to be the case in dominant tolerance induced by co-receptor and co-stimulation blockade (Lin et al. 2002). CBA/Ca

($H-2^k$) mice rendered tolerant to MHC-mismatched C57Bl/10 skin grafts were injected with CFSE-labelled $CD8^+$ T cells from a TCR transgenic mouse (on a CBA/Ca background) with specificity for the MHC Class I molecule K^b. These mice were then challenged with splenic dendritic cells from C57Bl/10 (the tolerated donor type). Evidence was obtained that these T cells proliferated normally, accumulated in normal numbers (indicating that the T cells had benefited from $CD4^+$ help), but that they failed to develop into T cells with effector function, lacking cytotoxicity, exhibiting low IFNγ production, and failing to reject grafts. These findings suggest that dominant tolerance mechanisms may indeed act downstream of the proliferative signals. This implies that a key function in differentiation of T cell effector function provides the most sensitive target for regulatory T cell activity, and that the elucidation of this mechanism should be a priority for research in this field.

8
What Are Regulatory T Cells Doing in the Tissues?

Although it may just be a fortuitous finding that regulatory T cells can localize to tolerated grafts, there is no reason to think that these T cells do not exert regulatory function within the tolerated tissue. We have proposed (Waldmann et al. 2004) that regulatory T cells interact with tissues to create a state of acquired immunological privilege which enables tissues to resist potentially damaging immune reactions. Recently, a similar idea has been proposed for the way that tumours may resist immunological control (Curiel et al. 2004). It has been proposed that tumour-derived chemokines such as CCL22, interacting with CCR4 receptors on regulatory T cells, selectively attract such T cells into tumour sites. Clearly transplanted tissues should not just be thought of as passive targets for immune attack, but as organs capable of interacting with the immune system to influence the types of immune response that can occur within them. The first example of one such mechanism of acquired privilege is that of inducing the expression of the enzyme indoleamine dioxygenase (IDO) in antigen-presenting cells. IDO by catabolism of tryptophan and/or generation of tryptophan metabolites can prevent local T cell function. In both published examples (Fallarino et al. 2003; Mellor et al. 2003, 2004), regulatory T cells (be they natural $CD4^+CD25^+$ or Tr1-like cells) mediate this effect through their surface CTLA4, interacting with complementary receptors on dendritic cells or monocytes. We speculate that this may be only one of many mechanisms of this kind, and have proposed that a number of others, e.g. interference with chemokine synthesis and function, should be sought (Fig. 3). An extension of this idea is that regulatory T cells set up a series of privileged microenvironments wherever they interact with antigen-presenting cells, and these microenvironments, be they in lymphoid tissues or in the graft, are responsible for ensuring acquired privilege and tissue protection. In so doing they perpetuate the processes of infectious tolerance.

9
Conclusions

It seems unlikely that the regulatory T cells that we have uncovered in transplantation tolerance arose for the purpose of graft protection (unless they play some crucial role in preventing abortion of the allogeneic foetus). More likely, they are by-products of mechanisms that evolved to guarantee self-tolerance. Whatever their physiological role, it is clear that the goal of drug minimization for the control of transplant rejection will be much facilitated by harnessing these cells and their regulatory mechanisms. Despite the protestations of some, regulatory T cells are here to stay, and harnessing their activity offers substantial optimism for the future of the field of transplantation.

References

Barthlott T, Kassiotis G, Stockinger B (2003) T cell regulation as a side effect of homeostasis and competition. J Exp Med 197:451–460

Bemelman F, Honey K, Adams E, Cobbold S, Waldmann H (1998) Bone marrow transplantation induces either clonal deletion or infectious tolerance depending on the dose. J Immunol 160:2645–2648

Billingham RE, Brent L, Medawar PB (1953) Actively acquired tolerance of foreign cells. Nature 172:603–606

Bommireddy R, Ormsby I, Yin M, Boivin GP, Babcock GF, Doetschman T (2003) TGF beta 1 inhibits Ca^{2+}-calcineurin-mediated activation in thymocytes. J Immunol 170:3645–3652

Chen TC, Cobbold SP, Fairchild PJ, Waldmann H (2004a) Generation of anergic and regulatory T cells following prolonged exposure to a harmless antigen. J Immunol 172:5900–5907

Chen TC, Waldmann H, Fairchild PJ (2004b) Induction of dominant transplantation tolerance by an altered peptide ligand of the male antigen Dby. J Clin Invest 113:1754–1762

Chen W, Jin W, Hardegen N, Lei K, Li L, Marinos N, McGrady G, Wahl S (2003) Conversion of peripheral $CD4^+CD25^-$ naive T cells to $CD4^+CD25^+$ regulatory T cells by TGF-beta induction of transcription factor Foxp3. J Exp Med 198:1875–1886

Chen ZK, Cobbold SP, Waldmann H, Metcalfe S (1996) Amplification of natural regulatory immune mechanisms for transplantation tolerance. Transplantation 62:1200–1206

Cobbold SP, Adams E, Marshall SE, Davies JD, Waldmann H (1996) Mechanisms of peripheral tolerance and suppression induced by monoclonal antibodies to CD4 and CD8. Immunol Rev 149:5–33

Cobbold SP, Adams E, Graca L, Waldmann H (2003a) Serial analysis of gene expression provides new insights into regulatory T cells. Semin Immunol 15:209–214

Cobbold SP, Nolan KF, Graca L, Castejon R, Le Moine A, Frewin M, Humm S, Adams E, Thompson S, Zelenika D, Paterson A, Yates S, Fairchild PJ, Waldmann H (2003b) Regulatory T cells and dendritic cells in transplantation tolerance: molecular markers and mechanisms. Immunol Rev 196:109–124

Cobbold SP, Castejon R, Adams E, Zelenika D, Graca L, Humm S, Waldmann H (2004) Induction of foxP3+ regulatory T cells in the periphery of T cell receptor transgenic mice tolerized to transplants. J Immunol 172:6003–6010

Curiel TJ, Coukos G, Zou L, Alvarez X, Cheng P, Mottram P, Evdemon-Hogan M, Conejo-Garcia JR, Zhang L, Burow M, Zhu Y, Wei S, Kryczek I, Daniel B, Gordon A, Myers L, Lackner A, Disis ML, Knutson KL, Chen L, Zou W (2004) Specific recruitment of regulatory T cells in ovarian carcinoma fosters immune privilege and predicts reduced survival. Nat Med 10:942–949

Davies JD, Leong LY, Mellor A, Cobbold SP, Waldmann H (1996a) T cell suppression in transplantation tolerance through linked recognition. J Immunol 156:3602–3607

Davies JD, Martin G, Phillips J, Marshall SE, Cobbold SP, Waldmann H (1996b) T cell regulation in adult transplantation tolerance. J Immunol 157:529–533

Fallarino F, Grohmann U, Hwang KW, Orabona C, Vacca C, Bianchi R, Belladonna ML, Fioretti MC, Alegre ML, Puccetti P (2003) Modulation of tryptophan catabolism by regulatory T cells. Nat Immunol 4:1206–1212

Gershon RK (1975) A disquisition on suppressor T cells. Transplant Rev 26:170–185

Gershon RK, Kondo K (1971) Infectious immunological tolerance. Immunology 21:903–914

Graca L, Honey K, Adams E, Cobbold SP, Waldmann H (2000) Cutting edge: anti-CD154 therapeutic antibodies induce infectious transplantation tolerance. J Immunol 165:4783–4786

Graca L, Cobbold SP, Waldmann H (2002a) Identification of regulatory T cells in tolerated allografts. J Exp Med 195:1641–1646

Graca L, Thompson S, Lin C, Adams E, Cobbold S, Waldmann H (2002b) Both CD4(+)CD25(+) and CD4(+)CD25(-) regulatory cells mediate dominant transplantation tolerance. J Immunol 168:5558–5565

Graca L, Le Moine A, Lin CY, Fairchild PJ, Cobbold SP, Waldmann H (2004) Donor-specific transplantation tolerance: the paradoxical behavior of CD4$^+$CD25$^+$ T cells. Proc Natl Acad Sci U S A 101:10122–10126

Groux H, O'Garra A, Bigler M, Rouleau M, Antonenko S, de Vries JE, Roncarolo MG (1997) A CD4$^+$ T-cell subset inhibits antigen-specific T-cell responses and prevents colitis. Nature 389:737–742

Hall BM, Jelbart ME, Gurley KE, Dorsch SE (1985) Specific unresponsiveness in rats with prolonged cardiac allograft survival after treatment with cyclosporine. Mediation of specific suppression by T helper/inducer cells. J Exp Med 162:1683–1694

Honey K, Cobbold SP, Waldmann H (1999) CD40 ligand blockade induces CD4$^+$ T cell tolerance and linked suppression. J Immunol 163:4805–4810

Hori S, Nomura T, Sakaguchi S (2003) Control of regulatory T cell development by the transcription factor foxp3. Science 299:1057–1061

Hsieh CS, Liang Y, Tyznik AJ, Self SG, Liggitt D, Rudensky AY (2004) Recognition of the peripheral self by naturally arising $CD25^+$ $CD4^+$ T cell receptors. Immunity 21:267–277

James MJ, Belaramani L, Prodromidou K, Datta A, Nourshargh S, Lombardi G, Dyson J, Scott D, Simpson E, Cardozo L, Warrens A, Szydlo RM, Lechler RI, Marelli-Berg FM (2003) Anergic T cells exert antigen-independent inhibition of cell-cell interactions via chemokine metabolism. Blood 102:2173–2179

Kingsley CI, Karim M, Bushell AR, Wood KJ (2002) $CD25^+CD4^+$ regulatory T cells prevent graft rejection: CTLA-4- and IL-10-dependent immunoregulation of alloresponses. J Immunol 168:1080–1086

Lee MKt, Moore DJ, Jarrett BP, Lian MM, Deng S, Huang X, Markmann JW, Chiaccio M, Barker CF, Caton AJ, Markmann JF (2004) Promotion of allograft survival by $CD4^+CD25^+$ regulatory T cells: evidence for in vivo inhibition of effector cell proliferation. J Immunol 172:6539–6544

Lin CY, Graca L, Cobbold SP, Waldmann H (2002) Dominant transplantation tolerance impairs $CD8^+$ T cell function but not expansion. Nat Immunol 3:1208–1213

Lombardi G, Sidhu S, Batchelor R, Lechler R (1994) Anergic T cells as suppressor cells in vitro. Science 264:1587–1589

Manavalan JS, Kim-Schulze S, Scotto L, Naiyer AJ, Vlad G, Colombo PC, Marboe C, Mancini D, Cortesini R, Suciu-Foca N (2004) Alloantigen specific $CD8^+CD28^-$ FOXP3+ T suppressor cells induce ILT3+ ILT4+ tolerogenic endothelial cells, inhibiting alloreactivity. Int Immunol 16:1055–1068

Marshall SE, Cobbold SP, Davies JD, Martin GM, Phillips JM, Waldmann H (1996) Tolerance and suppression in a primed immune system. Transplantation 62:1614–1621

Mellor AL, Baban B, Chandler P, Marshall B, Jhaver K, Hansen A, Koni PA, Iwashima M, Munn DH (2003) Cutting edge: induced indoleamine 2,3 dioxygenase expression in dendritic cell subsets suppresses T cell clonal expansion. J Immunol 171:1652–1655

Mellor AL, Chandler P, Baban B, Hansen AM, Marshall B, Pihkala J, Waldmann H, Cobbold S, Adams E, Munn DH (2004) Specific subsets of murine dendritic cells acquire potent T cell regulatory functions following CTLA4-mediated induction of indoleamine 2,3 dioxygenase. Int Immunol 16:1391–1401

Mueller DL (2004) E3 ubiquitin ligases as T cell anergy factors. Nat Immunol 5:883–890

Onodera K, Volk HD, Ritter T, Kupiec-Weglinski JW (1998) Thymus requirement and antigen dependency in the "infectious" tolerance pathway in transplant recipients. J Immunol 160:5765–5772

Piccirillo CA, Shevach EM (2004) Naturally-occurring $CD4^+CD25^+$ immunoregulatory T cells: central players in the arena of peripheral tolerance. Semin Immunol 16:81–88

Qin S, Cobbold SP, Pope H, Elliott J, Kioussis D, Davies J, Waldmann H (1993) "Infectious" transplantation tolerance. Science 259:974–977

Qin SX, Cobbold S, Benjamin R, Waldmann H (1989) Induction of classical transplantation tolerance in the adult. J Exp Med 169:779–794

Roncarolo MG, Gregori S, Levings M (2003) Type 1 T regulatory cells and their relationship with CD4$^+$CD25$^+$ T regulatory cells. Novartis Found Symp 252:115–127; discussion 127–131, 203–110

Sakaguchi S, Sakaguchi N, Asano M, Itoh M, Toda M (1995) Immunologic self-tolerance maintained by activated T cells expressing IL-2 receptor alpha-chains (CD25). Breakdown of a single mechanism of self-tolerance causes various autoimmune diseases. J Immunol 155:1151–1164

Scott D, Addey C, Ellis P, James E, Mitchell MJ, Saut N, Jurcevic S, Simpson E (2000) Dendritic cells permit identification of genes encoding MHC class II-restricted epitopes of transplantation antigens. Immunity 12:711–720

Scully R, Qin S, Cobbold S, Waldmann H (1994) Mechanisms in CD4 antibody-mediated transplantation tolerance: kinetics of induction, antigen dependency and role of regulatory T cells. Eur J Immunol 24:2383–2392

Stockinger B, Kassiotis G, Bourgeois C (2004) Homeostasis and T cell regulation. Curr Opin Immunol 16:775–779

Taams LS, Wauben MH (2000) Anergic T cells as active regulators of the immune response. Hum Immunol 61:633–639

Waldmann H (2002) Reprogramming the immune system. Immunol Rev 185:227–235

Waldmann H, Cobbold S (2004) Exploiting tolerance processes in transplantation. Science 305:209–212

Waldmann H, Qin S, Cobbold S (1992) Monoclonal antibodies as agents to reinduce tolerance in autoimmunity. J Autoimmun 5 Suppl A:93–102

Waldmann H, Graca L, Cobbold S, Adams E, Tone M, Tone Y (2004) Regulatory T cells and organ transplantation. Semin Immunol 16:119–126

Weiner HL (2001) Induction and mechanism of action of transforming growth factor-beta-secreting Th3 regulatory cells. Immunol Rev 182:207–214

Wise MP, Bemelman F, Cobbold SP, Waldmann H (1998) Linked suppression of skin graft rejection can operate through indirect recognition. J Immunol 161:5813–5816

Zelenika D, Adams E, Humm S, Lin CY, Waldmann H, Cobbold SP (2001) The role of CD4$^+$ T-cell subsets in determining transplantation rejection or tolerance. Immunol Rev 182:164–179

Zelenika D, Adams E, Humm S, Graca L, Thompson S, Cobbold SP, Waldmann H (2002) Regulatory T cells overexpress a subset of Th2 gene transcripts. J Immunol 168:1069–1079

Zelenika D, Adams E, Mellor A, Simpson E, Chandler P, Stockinger B, Waldmann H, Cobbold SP (1998) Rejection of H-Y disparate skin grafts by monospecific CD4$^+$ Th1 and Th2 cells: no requirement for CD8+ T cells or B cells. J Immunol 161:1868–1874

Zheng XX, Sanchez-Fueyo A, Sho M, Domenig C, Sayegh MH, Strom TB (2003) Favorably tipping the balance between cytopathic and regulatory T cells to create transplantation tolerance. Immunity 19:503–514

CD4⁺CD25⁺ Regulatory T Cells in Hematopoietic Stem Cell Transplantation

P. Hoffmann[1] · J. Ermann[2] · M. Edinger[3] (✉)

[1] Institute of Immunology, University Regensburg, Regensburg, Germany
[2] Department of Medicine, University of Tennessee, Memphis, Tennessee, USA
[3] Department of Hematology and Oncology, University Hospital Regensburg, Franz-Josef-Strauss-Allee 11, 93053 Regensburg, Germany
matthias.edinger@klinik.uni-regensburg.de

1	Introduction	266
2	Tolerance and Regulatory T Cells	268
3	CD4⁺CD25⁺ T_{reg} Cells as Modulators of Alloreactivity	268
4	Influence of CD4⁺CD25⁺ T_{reg} Cells on the Graft-Versus-Leukemia/Lymphoma Activity of Donor T Cells	272
5	Reconstitution of the T_{reg} Cell Compartment After Allogeneic Stem Cell Transplantation	275
6	Ex Vivo Expansion of CD4⁺CD25⁺ T_{reg} Cells for Allogeneic Stem Cell Transplantation	276
7	Prerequisites for the Use of CD4⁺CD25^{high} T_{reg} Cells in Clinical Stem Cell Transplantation	278
	References	279

Abstract Allogeneic hematopoietic stem cell transplantation (SCT) is a well-established treatment modality for malignant and nonmalignant hematologic diseases. High-dose radio- and/or chemotherapy eradicate the hematopoietic system of the patient and induce sufficient immunosuppression to enable donor stem cell engraftment. The replacement of the recipient's immune system with that of the donor significantly contributes to the success of this treatment, since donor immune cells facilitate stem cell engraftment, provide protection from infections, and eliminate residual malignant or nonmalignant host hematopoiesis, thereby protecting from disease relapse in patients transplanted for leukemia or lymphoma (graft-versus-leukemia effect, GVL). Mediators of these beneficial effects are mature T cells within the stem cell graft. However, donor T cells can also attack host tissues and induce a life-threatening syndrome called graft-versus-host disease (GVHD). The challenge of allogeneic SCT is to find a balance between beneficial and harmful T cell effects, which at present is only insufficiently achieved by the use of immunosuppressive drugs. In the future, it might be possible to replace or support such medications by using the intrinsic regulatory capacity of the transplanted immune system, as represented by T cell subpopulations with suppressive activity, such as $CD4^+CD25^+$ regulatory T (T_{reg}) cells. In various mouse model systems, these cells have been shown to suppress GVHD while preserving the GVL effect. As the characterization of their human counterparts is rapidly progressing, their application in allogeneic SCT might soon be explored in clinical trials.

1
Introduction

Allogeneic bone marrow or peripheral blood stem cell transplantation is the treatment of choice for a variety of malignant and nonmalignant diseases. Initially designed as organ-replacement therapy for patients with hematologic malignancies, it soon became evident that myeloablation by lethal irradiation and/or high-dose chemotherapy was not the only therapeutic mechanism, but that immunological interactions between donor and recipient cells were jointly responsible for the success of this treatment modality. Mature donor T cells co-transplanted with the stem cell graft play a central role in these immune-mediated effects and contribute to both the benefits and failures of allogeneic stem cell transplantation (SCT). The beneficial effect of donor T cells is documented by their ability to facilitate stem cell engraftment, to protect recipients from opportunistic infections and to eradicate residual host hematopoiesis (graft-versus-hematopoiesis effect), thereby promoting potent anti-tumor activity (graft-versus-leukemia/lymphoma effect, GVL) in patients who receive transplants for malignant diseases (Gratwohl et al. 2002). The negative aspect of co-transplanted donor T cells is their ability to cause immune-mediated organ injury in the recipient, a syndrome with various clinical manifestations generally termed graft-versus-host disease (GVHD). GVHD most frequently affects skin, gut, liver, and the lymphatic system, but can involve any other organ at various frequencies (Vogelsang et al. 2003). While mild forms of GVHD usually respond to immunosuppressive therapy, severe acute and chronic GVHD are still major causes of morbidity and mortality after allogeneic SCT and thus far restrict its widespread use. Thus, the holy grail of allogeneic SCT is the preservation of beneficial donor T cell effects while avoiding severe GVHD.

The pathophysiology of GVHD involves cellular as well as cytokine-mediated mechanisms (Ferrara 2000). Tissue damage and cytokine dysregulation caused by the conditioning of the patient provide a pro-inflammatory environment even before allogeneic T cells enter the body.

Host reactive donor T cells then respond to major or minor histocompatibility antigens consisting of mismatched HLA/peptide complexes (Daniel et al. 1998; Obst et al. 2000; Lechler et al. 2003) or matched HLA molecules loaded with host-specific peptides derived from polymorphic proteins, respectively (Goulmy 1997; Dickinson et al. 2002; Falkenburg et al. 2003). Residual host antigen-presenting cells (APC) play a crucial role for the early activation of donor T cells, since they present the relevant alloantigens and provide potent co-stimulation for the initiation of the alloresponse (Shlomchik et al. 1999; Teshima et al. 2002; Murai et al. 2003; Merad et al. 2004). Depending on the degree of HLA disparity and the (yet unknown) number of protein polymorphisms between donor and recipient, the precursor frequency of alloreactive T cells regularly exceeds that of T cells reacting to environmental antigens (Wang et al. 1996; Suchin et al. 2001). The combination of high precursor frequency, high T cell receptor (TCR) avidity, strong costimulation and a pro-inflammatory cytokine milieu results in the early activation and expansion of alloreactive T cells that further perpetuates the inflammatory process. Responding T cells differentiate into effector cells and either cause target tissue destruction directly or, by modulating the activity of other cell populations of the innate and adaptive immune system, indirectly (Ferrara et al. 1999).

Although donor T cell depletion from the graft reduces the incidence and severity of GVHD, a survival benefit for patients treated with T cell-depleted grafts has not yet been demonstrated due to frequent opportunistic infections (Hertenstein et al. 1995), increased graft rejection rates (Patterson et al. 1986), and high frequencies of tumor relapse (Champlin et al. 2000; Ho and Soiffer 2001). Therefore, several strategies are currently under investigation to reduce the risk of GVHD after allogeneic SCT without loss of the beneficial T cell effects. These include the co-transplantation of limited donor T cell numbers (Dazzi et al. 2000), in vivo blockade of co-stimulatory pathways after T cell transfer (Blazar et al. 1997), the in vitro depletion of host-reactive T cells before transfusion (Chen et al. 2002; Amrolia et al. 2003a; Michalek et al. 2003), or the selective co-transplantation of donor T cells specific for host hematopoietic cells (Amrolia et al. 2003a; Heemskerk et al. 2003), tumor antigens (Savage et al. 2004), or infectious pathogens (Heslop et al. 1994; Rauser et al. 2004), among others. Thus far, none of these experimental strategies is sufficiently reliable, practicable and safe to replace standard GVHD prophylaxis, i.e., unspecific immunosuppressive medication. The high complication rate after prolonged immunosuppression and frequent treatment failures continues to drive the search for improved transplantation strategies.

2
Tolerance and Regulatory T Cells

The majority of patients experience low-grade GVHD after allogeneic SCT, which is either self-limiting or rapidly responsive to therapy, and some patients never show any clinical signs of GVHD. In such patient groups, prophylactic or therapeutic immunosuppressionwithin a few months after SCT. Absence of GVHD after cessation of immunosuppression documents the development of a stable state of tolerance of the donor immune system toward the host. In fact, hematopoietic SCT is the most efficient way to induce tolerance to alloantigens, mainly by deletion of host-reactive T cells that develop from donor-derived precursors in the recipient's thymus (Ildstad and Sachs 1984; Salaun et al. 1990). Central tolerance mechanisms and the problems associated with the recovery of immune competence after transplantation have been reviewed elsewhere (Sprent and Kishimoto 2001; Sykes and Sachs 2001). In contrast, mature donor T cells within the stem cell graft are generally not tolerant toward recipient antigens and thus initiate GVHD, as detailed above. However, peripheral tolerance mechanisms that prevent autoimmunity or contribute to tolerance induction after solid organ transplantation are also operational in allogeneic SCT and eventually confine such alloaggression. These mechanisms include activation-induced cell death, clonal exhaustion, T cell anergy, or ignorance and peripheral deletion (Rocha and von Boehmer 1991; Tan et al. 1993; Sprent and Webb 1995; Guinan et al. 1999). In addition, active suppression of alloreactive cells has increasingly been recognized as a major means for the generation and maintenance of alloantigen-specific unresponsiveness, as studied extensively in a number of solid organ transplantation models (Cobbold et al. 2003). In experimental hematopoietic SCT, several cell populations have been implicated in these suppressive effects, such as NKT cells (Zeng et al. 1999, 2004), $CD4^-CD8^-$ (double negative) T cells (Zhang et al. 2000), cells containing "veto" activity (Bachar-Lustig et al. 2003), as well as regulatory T cell populations generated in vitro or in vivo by various manipulations (Roncarolo et al. 2001; Taylor et al. 2002a). In this review, we focus solely on recent findings concerning the subset of naturally occurring $CD4^+CD25^+$ regulatory T cells and discuss the prerequisites for their potential application in clinical bone marrow transplantation (BMT).

3
$CD4^+CD25^+$ T_{reg} Cells as Modulators of Alloreactivity

$CD4^+$ T cells that constitutively express the α-chain of the IL-2 receptor (CD25) have been identified in various species (mice, rats, and humans), where they constitute roughly 5%–10% of the CD4$^+$ T cell pool in peripheral blood and lymphoid organs. As described in detail in other contributions to this volume, CD4$^+$CD25$^+$ T$_{reg}$ cells are naturally occurring, thymus-derived cells that differ from nonregulatory T cells in their preferential expression of various molecules, such as intracellular cytotoxic T lymphocyte-associated antigen-4 (CTLA-4), glucocorticoid-induced TNF receptor family-related gene (GITR), and forkhead/winged-helix transcriptional regulator (Foxp3). Their most characteristic feature, however, is their functional behavior, i.e., their anergic state and suppressive activity (for recent reviews see Baecher-Allan et al. 2004; Piccirillo and Shevach 2004; Sakaguchi 2004). Anergy, i.e. the impaired proliferative response of T$_{reg}$ cells to standard T cell stimuli in vitro does not, however, indicate that these cells are generally insusceptible to activation. On the contrary, to gain suppressive function, CD4$^+$CD25$^+$ T$_{reg}$ cells require antigen-specific activation via their TCR. Once activated, they suppress the proliferation and cytokine secretion of co-cultured conventional CD4$^+$ and CD8$^+$ T cells antigen-nonspecifically (Thornton and Shevach 2000). In vivo, CD4$^+$CD25$^+$ T$_{reg}$ cells contribute to the maintenance of self-tolerance and thereby protect from a variety of autoimmune diseases (Sakaguchi 2000). They control the size of the peripheral T cell pool (Annacker et al. 2001) and modulate immune responses to infections (Belkaid et al. 2002), to tumors (Terabe and Berzofsky 2004) and to allogeneic organ grafts (Waldmann et al. 2004).

Mixed lymphocyte reactions (MLR) were among the first assay systems used for the functional characterization of CD4$^+$CD25$^+$ T$_{reg}$ cells. CD4$^+$CD25$^+$ T$_{reg}$ cells stimulated by MHC-mismatched MNCs did not respond with proliferation, but suppressed the proliferative response of conventional CD4$^+$ T cells (Jonuleit et al. 2001; Hoffmann et al. 2002a). These observations prompted several groups to study the potency of CD4$^+$CD25$^+$ T$_{reg}$ cells for the suppression of GVHD in animal models of allogeneic SCT. While the transplantation of purified bone marrow cells does not cause GVHD after MHC-mismatched transplantation in mice, the co-transplantation of "conventional" donor T cells rapidly induces GVHD. The severity of GVHD hereby depends on the degree of MHC disparity (major histocompatibility antigens), on the genetic background of donor and recipient strains (minor histocompatibility antigens), and on the number of transplanted T cells. In contrast, several independent studies using a variety of different models demonstrated that the transplantation of purified donor type CD4$^+$CD25$^+$ T$_{reg}$ cells into completely or partially MHC-mismatched bone marrow recipients did not induce signs of GVHD, even when large T cell numbers were used (Taylor et al. 2001; Edinger et al. 2003; Jones et al. 2003). In addition, neither residual host CD4$^+$CD25$^+$ T$_{reg}$ cells (e.g., after nonmyeloablative conditioning regimens), nor donor CD4$^+$CD25$^+$

T_{reg} cells within the BM graft interfered with stem cell engraftment, but rather facilitated hematopoietic reconstitution as well as the development of full donor chimerism (Hanash and Levy 2003; Jones et al. 2003; Taylor et al. 2003; Joffre et al. 2004). Thus, $CD4^+CD25^+$ T_{reg} cells are not inert, but are actively involved in immune-mediated mechanisms after allogeneic stem cell transplantation. This was most impressively demonstrated in studies where the co-transplantation of large numbers of donor-type $CD4^+CD25^+$ T_{reg} cells effectively suppressed GVHD induced by conventional ($CD25^-$) alloreactive T cells. $CD4^+CD25^+$ T_{reg} cells examined with respect to GVHD suppression were either freshly isolated and unmanipulated (Hoffmann et al. 2002) or in vitro activated and/or expanded, by either polyclonal anti-CD3 and IL-2 stimulation (Taylor et al. 2002b; Jones et al. 2003) or recipient type stimulator cells (Cohen et al. 2002). Suppression of GVHD was observed after T cell transfer between completely MHC-mismatched as well as selectively MHC class II-mismatched mouse strains and effects ranged from reduced loss of body weight and prolonged mean survival time to full protection from GVHD-associated lethality. Protection was only observed when donor (but not host) type $CD4^+CD25^+$ T_{reg} cells were used and occurred in $CD4^+$ as well as $CD8^+$ T cell-driven GVHD models. Interestingly, protection from GVHD was achieved even after delayed transfer of T_{reg} cells, provided the course of GVHD in the chosen model was not too aggressive (Jones et al. 2003). It thus seems that $CD4^+CD25^+$ T_{reg} cells not only prevent alloaggression after stem cell transplantation, but also modulate and potentially revert established disease, as recently also shown in a murine model of inflammatory bowel disease by Mottet et al. (2003).

The ability of donor $CD4^+CD25^+$ T_{reg} cells to potently protect from GVHD raised the question of where such host-protective donor T cells interact with alloaggressive T cells to prevent disease. In model systems of autoimmunity, migration of $CD4^+CD25^+$ T_{reg} cells to secondary lymphoid organs, especially draining lymph nodes of affected organs, appears decisive for efficient T_{reg} cell-mediated suppression in vivo. This was shown in the above-mentioned colitis experiments, but also in a number of experimental diabetes models (Green et al. 2002; Szanya et al. 2002). The most convincing of these studies by Walker and colleagues demonstrated the preferential accumulation and proliferation of TCR-transgenic $CD4^+CD25^+$ T_{reg} cells in draining lymph nodes of the pancreas expressing the relevant target antigen as a transgene (Walker et al. 2003). Secondary lymphoid organs also play a central role after allogeneic SCT. In an elegant series of experiments, Shlomchik et al. showed that only host but not donor type APC activate host-specific donor T cells to initiate lethal GVHD (Shlomchik et al. 1999). In complementary studies, Teshima et al. demonstrated that MHC expression on host APCs was necessary and sufficient to trigger GVHD, while MHC expression on GVHD target tissues was dispensable (Teshima et al. 2002). Thus, the encounter of donor T cells and professional APCs in secondary lymphoid organs, especially local lymph nodes (LN) and Peyer's patches in the gut, is crucial for GVHD induction (Murai et al. 2003).

Expression of CD62L (L-selectin), together with $\alpha_4\beta_7$-integrin, LFA-1, and chemokine receptor 7 (CCR7), is required for lymphocyte entry into LN via high endothelial venules (HEV). Li et al. reported that blockade of CD62L and CD49d (α_4-integrin) on donor T cells prevented the cells from entering LN (but not spleen) and ameliorated GVHD in two different mouse models (Li et al. 2001, 2004). CD62L and CCR7 are predominantly expressed on naïve, but not on memory T cells, and several reports described a reduced capacity of memory type (CD62L$^-$) T cells to induce GVHD (Anderson et al. 2003; Chen et al. 2004). Although the authors attributed this effect mainly to the skewed TCR repertoire of antigen-experienced T cells (that might lack allospecificities), it is likely that reduced GVHD was also the result of an impaired capacity of CD62L$^-$ cells to enter lymphatic organs. Mouse as well as human CD4$^+$CD25$^+$ T_{reg} cells are heterogeneous with respect to expression of CD62L (Szanya et al. 2002; Hoffmann et al. 2004) as well as other homing receptors (Lehmann et al. 2002). And although there is no difference in the suppressive activity of the CD62L$^+$ and the CD62L$^-$ subpopulations in vitro (Thornton and Shevach 2000; Szanya et al. 2002), only donor-type CD62L$^+$ T_{reg} cells conveyed protection from lethal GVHD after fully MHC-mismatched bone marrow transplantation (Hoffmann et al. 2002b; J. Ermann et al., 2005). Compared to CD62L$^+$ T_{reg} cells, CD62L$^-$ donor T_{reg} cells were impaired in their ability to migrate and/or expand in mesenteric LNs and in consequence less efficient in suppressing the expansion of co-transplanted conventional T cells. Thus, LN-homing capacity of donor CD4$^+$CD25$^+$ T_{reg} cells seems to be required for efficient protection from GVHD. These findings suggest that host APCs within lymphoid organs not only prime alloaggressive conventional donor T cells, but also allospecific donor T_{reg} cells such that they are sufficiently activated to gain suppressor activity. Thereby host APC probably provide the platform where the different T cell populations physically interact. Of note, these findings do not rule out additional suppressive activity within GVHD target organs. In fact, donor-derived CD4$^+$CD25$^+$ T_{reg} cells could be identified and isolated from liver and gut of recipient animals after allogeneic BMT (J. Ermann et al., unpublished results) and Graca et al. demonstrated potent T_{reg} cell-mediated suppression within the target tissue after allogeneic skin transplantation (Graca et al. 2002). However, in GVHD a hierarchy seems to exist among the various sites such that early suppression in secondary lymphoid organs, especially mesenteric LNs and Peyer's patches, is essential for protection from lethal disease. Suppression within GVHD target organs such as gut might occur later, through recruitment of T_{reg} cell subpopulations that were primed and expanded in lymphoid organs similar to disease-inducing conventional T cells. Activity of $CD4^+CD25^+$ T_{reg} cells in the periphery seems likely considering their heterogeneous chemokine receptor expression profile (Iellem et al. 2001; Sebastiani et al. 2001; Gavin et al. 2002; Szanya et al. 2002) as well as their differential display of tissue homing receptors other than CD62L and CCR7 (Lehmann et al. 2002, Huehn et al. 2004).

While cell contact seems to be required for suppression of conventional T cells by T_{reg} cells in vitro, the independence from soluble mediators is less stringent in vivo. It has been shown that cytokines contribute to T_{reg} cell-mediated suppression in several experimental disease models. In colitis, protection from disease by T_{reg} cells at least partially depends on IL-10 and TGF-β production (Read et al. 2000; Suri-Payer and Cantor 2001). In GVHD, the role of $CD4^+CD25^+$ T_{reg} cell-derived TGF-β has not been studied yet. However, IL-10 contributes to the protection from lethal GVHD, as $CD4^+CD25^+$ T_{reg} cells derived from $IL-10^{-/-}$ animals showed diminished capacity to inhibit GVHD-related lethality (Hoffmann et al. 2002a). The target cell populations for this IL-10 effect remain to be determined in detail, but it is plausible that T_{reg} cell-derived IL-10 ameliorates GVHD by altering APC function (Moore et al. 2001). In vitro, IL-10 treated DCs lose their potent pro-inflammatory effect and induce hyporesponsive conventional T cells with regulatory activity (Steinbrink et al. 1997; Jonuleit et al. 2000; Kubsch et al. 2003). In addition, inhibition of APC maturation as well as modulation of APC function via down-regulation of MHC as well as co-stimulatory molecules has recently been confirmed for mouse and human $CD4^+CD25^+$ T_{reg} cells (Cederbom et al. 2000; Misra et al. 2004). Thus, the protective effect of adoptively transferred T_{reg} cells in GVHD is probably the combined result of direct suppression of effector T cells in lymphoid organs as well as down-modulation of APC function with respect to presentation of alloantigens.

4
Influence of $CD4^+CD25^+$ T_{reg} Cells on the Graft-Versus-Leukemia/Lymphoma Activity of Donor T Cells

The high rate of leukemia relapse in patients transplanted with T cell-depleted grafts revealed the important contribution of donor T cells for the elimination of residual disease after allogeneic SCT. Final proof of principle was provided by the implementation of donor lymphocyte infusions (DLI) as a successful treatment strategy for patients suffering from disease relapse after hematopoietic SCT (Kolb et al. 1990). In chronic myeloid leukemia, 75% of relapsed patients achieve a complete remission within 6 months after DLI (Porter et al. 1999; Guglielmi et al. 2002). The target antigens for donor T cells on host-type leukemias are for the most part unidentified. Data from experimental as well as clinical studies suggest that the GVL effect, as seen after DLI, can be directed against broadly expressed major and minor histocompatibility antigens (Truitt and Johnson 1995; Riddell et al. 2002), but also against antigens restricted to host hematopoietic cells (Dickinson et al. 2002; Falkenburg et al. 2003) and eventually even against tumor-specific antigens (Molldrem et al. 2000). The frequent initiation of GVHD by DLI therapy suggests that it is often the broadly expressed host antigens that contribute to disease eradication. On the other hand, 50% of patients treated with DLI eradicate their leukemia without developing GVHD, suggesting that hematopoietic antigens are preferentially recognized and/or that hematopoietic cells are more susceptible to the graft-versus-host reaction. In line with these assumptions, a conversion of mixed chimeras to full donor chimerism is usually observed in patients successfully treated with DLI (Orsini et al. 2000; Serrano et al. 2000; Bader et al. 2004).

Since hematopoietic malignancies are the main indication for allogeneic SCT, several groups investigated whether suppression of GVHD by donor $CD4^+CD25^+$ T_{reg} cells would inevitably abrogate the GVL-effect of donor T cells. In one of these studies, in vivo bioluminescence imaging (Edinger et al. 2003a) was used for the real-time localization and quantification of tumor cells in living animals. This allowed dissecting the differential impact of donor $CD4^+CD25^+$ T_{reg} cells on GVHD and GVL activity of donor-derived conventional T cells after transfer into completely MHC-mismatched recipients (Edinger et al. 2003b). In this study it was shown that B cell lymphoma (BCL_1) -bearing mice that received a 1:1 ratio of T_{reg} cells and conventional T cells were protected from lethal GVHD and eradicated their lymphoma, whereas those that received only conventional donor T cells died rapidly from GVHD. In contrast, mice that received only $CD4^+CD25^+$ T_{reg} cells succumbed to lymphoma relapse, revealing the inability of these cells to mediate any GVL activity. These findings were confirmed in a second model, where active eradication of the host-type A20 leukemia from the bone marrow was observed when recipients were protected from lethal GVHD by high numbers of donor T_{reg} cells. Trenado et al. (2003) obtained similar results using the same GVHD/GVL model. However, in a C57BL/6 → (B6/D2) F_1 model with the P815 mastocytoma tumor, no GVL activity was observed in the presence of donor T_{reg} cells, suggesting that numerous factors contribute to clinical outcome in tumor-bearing hosts. Such factors may include the genetic disparity between donor and recipient, total numbers and/or ratios of transplanted conventional T cells and T_{reg} cells, the intensity of the conditioning regimen, and variables related to the malignancy itself, such as localization and growth kinetics, susceptibility to effector cell populations and their cytotoxic mechanisms, expression of co-stimulatory vs immunosuppressive molecules and other tumor escape mechanisms. Although such factors may preclude a precise prediction about the outcome of an individual transplantation procedure, they do not negate the concept that $CD4^+CD25^+$ T_{reg} cells suppress GVHD without causing generalized immune paralysis, since GVL activity can be maintained.

The ability of donor T_{reg} cells to protect from lethal GVHD without abrogating the GVL effect of donor T cells prompted studies for their therapeutic use. Jones and colleagues (Jones et al. 2003) induced a CD8 T cell-mediated form of GVHD in a minor histocompatibility-mismatch model (B10BR → CBA) and delayed the treatment of recipients with T_{reg} cells for up to 10 days after BMT. Even then, donor T_{reg} cells significantly ameliorated GVHD, demonstrating that they are not only able to inhibit the initiation of disease, but also to down-regulate an ongoing alloresponse. The early alloresponse in this model was sufficient to eradicate a host-type myeloid leukemia (MMCBA6), while its subsequent suppression by T_{reg} cells (at a time of subclinical GVHD) protected recipients from progression to lethal GVHD. In a second, more aggressive GVHD model of haploidentical BMT (C3H → (B6xC3H)F_1), the delayed transfer of donor T_{reg} cells was less effective. Here, the short time interval between BMT and death from GVHD did not provide a sufficient time window to prevent target organ destruction (Jones et al. 2003).

The putative paradox of maintained GVL activity despite GVHD suppression raised the question of how T_{reg} cells differentially influence responses of conventional T cells toward tumor cells and GVHD target tissues. After transfer into MHC-mismatched recipients, $CD4^+CD25^-$ and $CD8^+$ donor T cells dramatically expand within the first few days (Edinger et al. 2003b). This donor T cell expansion is a hallmark of the induction phase of acute GVHD and a prerequisite for disease progression finally leading to target organ destruction (Sprent et al. 1986; Ferrara 2000). When co-transplanted with donor T_{reg} cells, the expansion of alloaggressive T cells was inhibited by more than 70% at day 5 after MHC-mismatched BMT and by more than 90% after 7 days. Thus, donor T_{reg} cells interfered with the pathophysiology of acute GVHD by suppressing the increase of the host-reactive T cell pool (Li et al. 2001). However, the initial activation of conventional donor T cells as well as their capacity to produce cytokines or to exert cytolytic effects via the perforin/granzyme or Fas/FasL pathways in response to allogeneic stimulation was unaffected in vitro as well as in vivo (Edinger et al. 2003). These data indicated that a low level alloresponse still occurred in the presence of T_{reg} cells, which was sufficient to exert a graft-versus-leukemia effect (GVL), while the dramatic expansion of alloaggressive T cells required for the destruction of target organs such as the gut was sufficiently suppressed. Support for this hypothesis was provided by experiments in which tumor-bearing hosts received only limited numbers of donor T cells. In these experiments, 1×10^5 conventional C57BL/6 T cells still induced lethal GVHD in BALB/c recipients that was prevented by co-transplanted donor T_{reg} cells. However, full protection from tumor relapse was lost under these circumstances, since the few host reactive T cells, restricted in their ability to expand in the presence of T_{reg} cells, were unable to fully eradicate the tumor (Edinger et al. 2003). Taken together, these observations demonstrate that the balance between alloaggressive and host-protective immune mechanisms determines the outcome of GVL-permissive tolerance induction in allogeneic BMT by donor $CD4^+CD25^+$ T_{reg} cells.

5
Reconstitution of the T_{reg} Cell Compartment After Allogeneic Stem Cell Transplantation

Even before the role of donor $CD4^+CD25^+$ T_{reg} cells in GVHD was fully appreciated, Johnson and co-workers described the de-novo generation of immunosuppressive T cell populations from transplanted bone marrow. In experiments aimed at studying the pathophysiology of GVHD in animals that received delayed donor T cell infusions, they found a reduced incidence and severity of GVHD in reconstituted mice as compared to those receiving T cells at the time of BMT. Apart from other factors such as diminished tissue damage and pro-inflammatory cytokine levels late after conditioning, they revealed that immunosuppressive cells capable of ameliorating GVHD developed from bone marrow-derived precursors in a thymus-dependent process. These cells were of donor origin, $Thy1^+$, $TCR\alpha\beta^+$, and either $CD4^+CD8^-$ or DN (Johnson et al. 1999). Using bone marrow cells from knock-out strains, they recently proved that the generation of the suppressive $CD4^+$ subpopulation was rigorously dependent on expression of CD25 and CD28. As both molecules are critically required for the development of $CD4^+CD25^+$ T_{reg} cells (Salomon et al. 2000; Almeida et al. 2002; Malek et al. 2002), they concluded that the $CD4^+$ suppressor population represents bone marrow-derived donor $CD4^+CD25^+$ T_{reg} cells (Johnson et al. 2002).

A recent clinical study addressed the same issue. In this study, Foxp3 mRNA levels in MNC of BMT patients were quantified to monitor recovery of the regulatory T cell pool (Miura et al. 2004). The authors found impaired reconstitution of the T_{reg} cell compartment in patients with GVHD as compared to those without GVHD. In addition, diminished Foxp3 expression correlated with reduced T cell receptor excision circles (TREC), indicating that impaired thymic function was associated with lack of T_{reg} cell reconstitution in GVHD patients. Although these studies did not clarify whether the lack of T_{reg} cells was a cause or consequence of GVHD, they did suggest that donor type T_{reg} cells develop in a thymus-dependent manner after BMT and that dysfunction of the T_{reg} cell compartment might be involved in GVHD pathophysiology in humans. Therefore, the selective augmentation of T_{reg} cell reconstitution and/or function seems a promising strategy for immunomodulatory interventions after allogeneic BMT. Unfortunately, there is no biological or pharmacological reagent available yet that specifically targets T_{reg} cells in vivo to enhance their activity. Clinical trials currently in preparation therefore focus on the adoptive transfer of donor T_{reg} cells manipulated ex vivo.

6
Ex Vivo Expansion of $CD4^+CD25^+$ T_{reg} Cells for Allogeneic Stem Cell Transplantation

In contrast to murine T_{reg} cells that are sufficiently characterized by their co-expression of CD4 and CD25, human T_{reg} cells seem to be preferentially enriched in the $CD4^+CD25^{high}$ T cell population that constitutes merely 1%–3% of peripheral blood mononuclear cells (PBMCs). This paucity in human peripheral blood has thus far hampered the detailed characterization of $CD4^+CD25^{high}$ T_{reg} cells as well as their clinical application, clearly indicating the need for efficient ex vivo expansion protocols. Due to the anergic state of human and murine T_{reg} cells, in vitro expansion remained a problem until recently. A number of studies, however, have shown that the anergic state of murine $CD4^+CD25^+$ T_{reg} cells in vitro is not irreversible and that hypoproliferation might only poorly reflect their behavior in vivo. After transfer into lymphopenic hosts, for example, they show MHC class II-dependent homeostatic proliferation (Annacker et al. 2001; Almeida et al. 2002; Gavin et al. 2002), whereas in normal animals they expand locally in response to antigen-specific stimulation (Klein et al. 2003; Walker et al. 2003; Yamazaki et al. 2003) and to a certain degree even under steady-state conditions (Fisson et al. 2003). Limited in vitro proliferation of $CD4^+CD25^{+/high}$ T_{reg} cells was observed either after stimulation with allogeneic feeder cells combined with high-dose IL-2 (Levings et al. 2001; Taylor et al. 2002b; Jiang et al. 2003; Yamazaki et al. 2003) or by the combined stimulation via TCR and CD28 in the presence of IL-2 (Takahashi et al. 1998; Dieckmann et al. 2001; Ermann et al. 2001). For their long-term polyclonal in vitro expansion, however, human $CD4^+CD25^{high}$ T_{reg}

cells required optimized culture conditions where anti-CD3 and anti-CD28 antibodies were either presented by a FcγRII (CD32) -expressing fibroblast cell line, or by antibody-coated beads (T-cell expander) acting as artificial APCs. In such cultures, human CD4$^+$CD25^{high} T$_{reg}$ cells expanded on average 13,000-fold and 3,130-fold, respectively, within 3–4 weeks (Hoffmann et al. 2004). These and other studies (Godfrey et al. 2004) demonstrated that human CD4$^+$CD25^{high} T$_{reg}$ cells depend on strong co-stimulation and exogenous IL-2 for their large-scale expansion, but not on entirely different stimulatory signals as compared to conventional T cells. Helper cell-free expansion protocols are of particular interest with regard to potential clinical applications, as human CD4$^+$CD25$^+$ T$_{reg}$ cell expansion has to be achieved in line with good manufacturing practice (GMP) regulations. Importantly, in vitro expanded T$_{reg}$ cells do not lose but enhance their suppressive activity and maintain expression of lymph node homing receptors such as suggesting that their lymph node homing capacity is maintained (Godfrey et al. 2004; Hoffmann et al. 2004).

Trenado et al. recently concluded from murine studies that T$_{reg}$ cells primed by host hematopoietic cells show improved protection from GVHD as compared to T$_{reg}$ cells expanded in the presence of 3rd party stimulator cells (Trenado et al. 2003). Since T$_{reg}$ cells depend on specific TCR engagement to gain suppressive activity, it seems reasonable to preselect their TCR repertoire in vitro to achieve enhanced and specific suppressive activity after transfusion. For their clinical application, however, preselection of their TCR repertoire might not necessarily be beneficial. For example, donor T$_{reg}$ cells primed by recipient hematopoietic cells might result in loss of TCR specificities for minor alloantigens that are not expressed and/or presented by hematopoietic stimulator cells. On the other hand, suppressor cells primed by hematopoietic antigens might preferentially suppress the graft-versus-hematopoiesis effect of conventional donor T cells, which might increase the risk of graft rejection or disease relapse in patients transplanted for hematologic malignancies. Furthermore, allogeneic SCT today is predominantly carried out between MHC-matched donor and recipient pairs, a situation that might not provide sufficient stimulatory potential for the efficient expansion of antigen-specific T$_{reg}$ cells in vitro. Hence, the best strategy for T$_{reg}$ cell expansion for clinical applications awaits further clarification and it is crucial to compare alloantigen-primed T$_{reg}$ cells with polyclonally expanded T$_{reg}$ cells in GVHD models.

7
Prerequisites for the Use of CD4$^+$CD25^{high} T$_{reg}$ Cells in Clinical Stem Cell Transplantation

The potency of adoptively transferred donor CD4$^+$CD25$^+$ T$_{reg}$ cells to inhibit GVHD in experimental systems fueled the interest of clinicians in this approach. The fact that phenotypic, functional, and molecular characteristics of murine CD4$^+$CD25$^+$ T$_{reg}$ cells have all been confirmed for human CD4$^+$CD25^{high} T$_{reg}$ cells is encouraging for potential clinical trials. However, many hurdles have to be overcome before T$_{reg}$ cell administration can be evaluated in clinical SCT. One of the key technical issues thus far is their purification. Due to the lack of exclusive surface markers, CD25-specific reagents are used for T$_{reg}$ cell isolation. However, whether GMP-approved magnetic purification techniques will sufficiently separate the CD4$^+$CD25^{high} T$_{reg}$ cell population from the presumably nonregulatory CD4$^+$CD25^{intermediate} T cells in a clinical setting remains to be determined. Apart from their purity, the quantity of T$_{reg}$ cells within leukapheresis products of stem cell donors will determine the feasibility of this approach, since large numbers are required for protection from GVHD in murine models. Although the above-described expansion protocols permit the generation of sufficient human T$_{reg}$ cells for clinical trials, it will be crucial to show that their migration, function, and survival is not altered by their in vitro culture. The fact that in vitro-expanded murine T$_{reg}$ cells maintain their ability to protect from GVHD is encouraging in this regard (Taylor et al. 2002b; Jones et al. 2003; Trenado et al. 2003). However, monitoring T$_{reg}$ cell survival and function in humans is hampered by the lack of standardized functional assay systems and the inability to reliably distinguish transfused T$_{reg}$ cells from activated nonregulatory T cells by surface markers. Apart from such technical difficulties, clinical considerations represent even bigger challenges for the translation of preclinical findings into early clinical trials. In animal studies, T$_{reg}$ cell function in BMT was mainly examined in MHC-mismatch models. Since the majority of stem cell transplantations in humans are performed between HLA-matched donor–recipient pairs, it has to be determined whether HLA-identical host cells stimulate donor T$_{reg}$ cells with sufficient strength and frequency to induce their suppressive function. Similarly, the influence of different conditioning regimens, e.g., myeloablative vs reduced-intensity regimens, has not been addressed systematically in preclinical studies. In addition, drug-related effects on T$_{reg}$ cell performance require careful evaluation. For example, the influence of granulocyte colony stimulating factor (G-CSF) on T$_{reg}$ cell function has to be tested if mobilized peripheral blood stem cell products are to be used for their isolation. Even more important, the impact of drugs administered to the patient has to be investigated, especially if immunosuppressive medication is to be given in addition to T_{reg} cell transfusions. Thus, the best strategy for patient selection, dosage, and timing of T_{reg} cell administration is not solely deducible from animal studies, but requires carefully designed clinical trials.

In conclusion, there are still more questions than answers concerning the feasibility of human T_{reg} cell transfusions for the development of improved transplantation strategies. Their resolution will strongly depend on the joined efforts of clinicians and basic science researchers. The most important task, however, is the identification of the molecular mechanisms responsible for T_{reg} cell-mediated suppression. Once identified, it might be possible to develop pharmacological reagents that mimic T_{reg} cell function and that permit a much simpler approach to the specific modulation of immune responses to alloantigens.

References

Almeida AR, Legrand N et al (2002) Homeostasis of peripheral CD4+ T cells: IL-2R alpha and IL-2 shape a population of regulatory cells that controls CD4+ T cell numbers. J Immunol 169:4850–60

Amrolia PJ, Muccioli-Casadei G et al (2003a) Selective depletion of donor alloreactive T cells without loss of antiviral or antileukemic responses. Blood 102:2292–2299

Amrolia PJ, Reid SD et al (2003b) Allorestricted cytotoxic T cells specific for human CD45 show potent antileukemic activity. Blood 101:1007–1014

Anderson BE, McNiff J et al (2003) Memory CD4+ T cells do not induce graft-versus-host disease. J Clin Invest 112:101–108

Annacker O, Pimenta-Araujo R et al (2001) CD25+ CD4+ T cells regulate the expansion of peripheral CD4 T cells through the production of IL-10. J Immunol 166:3008–3018

Bachar-Lustig E, Reich-Zeliger S et al (2003) Anti-third-party veto CTLs overcome rejection of hematopoietic allografts: synergism with rapamycin and BM cell dose. Blood 102:1943–1950

Bader P, Kreyenberg H et al (2004) Increasing mixed chimerism is an important prognostic factor for unfavorable outcome in children with acute lymphoblastic leukemia after allogeneic stem-cell transplantation: possible role for pre-emptive immunotherapy? J Clin Oncol 22:1696–1705

Baecher-Allan C, Viglietta V et al (2004) Human CD4+CD25+ regulatory T cells. Semin Immunol 16:89–98

Belkaid Y, Piccirillo CA et al (2002) CD4+CD25+ regulatory T cells control Leishmania major persistence and immunity. Nature 420(6915):502–507

Blazar BR, Taylor PA et al (1997) Blockade of CD40 ligand-CD40 interaction impairs CD4+ T cell-mediated alloreactivity by inhibiting mature donor T cell expansion and function after bone marrow transplantation. J Immunol 158:29–39

Cederbom L, Hall H et al (2000) CD4+CD25+ regulatory T cells down-regulate costimulatory molecules on antigen-presenting cells. Eur J Immunol 30:1538–1543

Champlin RE, Passweg JR et al (2000) T-cell depletion of bone marrow transplants for leukemia from donors other than HLA-identical siblings: advantage of T-cell antibodies with narrow specificities. Blood 95:3996–4003

Chen BJ, Cui X et al (2002) Prevention of graft-versus-host disease while preserving graft-versus-leukemia effect after selective depletion of host-reactive T cells by photodynamic cell purging process. Blood 99:3083–3088

Chen BJ, Cui X et al (2004) Transfer of allogeneic CD62L- memory T cells without graft-versus-host disease. Blood 103:1534–1541

Cobbold SP, Graca L et al (2003) Regulatory T cells in the induction and maintenance of peripheral transplantation tolerance. Transpl Int 16:66–75

Cohen JL, Trenado A et al (2002) CD4(+)CD25(+) immunoregulatory T Cells: new therapeutics for graft-versus-host disease. J Exp Med 196:401–406

Daniel C, Horvath S et al (1998) A basis for alloreactivity: MHC helical residues broaden peptide recognition by the TCR Immunity 8:543–552

Dazzi F, Szydlo RM et al (2000) Comparison of single-dose and escalating-dose regimens of donor lymphocyte infusion for relapse after allografting for chronic myeloid leukemia. Blood 95:67–71

Dickinson AM, Wang XN et al (2002) In situ dissection of the graft-versus-host activities of cytotoxic T cells specific for minor histocompatibility antigens. Nat Med 8:410–414

Dieckmann D, Plottner H et al (2001) Ex vivo isolation and characterization of CD4(+)CD25(+) T cells with regulatory properties from human blood. J Exp Med 193:1303–1310

Edinger M, Cao YA et al (2003a) Revealing lymphoma growth and the efficacy of immune cell therapies using in vivo bioluminescence imaging. Blood 101:640–648

Edinger M, Hoffmann P et al (2003b) CD4(+)CD25(+) regulatory T cells preserve graft-versus-tumor activity while inhibiting graft-versus-host disease after bone marrow transplantation. Nat Med 9:1144–1150

Ermann J, Hoffmann P et al. (2005) Only the CD62L$^+$ subpopulation of CD4+CD25+ regulatory T cells protects from lethal acute GVHD. Blood 105:2220–2226

Ermann J, Szanya V et al (2001) CD4(+)CD25(+) T cells facilitate the induction of T cell anergy. J Immunol 167:4271–4275

Falkenburg JH, van de Corput L et al (2003) Minor histocompatibility antigens in human stem cell transplantation. Exp Hematol 31:743–751

Ferrara JL (2000) Pathogenesis of acute graft-versus-host disease: cytokines and cellular effectors. J Hematother Stem Cell Res 9:299–306

Ferrara JL, Levy R et al (1999) Pathophysiologic mechanisms of acute graft-vs.-host disease. Biol Blood Marrow Transplant 5:347–356

Fisson S, Darrasse-Jeze G et al (2003) Continuous activation of autoreactive CD4+ CD25+ regulatory T cells in the steady state. J Exp Med 198:737–746

Gavin MA, Clarke SR et al (2002) Homeostasis and anergy of CD4+CD25+ suppressor T cells in vivo. Nat Immunol 3:33–41

Godfrey WR, Ge YG et al (2004) In vitro-expanded human CD4(+)CD25(+) T-regulatory cells can markedly inhibit allogeneic dendritic cell-stimulated MLR cultures. Blood 104:453–461

Goulmy E (1997) Human minor histocompatibility antigens: new concepts for marrow transplantation and adoptive immunotherapy. Immunol Rev 157:125–140

Graca L, Cobbold SP et al (2002) Identification of regulatory T cells in tolerated allografts. J Exp Med 195:1641–1646

Gratwohl A, Brand R et al (2002) Graft-versus-host disease and outcome in HLA-identical sibling transplantations for chronic myeloid leukemia. Blood 100:3877–3886

Green EA, Choi Y et al (2002) Pancreatic lymph node-derived CD4(+)CD25(+) Treg cells: highly potent regulators of diabetes that require TRANCE-RANK signals. Immunity 16:183–191

Guglielmi C, Arcese W et al (2002) Donor lymphocyte infusion for relapsed chronic myelogenous leukemia: prognostic relevance of the initial cell dose. Blood 100:397–405

Guinan EC, Boussiotis VA et al (1999) Transplantation of anergic histoincompatible bone marrow allografts. N Engl J Med 340:1704–1714

Hanash AM, Levy RB (2003) Donor CD4+CD25+ T cells facilitate hematopoietic engraftment independent of host resistance and allo-antigen recognition (abstract) Blood 102:38a

Heemskerk MH, Hoogeboom M et al (2003) Redirection of antileukemic reactivity of peripheral T lymphocytes using gene transfer of minor histocompatibility antigen HA-2-specific T-cell receptor complexes expressing a conserved alpha joining region. Blood 102:3530–3540

Hertenstein B, Hampl W et al (1995) In vivo/ex vivo T cell depletion for GVHD prophylaxis influences onset and course of active cytomegalovirus infection and disease after BMT. Bone Marrow Transplant 15:387–393

Heslop HE, Brenner MK et al (1994) Administration of neomycin-resistance-gene-marked EBV-specific cytotoxic T lymphocytes to recipients of mismatched-related or phenotypically similar unrelated donor marrow grafts. Hum Gene Ther 5:381–397

Ho VT, Soiffer RJ (2001) The history and future of T-cell depletion as graft-versus-host disease prophylaxis for allogeneic hematopoietic stem cell transplantation. Blood 98:3192–204

Hoffmann P, Eder R et al (2004) Large-scale in vitro expansion of polyclonal human CD4(+)CD25high regulatory T cells. Blood 104:895–903

Hoffmann P, Edinger M et al (2002b) CD4+CD25+ regulatory T cells act in secondary lymphoid organs to protect from lethal acute GVHD (abstract) Blood 100:143a

Hoffmann P, Ermann J et al (2002a) Donor-type CD4(+)CD25(+) regulatory T cells suppress lethal acute graft-versus-host disease after allogeneic bone marrow transplantation. J Exp Med 196:389–399

Huehn J, Siegmund K et al (2004) Developmental stage phenotype, and migration distinguish naive- and effector/memory-like CD4+ regulatory T cells. J Exp Med 199:303–313

Iellem A, Mariani M et al (2001) Unique chemotactic response profile and specific expression of chemokine receptors CCR4 and CCR8 by CD4(+)CD25(+) regulatory T cells. J Exp Med 194:847–853

Ildstad ST, Sachs DH (1984) Reconstitution with syngeneic plus allogeneic or xenogeneic bone marrow leads to specific acceptance of allografts or xenografts. Nature 307(5947):168–170

Jiang S, Camara N et al (2003) Induction of allopeptide-specific human CD4+CD25+ regulatory T cells ex vivo. Blood 102:2180–2186

Joffre O, Gorsse N et al (2004) Induction of antigen-specific tolerance to bone marrow allografts with CD4+CD25+ T lymphocytes. Blood 103:4216–4221

Johnson BD, Becker EE et al (1999) Role of immunoregulatory donor T cells in suppression of graft-versus-host disease following donor leukocyte infusion therapy. J Immunol 163:6479–6487

Johnson BD, Konkol MC et al (2002) CD25+ immunoregulatory T-cells of donor origin suppress alloreactivity after BMT. Biol Blood Marrow Transplant 8:525–535

Jones SC, Murphy GF et al (2003) Post-hematopoietic cell transplantation control of graft-versus-host disease by donor CD4(+)25(+) T cells to allow an effective graft-versus-leukemia response. Biol Blood Marrow Transplant 9:243–256

Jonuleit H, Schmitt E et al (2000) Induction of interleukin 10-producing, nonproliferating CD4(+) T cells with regulatory properties by repetitive stimulation with allogeneic immature human dendritic cells. J Exp Med 192:1213–1222

Jonuleit H, Schmitt E et al (2001) Identification and functional characterization of human CD4(+)CD25(+) T cells with regulatory properties isolated from peripheral blood. J Exp Med 193:1285–1294

Klein L, Khazaie K et al (2003) In vivo dynamics of antigen-specific regulatory T cells not predicted from behavior in vitro. Proc Natl Acad Sci U S A 100:8886–8891

Kolb HJ, Mittermuller J et al (1990) Donor leukocyte transfusions for treatment of recurrent chronic myelogenous leukemia in marrow transplant patients. Blood 76:2462–2465

Kubsch S, Graulich E et al (2003) Suppressor activity of anergic T cells induced by IL-10-treated human dendritic cells: association with IL-2- and CTLA-4-dependent G1 arrest of the cell cycle regulated by p27Kip1. Eur J Immunol 33:1988–1997

Lechler RI, Garden OA et al (2003) The complementary roles of deletion and regulation in transplantation tolerance. Nat Rev Immunol 3:147–158

Lehmann J, Huehn J et al (2002) Expression of the integrin alpha Ebeta 7 identifies unique subsets of CD25+ as well as CD25− regulatory T cells. Proc Natl Acad Sci U S A 99:13031–13036

Levings MK, Sangregorio R et al (2001) Human CD25(+)CD4(+) t regulatory cells suppress naive and memory T cell proliferation and can be expanded in vitro without loss of function. J Exp Med 193:1295–1302

Li B, New JY et al (2004) Delaying acute graft-versus-host disease in mouse bone marrow transplantation by treating donor cells with antibodies directed at L-selectin and alpha4-integrin prior to infusion. Scand J Immunol 59:464–468

Li B, New JY et al (2001) Blocking L-selectin and alpha4-integrin changes donor cell homing pattern and ameliorates murine acute graft versus host disease. Eur J Immunol 31:617–624

Li XC, Strom TB et al (2001) T cell death and transplantation tolerance. Immunity 14:407–416

Malek TR, Yu A et al (2002) CD4 regulatory T cells prevent lethal autoimmunity in IL-2Rbeta-deficient mice. Implications for the nonredundant function of IL-2. Immunity 17:167–178

Merad M, Hoffmann P et al (2004) Depletion of host Langerhans cells before transplantation of donor alloreactive T cells prevents skin graft-versus-host disease. Nat Med 10:510–517

Michalek J, Collins RH et al (2003) Clinical-scale selective depletion of alloreactive T cells using an anti-CD25 immunotoxin. Neoplasma 50:296–299

Misra N, Bayry J et al (2004) Cutting edge: human CD4+CD25+ T cells restrain the maturation and antigen-presenting function of dendritic cells. J Immunol 172:4676–4680

Miura Y, Thoburn CJ et al (2004) Association of Foxp3 regulatory gene expression with graft-versus-host disease. Blood 104:2187–2193

Molldrem JJ, Lee PP et al (2000) Evidence that specific T lymphocytes may participate in the elimination of chronic myelogenous leukemia. Nat Med 6:1018–1023

Moore KW, de Waal Malefyt R et al (2001) Interleukin-10 and the interleukin-10 receptor. Annu Rev Immunol 19:683–765

Mottet C, Uhlig HH et al (2003) Cutting edge: cure of colitis by CD4+CD25+ regulatory T cells. J Immunol 170:3939–3943

Murai M, Yoneyama H et al (2003) Peyer's patch is the essential site in initiating murine acute and lethal graft-versus-host reaction. Nat Immunol 4:154–160

Obst R, Netuschil N et al (2000) The role of peptides in T cell alloreactivity is determined by self-major histocompatibility complex molecules. J Exp Med 191:805–812

Orsini E, Alyea EP et al (2000) Conversion to full donor chimerism following donor lymphocyte infusion is associated with disease response in patients with multiple myeloma. Biol Blood Marrow Transplant 6:375–386

Patterson J, Prentice HG et al (1986) Graft rejection following HLA matched T-lymphocyte depleted bone marrow transplantation. Br J Haematol 63:221–230

Piccirillo CA, Shevach EM (2004) Naturally-occurring CD4+CD25+ immunoregulatory T cells: central players in the arena of peripheral tolerance. Semin Immunol 16:81–88

Porter DL, Collins RH Jr et al (1999) Long-term follow-up of patients who achieved complete remission after donor leukocyte infusions. Biol Blood Marrow Transplant 5:253–261

Rauser G, Einsele H et al (2004) Rapid generation of combined CMV-specific CD4+ and CD8+ T-cell lines for adoptive transfer into recipients of allogeneic stem cell transplants. Blood 103:3565–3572

Read S, Malmstrom V et al (2000) Cytotoxic T lymphocyte-associated antigen 4 plays an essential role in the function of CD25(+)CD4(+) regulatory cells that control intestinal inflammation. J Exp Med 192:295–302

Riddell SR, Murata M et al (2002) Minor histocompatibility antigens—targets of graft versus leukemia responses. Int J Hematol 76 Suppl 2:155–161

Rocha B, von Boehmer H (1991) Peripheral selection of the T cell repertoire. Science 251:1225–1228

Roncarolo MG, Bacchetta R et al (2001) Type 1 T regulatory cells. Immunol Rev 182:68–79

Sakaguchi S (2000) Regulatory T cells: key controllers of immunologic self-tolerance. Cell 101:455–458

Sakaguchi S (2004) Naturally arising CD4+ regulatory T cells for immunologic self-tolerance and negative control of immune responses. Annu Rev Immunol 22:531–562

Salaun J, Bandeira A et al (1990) Thymic epithelium tolerizes for histocompatibility antigens. Science 247:1471–1474

Salomon B, Lenschow DJ et al (2000) B7/CD28 costimulation is essential for the homeostasis of the CD4+CD25+ immunoregulatory T cells that control autoimmune diabetes. Immunity 12:431–440

Savage P, Gao L et al (2004) Use of B cell-bound HLA-A2 class I monomers to generate high-avidity, allo-restricted CTLs against the leukemia-associated protein Wilms tumor antigen. Blood 103:4613–4615

Sebastiani S, Allavena P et al (2001) Chemokine receptor expression and function in CD4+ T lymphocytes with regulatory activity. J Immunol 166:996–1002

Serrano J, Roman J et al (2000) Molecular analysis of lineage-specific chimerism and minimal residual disease by RT-PCR of p210(BCR-ABL) and p190(BCR-ABL) after allogeneic bone marrow transplantation for chronic myeloid leukemia: increasing mixed myeloid chimerism and p190(BCR-ABL) detection precede cytogenetic relapse. Blood 95:2659–2665

Shlomchik WD, Couzens MS et al (1999) Prevention of graft versus host disease by inactivation of host antigen-presenting cells. Science 285:412–415

Sprent J, Kishimoto H (2001) The thymus and central tolerance. Philos Trans R Soc Lond B Biol Sci 356:609–616

Sprent J, Schaefer M et al (1986) Properties of purified T cell subsets. II. In vivo responses to class I vs. class II H-2 differences. J Exp Med 163:998–1011

Sprent J, Webb SR (1995) Intrathymic and extrathymic clonal deletion of T cells. Curr Opin Immunol 7:196–205

Steinbrink K, Wolfl M et al (1997) Induction of tolerance by IL-10-treated dendritic cells. J Immunol 159:4772–4780

Suchin EJ, Langmuir PB et al (2001) Quantifying the frequency of alloreactive T cells in vivo: new answers to an old question. J Immunol 166:973–981

Suri-Payer E, Cantor H (2001) Differential cytokine requirements for regulation of autoimmune gastritis and colitis by CD4(+)CD25(+) T cells. J Autoimmun 16:115–123

Sykes M, Sachs DH (2001) Mixed chimerism. Philos Trans R Soc Lond B Biol Sci 356:707–726

Szanya V, Ermann J et al (2002) The subpopulation of CD4+CD25+ splenocytes that delays adoptive transfer of diabetes expresses L-selectin and high levels of CCR7. J Immunol 169:2461–2465

Takahashi T, Kuniyasu Y et al (1998) Immunologic self-tolerance maintained by CD25+CD4+ naturally anergic and suppressive T cells: induction of autoimmune disease by breaking their anergic/suppressive state. Int Immunol 10:1969–1980

Tan P, Anasetti C et al (1993) Induction of alloantigen-specific hyporesponsiveness in human T lymphocytes by blocking interaction of CD28 with its natural ligand B7/BB1. J Exp Med 177:165–173

Taylor PA, Friedman TM et al (2002a) Tolerance induction of alloreactive T cells via ex vivo blockade of the CD40:CD40L costimulatory pathway results in the generation of a potent immune regulatory cell. Blood 99:4601–4609

Taylor PA, Lees CJ et al (2002b) The infusion of ex vivo activated and expanded CD4(+)CD25(+) immune regulatory cells inhibits graft-versus-host disease lethality. Blood 99:3493–3499

Taylor PA, Lees CJ et al (2003) Endogenous host or exogenous donor CD4+CD25+ cells promote donor BM engraftment: association with TGF-beta production and regulation of GITR signaling (abstract). Blood 102:37a

Taylor PA, Noelle RJ et al (2001) CD4(+)CD25(+) immune regulatory cells are required for induction of tolerance to alloantigen via costimulatory blockade. J Exp Med 193:1311–1318

Terabe M, Berzofsky JA (2004) Immunoregulatory T cells in tumor immunity. Curr Opin Immunol 16:157–162

Teshima T, Ordemann R et al (2002) Acute graft-versus-host disease does not require alloantigen expression on host epithelium. Nat Med 8:575–581

Thornton AM, Shevach EM (2000) Suppressor effector function of CD4+CD25+ immunoregulatory T cells is antigen nonspecific. J Immunol 164:183–190

Trenado A, Charlotte F et al (2003) Recipient-type specific CD4+CD25+ regulatory T cells favor immune reconstitution and control graft-versus-host disease while maintaining graft-versus-leukemia. J Clin Invest 112:1688–1696

Truitt RL, Johnson BD (1995) Principles of graft-vs.-leukemia reactivity. Biol Blood Marrow Transplant 1:61–68

Vogelsang GB, Lee L et al (2003) Pathogenesis and treatment of graft-versus-host disease after bone marrow transplant. Annu Rev Med 54:29–52

Waldmann H, Graca L et al (2004) Regulatory T cells and organ transplantation. Semin Immunol 16:119–126

Walker LS, Chodos A et al (2003) Antigen-dependent proliferation of CD4+ CD25+ regulatory T cells in vivo. J Exp Med 198:249–258

Wang XN, Proctor SJ et al (1996) Frequency analysis of recipient-reactive helper and cytotoxic T lymphocyte precursors using a combined single limiting dilution assay. Transpl Immunol 4:247–251

Yamazaki S, Iyoda T et al (2003) Direct expansion of functional CD25+ CD4+ regulatory T cells by antigen-processing dendritic cells. J Exp Med 198:235–247

Zeng D, Lan F et al (2004) Suppression of graft-versus-host disease by naturally occurring regulatory T cells. Transplantation 77:S9–S11

Zeng D, Lewis D et al (1999) Bone marrow NK1.1(–) and NK1.1(+) T cells reciprocally regulate acute graft versus host disease. J Exp Med 189:1073–1081

Zhang ZX, Yang L et al (2000) Identification of a previously unknown antigen-specific regulatory T cell and its mechanism of suppression. Nat Med 6:782–789

Naturally Arising CD25⁺CD4⁺ Regulatory T Cells in Tumor Immunity

T. Nomura · S. Sakaguchi (✉)

Department of Experimental Pathology, Institute for Frontier Medical Sciences, Kyoto University, 53 Shogoin-Kawahara-Cho, Sakyo-Ku, Kyoto 606–8507, Japan
shimon@frontier.kyoto-u.ac.jp

1	Introduction	287
2	Immunological Characteristics of Natural CD25⁺CD4⁺ T_R Cells	289
2.1	Suppressive Activity of CD25⁺CD4⁺ T_R Cells	289
2.2	Functional and Phenotypic Stability of Natural CD25⁺CD4⁺ T_R Cells	291
2.3	Control of CD25⁺CD4⁺ T_R Cell Development by *Foxp3*	291
3	CD25⁺CD4⁺ T_R Cells in Tumor Immunity	292
3.1	Induction of Tumor Immunity by Reducing Natural CD25⁺CD4⁺ T_R Cells	294
3.2	Attenuation of Immune Suppressive Activity of CD25⁺CD4⁺ T_R Cells Can Evoke Tumor Immunity	295
3.3	CD25⁺CD4⁺ T_R Cells and Tumor Immunity in Humans	296
4	Autoimmunity and Tumor Immunity	297
5	Conclusion and Perspective	297
References		299

Abstract Naturally arising regulatory T (T_R) cells, represented by CD25⁺CD4⁺ T_R cells, play an essential role in maintaining immunological self-tolerance. This T cell-mediated dominant control of the immune response not only inhibits the development of autoimmune disease, but also impedes effective immunosurveillance against autologous tumor cells. Attenuation of T_R cell-mediated immune suppression can therefore evoke effective tumor immunity in otherwise nonresponsive animals. This common regulatory mechanism for autoimmunity and tumor immunity can be exploited when devising a novel immunotherapy for cancer.

1
Introduction

There is substantial evidence from both animals and humans that the immune system controls cancer development; that is, a cancer immunosurveillance mechanism exists in normal individuals (Dunn et al. 2004). Recent studies have also shown that many cancer patients develop cytotoxic T lymphocytes (CTL) that can recognize tumor-associated antigens of autologous tumor cells, although they are not sufficiently strong to eradicate tumors in the majority of patients (Boon et al. 1994; Houghton 1994). A key issue in tumor immunology is therefore to understand the cellular and molecular basis of immunosurveillance against cancer, why cancer immunosurveillance is apparently not so effective in preventing cancer, and how it can be strengthened to prevent or treat cancer. A clue to these issues is the finding that many tumor antigens recognized by autologous CTLs are antigenically normal self-constituents. This indicates that a normal individual bears a T cell repertoire for tumor antigens as well as self antigens; i.e., tumor immunity is, in part, an autoimmunity. It also implies that the mechanisms that maintain immunologic tolerance to self-constituents may impede immunity against autologous tumor cells, and that manipulation of the immune system to break immunologic self-tolerance may provoke effective immune responses to autologous tumor cells.

T cells play key roles in mediating autoimmune disease as well as destroying tumor cells. It is now well established that, in addition to clonal deletion in the thymus or anergy induction in the periphery, there exists a T cell-mediated dominant mechanism of controlling self-reactive T cells; that is, a population of T cells actively suppresses the activation and expansion of self-reactive T cells (Sakaguchi 2004). Indeed, there are accumulating demonstrations that various autoimmune diseases can be produced in normal rodents by simply removing a particular $CD4^+$ T cell subpopulation defined by expression levels of certain cell surface molecules, and that reconstitution of the eliminated population can prevent autoimmune disease. CD25 is to date the most specific cell surface marker for such naturally occurring T_R cells that engage in the maintenance of natural self-tolerance. $CD25^+CD4^+$ T_R cells are unique in that the majority of them are naturally produced by the normal thymus as a functionally distinct and mature T cell subpopulation and persist in the periphery with stable regulatory functions (Asano et al. 1996; Itoh et al. 1999; Suri-Payer et al. 1998). Furthermore, recent studies have shown that the *Foxp3* gene, which encodes a transcription factor, specifically controls their development and function (Fontenot et al. 2003; Hori et al. 2003; Khattri et al. 2003).

T_R cells are heterogeneous in phenotype, function, and the way of generation. Some develop in the thymus as endogenous or natural T_R cells, which are represented by $CD25^+CD4^+$ T_R cells. Others are adaptive T_R cells that are induced in the periphery from mature T cells under particular in vivo or in vitro conditions for antigenic stimulation (Bluestone and Abbas 2003).

In this review, we focus on naturally arising $CD25^+CD4^+$ T_R cells because there is now substantial evidence that they play key roles in the control of autoimmunity and tumor immunity. We shall review the immunological properties of natural $CD25^+CD4^+$ T_R cells and their roles in immunologic self-tolerance and immunosurveillance against tumor cells. We also discuss how they can be exploited to provoke effective tumor immunity by breaching natural self-tolerance.

2
Immunological Characteristics of Natural $CD25^+CD4^+$ T_R Cells

2.1
Suppressive Activity of $CD25^+CD4^+$ T_R Cells

Upon in vitro T cell receptor (TCR) stimulation, $CD25^+CD4^+$ T_R cells from normal naive mice exert potent suppression on the activation/proliferation of other T cells (both $CD4^+$ T cells and $CD8^+$ T cells) in an antigen-nonspecific manner; i.e., once they are activated by a specific antigen, they suppress the proliferation of not only T cells with the same antigen specificity as the T_R cells, but also those specific for irrelevant antigens presented by the same antigen-presenting cells (APCs) (Takahashi et al. 1998; Thornton and Shevach 1998). This suppression, directly or indirectly, results in inhibition of IL-2 production by the T cells under suppression. In contrast with other regulatory T cells secreting immunoregulatory cytokines such as IL-10 and TGF-β, the $CD25^+CD4^+$ T_R cell-mediated suppression is not mediated by far-reaching or long-lasting humoral factors, such as IL-4, IL-10, or TGF-β, but is dependent, at least in vitro, on a cell-to-cell interaction among T_R cells, effector T cells, and APCs. This suppression is highly sensitive to antigenic stimulation. For example, when $CD25^+CD4^+$ T_R cells and $CD25^-CD4^+$ T cells are prepared from a TCR-transgenic mouse and stimulated with a specific peptide, the antigen concentration required for stimulating the former to exert suppression is much lower than that required for triggering the latter to proliferate. This high antigen sensitivity of $CD25^+CD4^+$ T_R cells is suited for the maintenance of self-tolerance but potentially a hindrance to provoking effective tumor immunity.

$CD25^+CD4^+$ T_R cells constitutively express CTLA-4 as an essential co-stimulatory molecule for their activation (Read et al. 2000; Takahashi et al. 2000). In an in vitro proliferation assay, blocking CTLA-4 with a Fab fragment of anti-CTLA-4 monoclonal antibody (mAb) abrogated the suppression by $CD25^+CD4^+$ T_R cells. In addition, $CD25^+CD4^+$ T_R cells from normal mice suppressed the activation of $CD25^-CD4^+$ T cells from CTLA-4 deficient mice in vitro, and Fab anti-CTLA-4 mAb abrogated this suppression. These data suggest that engagement of CTLA-4 on $CD25^+CD4^+$ T_R cells transduces a costimulatory signal for activating them; failure to activate $CD25^+CD4^+$ T_R cells by blocking CTLA-4 expressed on them, therefore, results in attenuated suppression on self-reactive T cells. Indeed, administration of anti-CTLA-4 mAb in normal mice elicited autoimmune disease similar to the one produced by depleting natural T_R cells. Interestingly, $CD25^+CD4^+$ T cells from CTLA-4-deficient mice can also suppress other T cells in vitro. This is presumably because CTLA-4-deficient $CD25^+CD4^+$ T_R cells are somehow intrinsically activated already, and hence can exert suppression. It is also well substantiated that activated T cells in general express CTLA-4 and interaction with B7 molecules transduces a negative signal to activated T cells. Blockade of CTLA-4 on activated T cells therefore sustains their activated state and effector activity. Taken together, it is likely that CTLA-4 possesses two roles in immunoregulation: one is to transduce a braking signal to activated effector T cells, the other to activate $CD25^+CD4^+$ T_R cells. The outcome of these two effects is the same, i.e., attenuation of immune responses. Blockade of the two events simultaneously therefore enhances immune responses synergistically.

$CD25^+CD4^+$ T_R cells also predominantly express glucocorticoid-induced tumor necrosis factor-related gene (GITR) (McHugh et al. 2002; Shimizu et al. 2002), which encodes a member of the tumor necrosis factor (TNF) receptor superfamily. Every T cell also expresses GITR at a low level, and T-cell activation upregulates the expression. Interestingly, addition of a monoclonal or polyclonal antibody to GITR abrogates $CD25^+CD4^+$ T_R cell-mediated suppression in vitro. Whole Ig molecules of agonistic anti-GITR mAb abrogated in vitro $CD25^+CD4^+$ T_R cell-mediated suppression, whereas Fab anti-GITR did not. Furthermore, administration of anti-GITR mAb produced autoimmune disease similar to the one produced by anti-CTLA-4 treatment (Shimizu et al. 2002). These results, taken together, indicate that ligation of the GITR molecule expressed on $CD25^+CD4^+$ T_R cells transduces a signal that attenuates their suppressive activity. Alternatively, ligation of GITR on activated T cells and not T_R cells renders them resistant to suppression (Stephens et al. 2004). It remains to be determined how GITR ligand physiologically transduces a signal to GITR-expressing T_R cells or non-T_R cells, or both.

Thus, the attenuation of the suppressive function of natural T_R cells with anti-CTLA-4 or anti-GITR mAb not only induces autoimmunity but also may enhance immune responses to autologous tumor cells in otherwise unresponsive individuals.

2.2
Functional and Phenotypic Stability of Natural CD25$^+$CD4$^+$ T$_R$ Cells

Another unique property of naturally arising CD25$^+$CD4$^+$ T$_R$ cells is their anergy to TCR stimulation. Purified CD25$^+$CD4$^+$ T$_R$ cells from normal mice hardly proliferate in response to in vitro antigenic stimulation, and fail to transcribe the IL-2 gene, which is the hallmark of T cell anergy. Importantly, this anergic state is tightly coupled with their suppressive activity. For example, when CD25$^+$CD4$^+$ T$_R$ cells are stimulated by antigen in the presence of high-dose exogenous IL-2 or agonistic anti-CD28 mAb, they can proliferate and at the same time lose their suppressive activity; upon removal of IL-2 or anti-CD28 mAb, they spontaneously revert to the original anergic state and reacquire suppressive activity (Kuniyasu et al. 2000; Takahashi et al. 1998). This indicates that the anergic and suppressive state is the basal and default condition for CD25$^+$CD4$^+$ T$_R$ cells, at least in vitro. It also suggests that a functional breach of their anergic and suppressive state may elicit autoimmunity and also enhance tumor immunity.

Phenotypically, natural CD25$^+$CD4$^+$ T$_R$ cells show an "activated" or "antigen-primed" phenotype already in the thymus and this phenotype is stably maintained in the periphery; e.g., they are CD25$^+$, CD45RB^{low}, CD44^{high}, and CD5^{high}. This suggests that the majority of CD25$^+$CD4$^+$ T$_R$ cells could be inherently reactive with self-antigens and continuously activated by them in the normal internal environment.

2.3
Control of CD25$^+$CD4$^+$ T$_R$ Cell Development by *Foxp3*

Another feature of natural CD25$^+$CD4$^+$ T$_R$ cells is that their generation is in part developmentally and genetically controlled. Recent studies showed that *Foxp3*, a gene encoding a transcription factor of the forkhead/winged-helix family, plays a key role in their development and function. *Foxp3* was originally identified as the disease gene of fatal autoimmune/inflammatory disease of scurfy mice (Brunkow et al. 2001). Subsequently, mutations in *FOXP3* (the human ortholog of murine *Foxp3*) were found in patients with immune dysregulation, polyendocrinopathy, enteropathy, X-linked (IPEX) syndrome, which phenotypically and pathologically resembles autoimmune/inflammatory diseases that develop in rodents following the removal of natural CD25$^+$CD4$^+$ T$_R$ cells (Bennett et al. 2001; Chatila et al. 2000; Wildin et al. 2001). It was indeed shown that CD25$^+$CD4$^+$ T$_R$ cells in the thymus and periphery predominantly expressed *Foxp3* mRNA, whereas B cells, CD8$^+$ T cells, CD4$^+$CD8$^+$, or CD4$^-$CD8$^+$ thymocytes did not (Hori et al. 2003; Khattri et al. 2003). The *Foxp3* expression levels in CD25$^+$CD4$^+$ T$_R$ cells were approximately 100-fold higher than that in CD25⁻CD4⁺ T cells. Activation of CD25⁻CD4⁺ T cells, Th1, or Th2 cells failed to induce *Foxp3* expression, in contrast with their expression of CD25, CTLA-4, and GITR, which are generally expressed on any activated T cells (Hori et al. 2003). Importantly, retroviral transduction of *Foxp3/FOXP3* into CD25⁻CD4⁺ T cells converted them to CD25⁺CD4⁺ T_R-like cells (Hori et al. 2003, Yagi et al. 2004). Such *Foxp3*-transduced T cells showed hypoproliferation and low production of cytokines in response to in vitro antigenic stimulation, and suppressed the activation of co-cultured CD25⁻CD4⁺ naive T cells in a similar manner to natural T_R cells. *Foxp3*-transduced T cells were also able to negatively control self-reactive T cells in vivo; for example, co-transfer of *Foxp3*-transduced T cells inhibited the development of inflammatory bowel disease and autoimmune gastritis that can be induced in SCID mice by the transfer of CD25⁻CD45RB^{high}CD4⁺ T cells from normal mice. *Foxp3* is also indispensable for the development of CD25⁺CD4⁺ T_R cells, as bone marrow cells from *Foxp3*-deficient mice failed to give rise to CD25⁺CD4⁺ T_R cells (Fontenot et al. 2003).

These results taken together indicate that *FOXP3/Foxp3* is a master control gene for the development and function of CD25⁺CD4⁺ T_R cells. Furthermore, *FOXP3/Foxp3* is a highly specific marker for natural T_R cells.

3
CD25⁺CD4⁺ T_R Cells in Tumor Immunity

The findings on self-tolerance and autoimmunity controlled by CD25⁺CD4⁺ T_R cells indicate that elimination of this regulatory population may provoke specific immune responses to syngeneic tumors as a "quasi-autoimmune" response. To examine this possibility, we transferred to BALB/c athymic nude mice splenic cell suspensions depleted of CD25⁺ cells and subsequently

Fig. 1A, B Induction of autoimmune disease and tumor immunity in T cell-deficient mice. **A** Transfer of T cell suspensions depleted of CD25⁺ cells induces autoimmune diseases and also tumor immunity in the recipient a nude mice, without deliberate immunization. **B** Tumor growth was monitored for BALB/c nude mice subcutaneously transplanted with 1.5×10^5 RLmale1 cells (*arrow*) immediately after intravenous transfer of 3×10^7 whole spleen cells (*upper panel*), or 3×10^7 CD25⁻ spleen cells (*middle panel*), or mixture of CD25⁻ spleen cells (3×10^7) and CD4⁺ spleen cells (1×10^7) (*lower panel*). The CD25⁻ spleen cell-transferred nude mice having rejected the tumors were re-challenged on day 60 (*arrow*) with a ten times larger dose (1.5×10^6) of RLmale1 cells (*middle panel*). Insets show staining of each cell inoculum with CD4 (*ordinate*) and CD25 (*abscissa*), and percentages of cells in each quadrant

transplanted BALB/c-derived RLmale1 leukemia cells (Shimizu et al. 1999) (Fig. 1A). In the majority of mice, the tumors first grew and then regressed within a month, allowing the hosts to survive more than 80 days after tumor inoculation (Fig. 1B, middle panel), whereas all the nude mice transferred with nondepleted spleen cells (Fig. 1B, upper panel) or the mixture of an

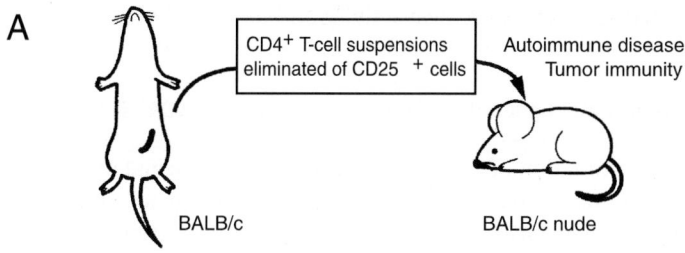

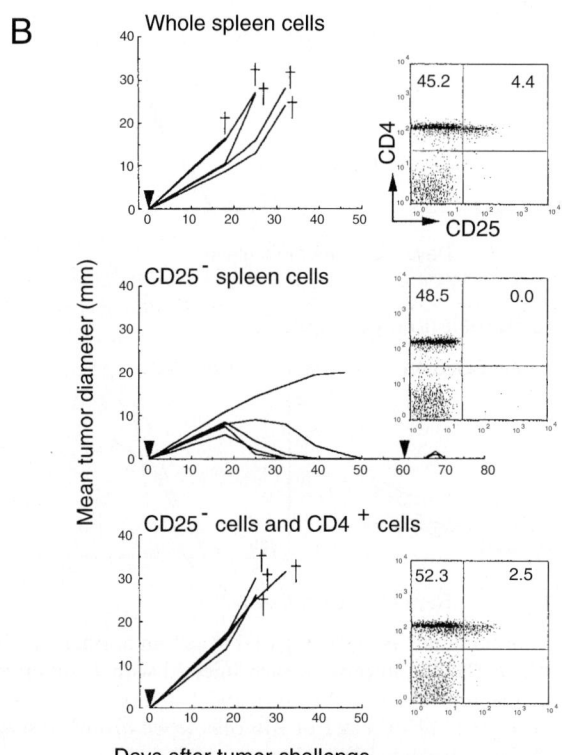

Days after tumor challenge

equal number of CD25⁻ cells and CD4⁺ T cells died of tumor progression (Fig. 1B, lower panel). Upon re-challenge with a larger dose of RLmale1, the CD25⁻ cell-transferred nude mice rejected the tumor cells more rapidly and vigorously than the primary rejection, indicating that they had become immune to the tumor cells (Fig. 1B, middle panel). The results indicate that tumor immunity can be evoked by reducing the number of natural T_R cells or by attenuating their suppressive activity.

3.1
Induction of Tumor Immunity by Reducing Natural $CD25^+CD4^+$ T_R Cells

Transient elimination of $CD25^+CD4^+$ T_R cells from normal mice by administering anti-CD25 mAb can also elicit immunity to syngeneic tumors (Shimizu et al. 1999). When anti-CD25 mAb (PC61) were administered twice (on 4 and 2 days before tumor inoculation) to BALB/c or C57BL/6 mice, the number of

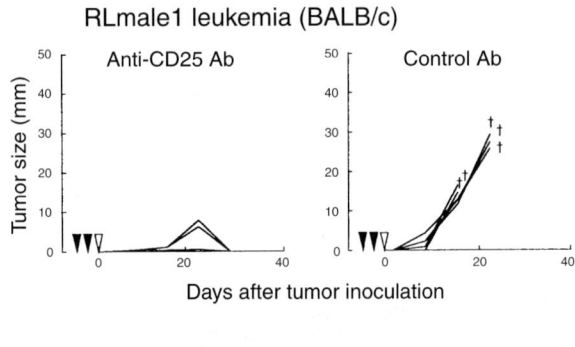

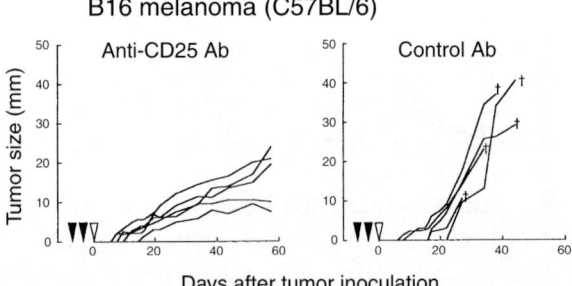

Fig. 2 Induction of tumor immunity by depleting $CD25^+$ cells in normal mice in vivo. Eight-week-old BALB/c or C57BL6 mice were each injected with 1 mg of purified PC61 (anti-CD25 depleting mAb) intravenously on 4 and 2 days (*filled arrows*) before subcutaneous inoculation of 1×10^5 Rlmale1 or B16 cells (*open arrow*), respectively. Tumor growth was monitored for individual mice

peripheral $CD25^+CD4^+$ T_R cells reduced to a quarter of control mice for nearly 1 month. In the majority of PC61-treated BALB/c mice, the subsequently inoculated RLmale1 cells first grew and then regressed within 1 month, whereas all the BALB/c mice treated with normal rat immunoglobulin as a control died of tumor progression within 1 month (Fig. 2, upper panels). Likewise, PC61 treatment of C57BL/6 mice significantly suppressed the growth of B16 melanoma cells when compared with control C57BL/6 mice treated with normal rat IgG, allowing the former to survive longer (>60 days) compared with the latter (<40 days) (Fig. 2, lower panels). This anti-CD25 treatment was also effective in eradicating a variety of tumors in other mouse strains (Onizuka et al. 1999).

Tumor effector cells can also be generated in vitro from normal spleen cells by simply eliminating $CD25^+CD4^+$ T_R cells. During this in vitro induction of tumor immunity, $CD25^-CD4^+$ T cells responding to self-peptides/class II MHC molecules expressed on syngeneic APCs spontaneously proliferated following removal of $CD25^+CD4^+$ T_R cells. A large amount of IL-2 produced by such $CD4^+$ self-reactive T cells generated natural killer-like tumor effector cells as lymphokine-activated killer (LAK) cells that were capable of indiscriminately killing various tumor cells (Shimizu et al. 1999).

3.2
Attenuation of Immune Suppressive Activity of $CD25^+CD4^+$ T_R Cells Can Evoke Tumor Immunity

The finding that blockade of CTLA-4 or signaling through GITR can attenuate $CD25^+CD4^+$ T_R cell-mediated suppression indicates that these treatments may also enhance tumor immunity (Shimizu et al. 2002). When DTA-1 anti-GITR mAb, which is nondepleting, was administered after the inoculation of Meth-A, a methylcholanthrene-induced sarcoma of BALB/c origin, the growth of tumor cells was significantly inhibited even when the treatment was commenced after tumor grew to a visible mass (Ko et al., manuscript in preparation). Interestingly, examination of *Foxp3* expression in tumor masses revealed that the number of *Foxp3*-expressing cells was decreased to a larger degree compared with other tumor infiltrating T cells in the DTA-1 treated mice. This indicates that DTA-1 treatment enhanced the activation and proliferation of tumor effector cells by abrogating T_R cell-mediated suppression, inhibited infiltration of T_R cells to the tumor mass, or both.

In vivo administration of anti-CTLA-4 antibody also enhances tumor immunity (Leach et al. 1996). This effect has been attributed to the possible hindrance of CTLA-4-induced negative signals to activated effector T cells mediating anti-tumor immune responses (for a recent review see Chen 2004).

Another possibility, which is not mutually exclusive, is the blockade of CTLA-4 molecules expressed on $CD25^+CD4^+$ T_R cells and consequent interference with T cell-mediated immunoregulation, as in the case of induction of autoimmunity by anti-CTLA-4 antibody treatment (Luhder et al. 1998; Perrin et al. 1996).

Taken together, reduction of natural $CD25^+CD4^+$ T_R cells or attenuation of immunosuppressive function of $CD25^+CD4^+$ T_R cells can break immunological unresponsiveness to syngeneic tumors both in vivo and in vitro, leading to spontaneous development of tumor-specific as well as tumor-nonspecific effector cells.

3.3
$CD25^+CD4^+$ T_R Cells and Tumor Immunity in Humans

T cells reactive with normal self-constituents or tumor-associated antigens are present in the peripheral blood of normal individuals. For example, peripheral blood $CD4^+$ T cells show in vitro proliferative responses to self-antigens such as human heat shock protein-60 (hHSP60) and myelin oligodendrocyte glycoprotein (MOG) when $CD25^+CD4^+$ T_R cells are removed before culture (Taams et al. 2002; Wing et al. 2003). Direct visualization of self-reactive T cells in healthy individuals was achieved by using class II tetramers loaded with the diabetes-associated antigen glutamic acid decarboxylase (GAD) 65, the vitiligo and melanoma-associated antigen tyrosinase, or the cancer/testis antigen NY-ESO-1 (Danke et al. 2004). Following removal of $CD25^+CD4^+$ T_R cells and stimulation with antigens, tetramer positive T cells became easily detected in vitro. T cells specific for tumor-associated antigens, most of which are normal self-constituents, can also be detected in the peripheral blood, within tumors, and in draining lymph nodes of cancer patients (Boon et al. 1994; Houghton, 1994). Despite the presence of such tumor-reactive T cells, it is rare to observe spontaneous regression of cancers. Although it remains to be determined whether cancer cells may somehow escape immune attack, or the immune system protects cancers from the attack, it is likely that naturally present $CD25^+CD4^+$ T_R cells play a role in suppressing the development of effective tumor immunity. A recent clinical study indeed showed that ovarian or gastric carcinomas with intra-tumor accumulation of $CD25^+CD4^+FOXP3^+$ T cells, supposedly $CD25^+CD4^+$ T_R cells, were associated with poor prognosis (Curiel et al. 2004; Sasada et al. 2003). Further study is needed to determine the role of natural T_R cells in tumor immunity in humans.

4
Autoimmunity and Tumor Immunity

Removal of $CD25^+CD4^+$ T_R cells may elicit autoimmunity in addition to provoking tumor immunity. This raises the issue of how tumor immunity can be evoked without autoimmunity by manipulating natural T_R cells. It is of note in this regard that the intensity and the range of autoimmune responses (i.e., the severity, the incidence, and the spectrum of autoimmune diseases) elicited by removal of T_R cells depend on the degree and duration of depleting $CD25^+CD4^+$ T_R cells, and, more importantly, the genetic background of the hosts (Sakaguchi et al. 1995, 1996). For example, in genetically autoimmune-prone BALB/c mice, generation of effective tumor immunity can be achieved without deleterious autoimmunity by limiting the period of depleting $CD25^+CD4^+$ T_R cells, whereas, in genetically autoimmune-resistant C57BL/6 mice, complete depletion of $CD25^+CD4^+$ T_R cells leads to tumor rejection without producing autoimmune disease (S. Yamazaki et al., unpublished results). Thus, autoimmunity and tumor immunity evoked by abrogation of the T_R-mediated immunoregulation can be differentiated by the duration or degree of T_R cell-depletion required for induction of autoimmunity or tumor immunity, and by host genetic factors that determine susceptibility or resistance to autoimmune disease. In addition, effector T cells involved in autoimmunity and tumor immunity may be different; for example, $CD8^+$ CTLs may play a more important role in tumor immunity than autoimmunity.

5
Conclusion and Perspective

It has been postulated since the 1970s that one of the elements that impedes the generation of effective tumor immunity in tumor-bearing hosts may be concomitant development of a T cell population suppressing the generation or action of tumor-killing effector cells. Although some of such suppressor T cells were previously shown to be $CD4^+$, they eluded further characterization and manipulation because of the lack of reliable markers specific for them (Awwad and North 1988). There is now accumulating evidence that such suppressive T cells, at least in part, can be naturally present $CD25^+CD4^+$ T_R cells (Fig. 3). The $CD25^+CD4^+$ T_R cells, however, bear several characteristics distinct from the suppressor T cells concomitantly induced by sensitization to tumor antigens. First, natural T_R cells are present before the appearance of tumor cells; that is, removal of $CD25^+CD4^+$ T_R cells before tumor development is effective in evoking specific tumor immunity. This means that they are physiologically

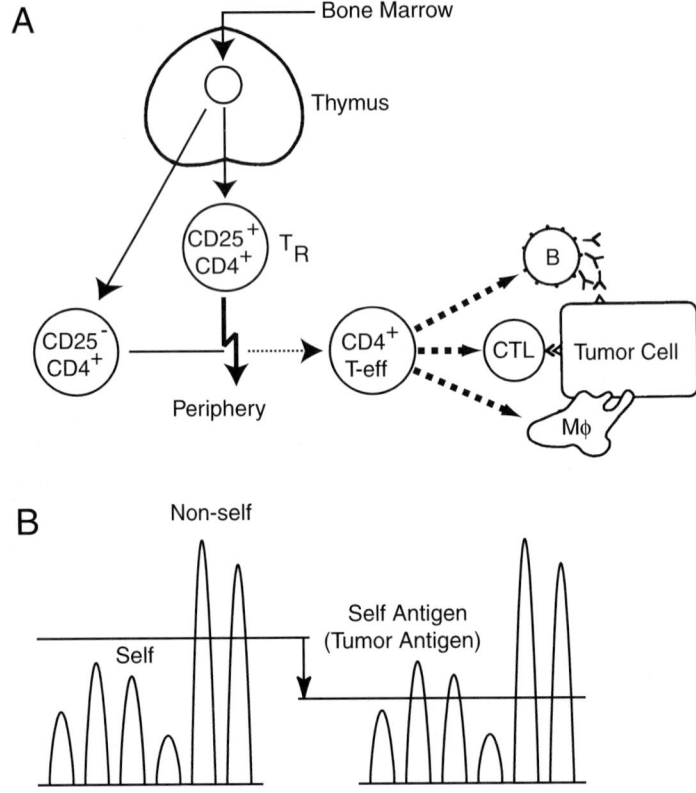

Fig. 3A, B Dominant suppression of tumor immunity by $CD25^+CD4^+$ T_R cells. **A** Although highly self-reactive T cells are eliminated during their thymic generation, the normal thymus continuously produces potentially pathogenic self-reactive $CD4^+$ T cells that persist in a $CD25^-$ quiescent state in the periphery. The normal thymus also continuously produces naturally anergic and suppressive $CD25^+CD4^+$ T_R cells that dominantly suppress the activation and expansion of $CD4^+$ self-reactive effector T cells from their $CD25^-$ dormant state. When $CD25^+CD4^+$ T_R cells are reduced in number or functionally impaired, $CD25^-$ self-reactive T cells become activated, expand, and differentiate to $CD25^+$-activated effector T cells (*dotted thin arrow*), which help B cells to form antibodies, conduct cell-mediated tumor immunity by recruiting inflammatory cells, including activated macrophages ($M\phi$), and help activation and expansion of $CD8^+$ cytotoxic lymphocytes (*CTLs*) (*dotted thick arrows*). **B** Immune responsiveness to self and non-self depicted as a continuum. The *upper horizontal line* indicates the level of immunoregulation by T_R cells. The *peaks above the line* represent overt immune responses to non-self antigens. When the level goes down, immune responses to certain self-antigens (including tumor antigens) become apparent. The peaks representing immune responses to self-antigens are depicted as being lower than those to non-self-antigens, because T cells bearing high-avidity T cell receptors for the self antigens are supposed to be deleted in the thymus

impeding natural immunosurveillance and depletion/reduction of this population can augment immunosurveillance against cancer. Second, they are engaged in the maintenance of natural self-tolerance; therefore their removal can elicit not only tumor immunity but also autoimmunity. Third, natural $CD25^+CD4^+$ T_R cells are continuously produced by the normal thymus, constantly replenishing a fraction of the T-cell compartment (Itoh et al. 1999). This means that elimination of T_R cells for induction of tumor immunity may not impair immune function for a long period of time, and recovery of T_R cells may prevent the development of serious autoimmune disease.

Manipulation of natural $CD25^+CD4^+$ T_R cells is thus instrumental for cancer immunotherapy. For example, administration of anti-CD25, anti-CTLA-4, or anti-GITR antibody, or their combination, to cancer-bearing hosts for a limited period may evoke or enhance tumor immunity. Removal of T_R cells prior to in vitro culture of lymphocytes from cancer patients with high-dose IL-2 may lead to production of more potent or larger numbers of cytotoxic cells, including CTLs and NK cells (Rosenberg and Lotze 1986). Furthermore, monitoring FoxP3 expression in tumor tissue may be informative in assessing local tumor immunity.

Acknowledgements We thank Dr. Zoltan Fehervari for discussion and critically reading the manuscript.

References

Asano M, Toda M, Sakaguchi N, Sakaguchi S (1996) Autoimmune disease as a consequence of developmental abnormality of a T cell subpopulation. J Exp Med 184:387–396

Awwad M, North RJ (1988) Immunologically mediated regression of a murine lymphoma after treatment with anti-L3T4 antibody. A consequence of removing L3T4+ suppressor T cells from a host generating predominantly Lyt-2+ T cell-mediated immunity. J Exp Med 168:2193–2206

Bennett CL, Christie J, Ramsdell F, Brunkow ME, Ferguson PJ, Whitesell L, Kelly TE, Saulsbury FT, Chance PF, Ochs HD (2001) The immune dysregulation, polyendocrinopathy, enteropathy, X-linked syndrome (IPEX) is caused by mutations of FOXP3. Nat Genet 27:20–21

Bluestone JA, Abbas AK (2003) Natural versus adaptive regulatory T cells. Nat Rev Immunol 3:253–257

Boon T, Cerottini JC, Van den Eynde B, van der Bruggen P, Van Pel A (1994) Tumor antigens recognized by T lymphocytes. Annu Rev Immunol 12:337–365

Brunkow ME, Jeffery EW, Hjerrild KA, Paeper B, Clark LB, Yasayko SA, Wilkinson JE, Galas D, Ziegler SF, Ramsdell F (2001) Disruption of a new forkhead/winged-helix protein, scurfin, results in the fatal lymphoproliferative disorder of the scurfy mouse. Nat Genet 27:68–73

Chatila TA, Blaeser F, Ho N, Lederman HM, Voulgaropoulos C, Helms C, Bowcock AM (2000) JM2, encoding a fork head-related protein, is mutated in X-linked autoimmunity-allergic disregulation syndrome. J Clin Invest 106:R75–81

Chen L (2004) Co-inhibitory molecules of the B7-CD28 family in the control of T-cell immunity. Nat Rev Immunol 4:336–347

Curiel TJ, Coukos G, Zou L, Alvarez X, Cheng P, Mottram P, Evdemon-Hogan M, Conejo-Garcia JR, Zhang L, Burow M, Zhu Y, Wei S, Kryczek I, Daniel B, Gordon A, Myers L, Lackner A, Disis ML, Knutson KL, Chen L, Zou W (2004) Specific recruitment of regulatory T cells in ovarian carcinoma fosters immune privilege and predicts reduced survival. Nat Med 10:942–949

Danke NA, Koelle DM, Yee C, Beheray S, Kwok WW (2004) Autoreactive T cells in healthy individuals. J Immunol 172:5967–5972

Dunn GP, Old LJ, Schreiber RD (2004) The immunobiology of cancer immunosurveillance and immunoediting. Immunity 21:137–148

Fontenot JD, Gavin MA, Rudensky AY (2003) Foxp3 programs the development and function of CD4+CD25+ regulatory T cells. Nat Immunol 4:330–336

Hori S, Nomura T, Sakaguchi S (2003) Control of regulatory T cell development by the transcription factor Foxp3. Science 299:1057–1061

Houghton AN (1994) Cancer antigens: immune recognition of self and altered self. J Exp Med 180:1–4

Itoh M, Takahashi T, Sakaguchi N, Kuniyasu Y, Shimizu J, Otsuka F, Sakaguchi S (1999) Thymus and autoimmunity: production of CD25+CD4+ naturally anergic and suppressive T cells as a key function of the thymus in maintaining immunologic self-tolerance. J Immunol 162:5317–5326

Khattri R, Cox T, Yasayko SA, Ramsdell F (2003) An essential role for Scurfin in CD4+CD25+ T regulatory cells. Nat Immunol 4:337–342

Kuniyasu Y, Takahashi T, Itoh M, Shimizu J, Toda G, Sakaguchi S (2000) Naturally anergic and suppressive CD25(+)CD4(+) T cells as a functionally and phenotypically distinct immunoregulatory T cell subpopulation. Int Immunol 12:1145–1155

Leach DR, Krummel MF, Allison JP (1996) Enhancement of antitumor immunity by CTLA-4 blockade. Science 271:1734–1736

Luhder F, Hoglund P, Allison JP, Benoist C, Mathis D (1998) Cytotoxic T lymphocyte-associated antigen 4 (CTLA-4) regulates the unfolding of autoimmune diabetes. J Exp Med 187:427–432

McHugh RS, Whitters MJ, Piccirillo CA, Young DA, Shevach EM, Collins M, Byrne MC (2002) CD4(+)CD25(+) immunoregulatory T cells: gene expression analysis reveals a functional role for the glucocorticoid-induced TNF receptor. Immunity 16:311–323

Onizuka S, Tawara I, Shimizu J, Sakaguchi S, Fujita T, Nakayama E (1999) Tumor rejection by in vivo administration of anti-CD25 (interleukin-2 receptor alpha) monoclonal antibody. Cancer Res 59:3128–3133

Perrin PJ, Maldonado JH, Davis TA, June CH, Racke MK (1996) CTLA-4 blockade enhances clinical disease and cytokine production during experimental allergic encephalomyelitis. J Immunol 157:1333–1336

Read S, Malmstrom V, Powrie F (2000) Cytotoxic T lymphocyte-associated antigen 4 plays an essential role in the function of CD25(+)CD4(+) regulatory cells that control intestinal inflammation. J Exp Med 192:295–302

Rosenberg SA, Lotze MT (1986) Cancer immunotherapy using interleukin-2 and interleukin-2-activated lymphocytes. Annu Rev Immunol 4:681–709

Sasada T, Kimura M, Yoshida Y, Kanai M, Takabayashi A (2003) CD4+CD25+ regulatory T cells in patients with gastrointestinal malignancies: possible involvement of regulatory T cells in disease progression. Cancer 98:1089–1099

Sakaguchi S (2004) Naturally arising CD4+ regulatory t cells for immunologic self-tolerance and negative control of immune responses. Annu Rev Immunol 22:531–562

Sakaguchi S, Sakaguchi N, Asano M, Itoh M, Toda M Immunologic self-tolerance maintained by activated T cells expressing IL-2 receptor alpha-chains (CD25). Breakdown of a single mechanism of self-tolerance causes various autoimmune diseases. (1995) J Immunol 155:1151–1164

Sakaguchi S, Toda M, Asano M, Itoh M, Morse SS, Sakaguchi N (1996) T cell-mediated maintenance of natural self-tolerance: its breakdown as a possible cause of various autoimmune diseases. J Autoimmun 9:211–220

Shimizu J, Yamazaki S, Sakaguchi S (1999) Induction of tumor immunity by removing CD25+CD4+ T cells: a common basis between tumor immunity and autoimmunity. J Immunol 163:5211–5218

Shimizu J, Yamazaki S, Takahashi T, Ishida Y, Sakaguchi S (2002) Stimulation of CD25(+)CD4(+) regulatory T cells through GITR breaks immunological self-tolerance. Nat Immunol 3:135–142

Stephens GL, McHugh RS, Whitters MJ, Young DA, Luxenberg D, Carreno BM, Collins M, Shevach EM (2004) Engagement of glucocorticoid-induced TNFR family-related receptor on effector T cells by its ligand mediates resistance to suppression by CD4+CD25+ T cells. J Immunol 173:5008-5020

Suri-Payer E, Amar AZ, Thornton AM, Shevach EM (1998) CD4+CD25+ T cells inhibit both the induction and effector function of autoreactive T cells and represent a unique lineage of immunoregulatory cells. J Immunol 160:1212–1218

Taams LS, Vukmanovic-Stejic M, Smith J, Dunne PJ, Fletcher JM, Plunkett FJ, Ebeling SB, Lombardi G, Rustin MH, Bijlsma JW, Lafeber FP, Salmon M, Akbar AN (2002) Antigen-specific T cell suppression by human CD4+CD25+ regulatory T cells. Eur J Immunol 32:1621–1630

Takahashi T, Kuniyasu Y, Toda M, Sakaguchi N, Itoh M, Iwata M, Shimizu J, Sakaguchi S (1998) Immunologic self-tolerance maintained by CD25+CD4+ naturally anergic and suppressive T cells: induction of autoimmune disease by breaking their anergic/suppressive state. Int Immunol 10:1969–1980

Takahashi T, Tagami T, Yamazaki S, Uede T, Shimizu J, Sakaguchi N, Mak TW, Sakaguchi S (2000) Immunologic self-tolerance maintained by CD25(+)CD4(+) regulatory T cells constitutively expressing cytotoxic T lymphocyte-associated antigen 4. J Exp Med 192:303–310

Thornton AM, Shevach EM (1998) CD4+CD25+ immunoregulatory T cells suppress polyclonal T cell activation in vitro by inhibiting interleukin 2 production. J Exp Med 188:287–296

Wildin RS, Ramsdell F, Peake J, Faravelli F, Casanova JL, Buist N, Levy-Lahad E, Mazzella M, Goulet O, Perroni L, Bricarelli FD, Byrne G, McEuen M, Proll S, Appleby M, Brunkow ME (2001) X-linked neonatal diabetes mellitus, enteropathy and endocrinopathy syndrome is the human equivalent of mouse scurfy. Nat Genet 27:18–20

Wing K, Lindgren S, Kollberg G, Lundgren A, Harris RA, Rudin A, Lundin S, Suri-Payer E (2003) CD4 T cell activation by myelin oligodendrocyte glycoprotein is suppressed by adult but not cord blood CD25+ T cells. Eur J Immunol 33:579–587

Yagi H, Nomura T, Nakamura K, Yamazaki S, Kitawaki T, Hori S, Maeda M, Onodera M, Uchiyama T, Fujii S, Sakaguchi S (2004) Crucial role of FOXP3 in the development and function of human CD25+CD4+ regulatory cells. Int Immunol 16:1643–1656

Phenotypic and Functional Differences Between Human $CD4^+CD25^+$ and Type 1 Regulatory T Cells

M. K. Levings[1] (✉) · M. G. Roncarolo[2]

[1] Department of Surgery, University of British Columbia and Immunity and Infection Research Centre, Vancouver Coastal Health Research Institute, 2660 Oak St., Vancouver B.C., V6H 3Z6, Canada
mlevings@interchange.ubc.ca

[2] San Raffaele Telethon Institute for Gene Therapy (HSR-TIGET) & Università Vita-Salute San Raffaele, 20132 Milan, Italy

1	Introduction	304
2	Tr1 Cells	304
2.1	Origins	305
2.2	Phenotype	306
2.3	Mechanisms of Action and Functions	307
2.4	In Vivo Evidence for Tr1 Cells in Humans	308
3	Naturally Occurring Human $CD4^+CD25^+$ Tr Cells	311
3.1	Origins	311
3.2	Phenotype	312
3.3	Functions	313
3.4	Mechanisms of Action	314
3.5	In Vivo Evidence for $CD4^+CD25^+$ Tr Cells in Humans	315
4	Peripheral Generation of $CD4^+CD25^+$ Tr Cells	315
5	Networks of Tr1 and $CD4^+CD25^+$ Tr Cells	316
6	Therapeutic Opportunities	317
References		318

Abstract T regulatory (Tr) cells have an essential role in the induction and maintenance of tolerance to both and foreign self-antigens. Many types of T cells with regulatory activity have been described in mice and humans, and those within the $CD4^+$ subset have been extensively characterized. $CD4^+$ Type-1 regulatory T (Tr1) cells produce high levels of IL-10 and mediate IL-10-dependent suppression, whereas the effects of naturally occurring $CD4^+CD25^+$ Tr cells appear to be cell-contact-dependent. Tr1 cells arise in the periphery upon encountering antigen in a tolerogenic environment. In contrast, it appears that $CD4^+CD25^+$ Tr cells can either arise directly in the thymus or be induced by antigen in the periphery. We have been interested in defining the phenotype and function of different subsets of CD4$^+$ Tr cells present in human peripheral blood, with the ultimate aim of designing therapeutic strategies to harness their immunoregulatory effects. This review will discuss the similarities and differences between human Tr1 and naturally occurring CD4$^+$CD25$^+$ Tr cells, as well as evidence that indicates that they have nonoverlapping, but synergistic roles in immune homeostasis.

Abbreviations

Ag	Antigen
APCs	Antigen-presenting cells
DCs	Dendritic cells
GITR	Glucocorticoid-induced TNFR superfamily member 18
GVHD	Graft versus host disease
SIT	Specific immunotherapy
Tr	T regulatory
Tr1	Type-1 T regulatory

1
Introduction

T regulatory (Tr) cells have an essential role in the induction and maintenance of tolerance to both and foreign self-antigens (Ags). Many types of T cells with regulatory activity have been described in mice and humans [83, 85, 90, 107], and those within the CD4$^+$ subset have been extensively characterized. CD4$^+$ Type-1 T regulatory (Tr1) cells arise in the periphery upon encountering Ag in a tolerogenic environment via a process that requires IL-10. Tr1 cells produce high levels of IL-10 themselves, and mediate IL-10-dependent suppression of T cell responses. In contrast, CD4$^+$CD25$^+$ Tr cells can either arise directly in the thymus (the so-called naturally occurring subset) or be induced by Ag in the periphery. Naturally occurring CD4$^+$CD25$^+$ Tr cells do not produce IL-10, and mediate cell-contact-dependent suppression. We have been interested in better defining the phenotype and function of these different subsets of CD4$^+$ Tr cells present in human peripheral blood, with the ultimate aim of designing therapeutic strategies that harness their immunoregulatory effects. In this review, we will discuss the similarities and differences between human Tr1 and CD4$^+$CD25$^+$ Tr cells, and evidence that indicates that they have nonoverlapping, but nevertheless synergistic roles in immune homeostasis.

2
Tr1 Cells

Tr1 cells were first defined in in vitro differentiation systems that involved priming CD4$^+$ T cells in the presence of exogenous IL-10 [40]. These IL-

10-anergized T cells appear to undergo two stages of differentiation. First, they become nonresponsive and fail to proliferate or produce cytokines in response to Ag-specific or polyclonal activation [24, 40]. In this intermediate stage, although the T cells have already acquired the capacity to suppress naive T-cell responses, this function is not dependent on production of immunosuppressive cytokines, but is cell-contact-dependent [24]. A second stage of differentiation occurs following forced proliferation in vitro [42], and likely following repeated Ag exposure in vivo. The previously anergic cells regain some ability to proliferate, and acquire a unique profile of cytokine production (IL-2$^{-/low}$, IL-4$^-$, IL-5$^+$, IL-10$^+$, TGF-β^+), which is distinct from those of classical Th0, Th1, or Th2 cells [42]. In addition to IL-10 and TGF-β, human Tr1 cells also produce IFN-γ, although at levels that are at least 1 log lower than those produced by Th1 cells [8, 62]. In contrast, murine Tr1 cells usually do not produce IFN-γ [42]. The finding that these fully differentiated Tr1 cells mediate IL-10- and TGF-β-dependent suppression in vitro and in vivo, in both Th1 and Th2-mediated diseases [60, 82], sparked intensive interest in better defining their origins, phenotype, and potential clinical application.

2.1
Origins

In addition to T-cell priming in the presence of exogenous IL-10, many other methods can be used to promote the differentiation of Tr1 cells. Indeed, in the absence of antigen presenting cells (APCs), IL-10 alone is relatively inefficient at generating Tr1 cells, and addition of IFN-α can enhance its effects [62]. This was recently confirmed in vivo upon treatment with G-CSF, which appears to induce Tr1 cells via induction of IL-10 and IFN-α [84]. Stimulation of T cells in the presence of immunosuppressants such as vitamin D3 and dexamethasone has a similar Tr1-inducing effect, which depends on induction of autocrine IL-10 [12]. Interestingly, co-stimulation via CD2 [105] or with antibodies against CD46, a receptor that binds and inactivates complement C3b [52], also results in the generation of Tr1 cells. A general conclusion from these studies conducted in the absence of APCs, is that IL-10, be it from an autocrine, paracrine, or exogenous source, is necessary, but probably not sufficient, for the differentiation of Tr1 cells.

Many groups have investigated the capacity of different subsets of APCs to prime Tr1 cells. We recently studied the capacity of immature dendritic cells (DCs) to drive the differentiation of Tr1 cells upon repeated stimulation of naive peripheral blood CD4$^+$ T cells. Allogeneic immature DCs prime Tr1 cells via an IL-10-dependent mechanism, and the resulting cells suppress proliferation and cytokine production by an IL-10- and TGF-β-dependent mechanism [61]. Induction of Tr1 cells by immature DCs does not require the presence of CD4$^+$CD25$^+$ Tr cells, and the resulting cells do not express high levels of CD25, providing further evidence that Tr1 and CD4$^+$CD25$^+$ Tr cells are distinct subsets (see also below). In contrast, when immature DCs are used to prime CD4$^+$ T cells isolated from cord blood, although the resulting T cells do produce IL-10, they do not mediate cytokine-dependent suppression [48]. The reason for this difference is not clear, but may be related to the fact that CD4$^+$ T cells from cord blood contain proportionally more CD4$^+$CD25$^+$ Tr cells and IL-10-producing cells than do adult peripheral blood T cells [62, 111], and therefore CD4$^+$CD25$^+$ Tr cells could have contaminated the cultures.

In addition to immature DCs, DCs that have developed and/or been activated in the presence of a variety of tolerogenic stimuli, including IL-10 itself [106], vitamin D3 [77], cholera toxin [58], or *Bordetella pertussis* toxin [71], all promote the differentiation of Tr1 cells. Although these agents seem to have little in common, they all in fact lead to suppression or inhibition of NFκB activation. In the absence of functional NFκB activity, IL-12 secretion would be inhibited, resulting in DCs that could predominantly secrete IL-10. In support of this concept, DCs that are genetically deficient for RelB (an NFκB family member) and lack expression of CD40, efficiently drive Tr1 differentiation [70]. Moreover, T cells primed with DCs previously treated with a proteasome inhibitor, which inhibits the degradation of IkB (and thus activation of NFkB), become Tr-like cells [113]. Thus, in the absence of a "normal" inflammatory response, Ag-loaded DCs might by default generate regulatory rather than effector T cells. Key open questions in this scenario include: where would priming of Tr1 cells take place in vivo? and would the resulting Tr1 cells always be phenotypically and functionally identical regardless of the tolerizing stimuli? Careful studies on the trafficking of tolerogenic DCs, the sites of DC–T cell interaction, and definition of molecular markers for Tr1 cells will be required to address these questions.

2.2
Phenotype

Currently, the defining phenotype of Tr1 cells is solely based on cytokine production, with the most consistent finding being T cells that secrete IL-10, but not IL-4, and very little, if any, IL-2. An unresolved question is whether co-secretion of TGF-β should also be included as part of the definition of Tr1 cells. Many reports describe a role for both IL-10 and TGF-β in their suppressive effects [26, 42, 116], whereas others describe an exclusive role for IL-10 [30]. Suppressive phenomena that are entirely dependent on T-cell-derived TGF-β have been attributed to either Th3 [23] or CD4$^+$CD25$^+$ Tr cells [74]. Until more reliable molecular markers of these different subsets of Tr cells are found, we would argue that suppressive effects mediated by T-cell-derived IL-10 should be attributed to Tr1 cells, regardless of the presence or absence of TGF-β.

Like most Tr cells, Tr1 cells proliferate poorly following polyclonal or Ag-specific activation, but their proliferation can be significantly enhanced by exogenous IL-2 and/or IL-15 [8]. Despite this low proliferative capacity, Tr1 cells express normal levels of T-cell activation markers such as CD25, CD40L, CD69, HLA-DR, and CTLA-4 [8]. It should be noted that since Tr1 cells upregulate CD25 normally when activated, they could potentially fall into the CD25$^+$ pool. An important distinction from bona fide CD4$^+$CD25$^+$ Tr cells is that they do not continue to express high levels of CD25 in the resting phase. Thus, cells that are found to be IL-10$^+$ and CD25$^+$ should be re-analyzed for expression levels of CD25 after in vitro culture and entry into resting phase.

The difficulties associated with defining Tr1 cells solely on the basis of cytokine production have led to many studies designed to identify specific cell-surface markers. In the resting state, Tr1-cell clones constitutively express high levels of the IL-2/-15Rβ and γ common chains [8], and a vast repertoire of chemokine receptors, including some previously associated with the Th1 or Th2 phenotypes [89]. Notably, expression levels of FoxP3 (a transcription factor associated with CD4$^+$CD25$^+$ Tr cells, see below) in Tr1 cells do not differ from those in normal activated CD4$^+$ T cells ([102, 107] and our unpublished data). The group of Waldmann et al. has performed extensive serial analysis of gene expression (SAGE) experiments on murine Tr1 clones, and reported that prepro-enkephalin, GM2 ganglioside activator protein, glucocorticoid-induced TNFR superfamily member 18 (GITR), and integrin αEβ7 (CD103) are all potential markers of Tr1 cells [114]. Further work to validate the specificity of these molecules, and to identify more Tr1-specific genes is required.

2.3
Mechanisms of Action and Functions

Tr1 cells regulate the responses of naive and memory T cells in vitro and in vivo and can suppress both Th1 and Th2 cell-mediated pathologies [39, 82]. Via production of suppressive cytokines, Tr1 cells exert suppressive effects on a variety of cell types in addition to T cells. For example, supernatants from activated Tr1 cells strongly reduce the capacity of DCs to induce alloAg-specific proliferation [22, 59]. Tr1-cell clones also suppress the production of immunoglobulins by B cells [54]. Furthermore, via local secretion of IL-10, it is likely that Tr1 cells will also educate naive CD4$^+$ T cells to become Tr1 cells. Data indicating that TGF-β is a differentiation/growth factor for CD4$^+$CD25$^+$

Tr cells [112], suggest that Tr1 cells may also be able to promote different Tr-cell subsets.

Evidence from both murine and human studies indicates that the major function of Tr1 cells is to control homeostasis of the response to foreign Ags in the periphery. Although Tr1 cells can also recognize self-Ags [43, 54] and tumor Ags [109], a majority of studies have reported IL-10-dependent regulation of responses to allergens, pathogens and alloAgs. Tr1 cells seem to be of particular importance in mucosal tissues, where foreign Ags are first encountered. Indeed, mucosal tissues may contain specialized subsets of dendritic cells that are dedicated to priming Tr1 cells [3, 4]. Also of particular interest is the remarkable ability of many bacteria [57, 71], parasites [88], and viruses [69, 66] to actively promote the generation of Tr1 cells. Study of the mechanisms that pathogens have evolved over millions of years to promote the generation of Tr1 cells will undoubtedly lead to new therapeutic strategies to induce their generation in clinically relevant situations.

2.4
In Vivo Evidence for Tr1 Cells in Humans

Following widespread revival of the concept of active suppression and armed with a phenotype (i.e., IL-10 production in the absence of IL-2 or IL-4) and the in vitro suppression assay, many groups have designed studies aimed at assessing the quantitative and qualitative presence of Tr1 cells in a variety of disease settings. Unfortunately, due to the ease of using CD25 as a marker to track and isolate Tr cells ex vivo, it is sometimes hard to dissect whether an effect attributed to IL-10$^+$CD25$^+$ Tr cells involves classical Tr1 cells, naturally occurring CD4$^+$CD25$^+$ Tr cells, Ag-induced CD4$^+$CD25$^+$ Tr cells, or some combination of these three cell types. Recent data that indicate CD4$^+$CD25$^+$ Tr cells may have a role in inducing both IL-10 and/or TGF-β-producing cells [30, 92] strongly suggest that the latter case may often be true. Table 1 highlights some recent reports that have found IL-10-producing Tr1 cells specific for a variety of Ags in humans. There is also an impressive number of studies that have found evidence of functional Tr1 cells in a variety of murine models (reviewed in [39, 41, 60, 82]). A general conclusion from these studies is that Tr1 cells are undoubtedly present naturally in vivo in both mice and humans, and regulate responses to a wide variety of Ags. However, thus far, it has been difficult to conduct quantitative studies that correlate relative numbers of Tr1 cells with clinical status.

Table 1 Summary of some recent studies that show quantitative and/or functional changes in Tr1 or CD4$^+$CD25$^+$ Tr cells in a variety of human diseases (*continued on next page*)

	Tr1/CD25	Ag specificity	Comments	Reference(s)
Autoimmunity				
Hemolytic anemia	Tr1	RhD	Mapped Tr1-specific epitopes	[43]
Multiple sclerosis	CD25	Unknown	Numbers not affected by treatment with Copaxone or IFN-α	[80]
	CD25	Unknown	Although numbers are normal, suppressive function abnormal	[103]
Systemic lupus erythematosus	CD25	Unknown	Decreased numbers in patients' PBMCs; no functional data	[65]
Rheumatoid arthritis	CD25	Unknown	Synovial fluid from patients contains functional Tr cells	[20,29]
Autoimmune polyglandular syndrome type II	CD25	Unknown	Although numbers are normal, suppressive function abnormal	[56]
Pemphigus Vulgaris	Tr1	Desmoglein 3	Classical Ag-specific Tr1 clones found in healthy donors	[100]
Myasthenia Gravis	CD25	Unknown	Normal numbers in thymus, but severely compromised function	[11]
Cancer				
Hodgkin's lymphoma	Tr1 and CD25	Unknown	Suppression in vitro largely IL-10-dependent	[68]
Gastrointestinal and esophageal malignancies	CD25, possibly Tr1	Unknown	Higher proportion in PBMCs and ascites correlates with poor prognosis	[45,87]
Melanoma	CD25 and Tr1	LAGE1	Ag-specific clones produce high levels of IL-10, but mediate contact-dependent suppression	[109]
	CD25, possibly Tr1	Unknown	Twofold increased frequency in metastatic lymph nodes	[104]
Ovarian carcinoma	CD25	Her2	Tr cells traffic to the tumor via CCR4-CCL22 interactions; their presence predicts poor survival	[28]

Table 1 (*continued*)

	Tr1/CD25	Ag specificity	Comments	Reference(s)
Infectious diseases				
EBV	Tr1	LMP1	IL-10-dependent suppression	[69]
Onchocerciasis (river blindness)	Tr1	Onchocerca Ags	Classical Ag-specific Tr1-cell clones found in chronically infected patients	[88]
Hepatitis C	Tr1	HCV core protein	HCV core-specific Tr1 cell clones isolated from chronically infected patients	[66]
HIV and CMV	CD25	viral Ags	Depletion of CD25$^+$ cells enhances in vitro responses to viral Ags	[1]
Allergy				
Cat allergy	Tr1	FelD1	Tr1 cells present in normal and allergic subjects, but increase following SIT	[81]
Grass pollen allergy	Tr1 and CD25	Phleum pratense	Increase in numbers of CD25$^+$IL-10$^+$ T cells following SIT	[36]
House dust and birch pollen allergies	Tr1 and CD25	Der p1 and Bet v1	Tr1 cells present in normal donors and increase following SIT in allergic patients	[50]
Allergic rhinitis	CD25	Grass or birch pollen extracts	No difference in numbers between normal donors and allergic patients	[15]
Nickel allergy	CD25	Nickel	Present in normal PBMCs, allergic patients not investigated	[21]
	Tr1	Nickel	Nickel-specific Tr1 clones	[22]
Celiac disease	Tr1	Gliadin	Tr1 clones isolated from mucosa of patients in remission	[37]
Transplantation				
Allogeneic hematopoietic stem cell transplantation	CD25	Unknown	Patients with chronic GVHD had elevated numbers of functional CD4$^+$CD25$^+$ T cells; did not assess alloAg-specific suppression	[25]
	CD25	Unknown	Patients with GVHD received grafts containing significantly higher frequencies of CD4$^+$CD25$^+$ T cells	[91]
	Tr1	Host alloAg	Donor-derived Tr1 cell clones specific for host alloAgs isolated ex vivo	[7]

3
Naturally Occurring Human CD4$^+$CD25$^+$ Tr Cells

Like their murine counterparts, CD4$^+$CD25$^+$ Tr cells isolated from human peripheral blood constitutively express the IL-2Rα chain [10, 78, 86]. However, in contrast to mice, where a distinct population of CD25$^+$CD4$^+$ cells can be identified by flow cytometry, human peripheral blood mononuclear cells (PBMCs) reveal a continuum of CD25 expression, with up to 20% of cells being positive if gates are set based on control antibodies. However, only the brightest CD25$^+$ cells (~3% of CD4$^+$ cells) are highly enriched for Tr activity, and the intermediate CD25$^+$ population contains a highly variable mixture of Tr cells and activated effector cells [9, 10]. Thus, in the human system, FACS sorting must be employed if long-term Tr cell lines and/or clones are to be generated. In fact, even the CD4$^+$CD25^{bright} population does not contain Tr cells exclusively [64]. To accurately asses the purity of Tr cells within a population of CD25$^+$ cells, they must be allowed to rest in vitro; only true CD4$^+$CD25$^+$ Tr cells will maintain very high levels of CD25 expression in this phase [64].

3.1
Origins

Although it is clear that naturally occurring CD4$^+$CD25$^+$ Tr cells arise in the thymus, the cells, signals, and Ags that stimulate their development are poorly characterized. In humans, CD4$^+$CD25$^+$ Tr cells are present in the thymus, particularly in the perivascular areas of fibrous septa [5], and these cells share many phenotypic and functional similarities with their peripheral counterparts. Moreover, patients with thymic hypoplasia (DiGeorge syndrome) have low numbers of peripheral CD4$^+$CD25$^+$ Tr cells, supporting the concept that they are thymically derived [94]. Whether or not CD4$^+$CD25$^+$ Tr cells exclusively recognize self-Ags, or posses a repertoire broad enough to include foreign Ags, remains unclear. Analysis of V gene region diversity in human cell populations does not reveal any significant differences between that CD4$^+$CD25$^+$ Tr cells and nonsuppressive controls [51, 96], suggesting the Tr cells do not recognize a specialized subset of Ags. A definitive answer to this question is crucial to the therapeutic approach in settings such as allergy, since it determines whether it would be feasible simply to expand a pre-existing pool of Ag-specific CD4$^+$CD25$^+$ Tr cells, or whether, as for Tr1 cells, de novo differentiation would be required.

3.2
Phenotype

In addition to CD25, CD4$^+$CD25$^+$ Tr cells isolated from peripheral blood constitutively express high levels of CTLA4, GITR, CD71, HLA-DR, CD45RO, IL-2Rβ (CD122), IL-2Rγ (CD132), PD-L1, and ICOS [10]. In contrast to murine cells, human CD4$^+$CD25$^+$ Tr cells do not express high levels of the integrin CD103 ([92] and our unpublished data), but high expression of the chemokine receptors CCR4 and CCR8 may be functionally relevant [46]. Unfortunately, none of these markers have proven to be truly specific for CD4$^+$CD25$^+$ Tr cells and their expression is merely indicative of an apparently constitutive state of T cell activation. Indeed, CD4$^+$CD25$^+$ Tr cells have short telomeres, suggesting that these cells have experienced repeated episodes of Ag-specific stimulation in vivo [96].

The cytokine production phenotype of human CD4$^+$CD25$^+$ Tr cells has been intensively studied. A majority of studies have failed to detect significant production of IL-10 in vitro [31, 49, 63]. In contrast, human CD4$^+$CD25$^+$ Tr cells can secrete TGF-β, although at levels that are not significantly different from nonsuppressive cells [64]. We failed to detect membrane bound TGF-β on suppressive CD4$^+$CD25$^+$ Tr cell clones, and instead found evidence that positive staining of freshly isolated cells was due to an artifact of purification by magnetic beads [64]. The phenotype of human CD4$^+$CD25$^+$ Tr cells in terms of other Th cytokines is quite remarkable: they fail to produce detectable levels of IL-2, IL-4, IL-5, IL-10 or IFN-γ [9, 64]. In fact, they are the only human T cell clones that we have found not to produce IFN-γ. Thus, a crucial difference between Tr1 and CD4$^+$CD25$^+$ Tr cells lies in their cytokine production profiles.

Despite their inability to produce IL-2, this cytokine is a key growth factor for CD4$^+$CD25$^+$ Tr cells both in vitro and in vivo. As for Tr1 cells, IL-15 can completely replace IL-2 as a growth and survival factor for CD4$^+$CD25$^+$ Tr cells in vitro [31]; however, data from IL-2$^{-/-}$ mice indicate that in vivo this is not the case [79]. In human cell cultures, IL-4 cannot replace IL-2 as a growth factor (our unpublished data), whereas in mouse cultures it can [98]. This may be due to differential receptor expression and/or signaling. IL-2 or IL-15 can also rescue CD4$^+$CD25$^+$ Tr cells from apoptosis, likely via induction of Bcl-2 expression [95] and allowing exit from cell cycle arrest in the G1/G0 phase [49]. Interestingly, IL-2-induced activation of the PI3'kinase/Akt pathway appears to be defective in CD4$^+$CD25$^+$ Tr cells [16], which may provide an explanation for their poor proliferative capacity, at least in vitro. Evidence that CD4$^+$CD25$^+$ Tr cells are not anergic in vivo [33] suggests that current in vitro culture conditions may still be lacking essential growth factors(s).

A major advance in the study of CD4$^+$CD25$^+$ Tr cells came with the finding that a transcription factor known as FoxP3 may not only be a novel Tr-cell marker, but it may also be necessary for their development [34, 44, 53]. Thus, when mouse CD4$^+$ T cells are forced to overexpress Foxp3, they adopt a phenotype virtually identical to naturally occurring CD25$^+$CD4$^+$ Tr cells [34, 44]. These "artificial" Tr cells are even able to suppress autoimmune bowel disease in vivo. Notably, both mice and humans deficient for FoxP3 rapidly develop systemic autoimmunity, which correlates with the notion that FoxP3 is required for the development and/or function of CD4$^+$CD25$^+$ Tr cells [17, 110]. This finding also supports the hypothesis that the primary role of CD4$^+$CD25$^+$ Tr cells is controlling responses to self-Ags.

Like murine cells, human CD4$^+$CD25$^+$ Treg cells express significantly more FoxP3 mRNA and protein than do CD4$^+$CD25$^-$ T cells [108]. However, expression of FoxP3 can also be induced upon TCR-mediated activation of normal human CD4$^+$CD25$^-$ Tr cells. Indeed, induction of FoxP3 in effector CD4$^+$ T cells may be a natural mechanism that allows the peripheral induction of Tr cells [108].

3.3
Functions

All published reports agree that human CD4$^+$CD25$^+$ Tr cells potently suppress the proliferation and effector functions of both CD4$^+$ and CD8$^+$ T cells. Interestingly, there may be an age-dependent loss of this suppressive activity, possibly correlated with decreased thymic function [99]. The effectiveness of CD4$^+$CD25$^+$ Tr cells in vivo is likely related to the state of activation of their targets, since when strongly stimulated by polyclonal [10] or Ag-specific activation [76], their targets become transiently resistant to suppression. CD4$^+$CD25$^+$ Tr cells that are fully functional in vitro, are found in inflamed tissues (see Table 1), but whether they would be functional in vivo in an environment full of pro-inflammatory cytokines and T cell stimuli is an important, and as yet unanswered, question.

Originally, it was hypothesized that the major role of naturally occurring CD4$^+$CD25$^+$ Tr cells was to regulate tolerance to self-Ags. In fact, a recent study suggests they may recognize epitopes within the TCR itself [18]. However, a growing body of literature suggests that, like Tr1 cells, they may also be key regulators of tolerance to foreign Ags [79]. This is illustrated in Table 1, where several recent reports of isolation of CD4$^+$CD25$^+$ Tr cells specific for foreign Ags (e.g., allergens and viruses) are summarized. However, since any activated Tr cell could be in the CD25$^+$ pool in vivo, experiments that truly define the nature of the TCR repertoire of these naturally occurring Tr cells are required before conclusions about Ag specificity can be drawn.

Human $CD4^+CD25^+$ Tr cells potently suppress IL-2, IFN-γ, and IL-13 production by $CD4^+$ T cells [9], although some evidence indicates that Th2 cells may be less susceptible than Th1 cells to their suppressive effects [27]. Human $CD4^+CD25^+$ Tr cells can also potently inhibit the cytotoxic activity of $CD8^+$ T cells by down-regulating perforin and granzyme B [19], and $Va24^+NKT$ cell proliferation and cytokine production [6]. Presumably, these actions allow $CD4^+CD25^+$ Tr cells to control adaptive immune responses by multiple mechanisms.

3.4
Mechanisms of Action

Almost 10 years after their initial description, the mechanism(s) by which $CD4^+CD25^+$ Tr cells achieve these remarkable effects remain unclear. Some reports indicate that they may act by down-regulating the function of APCs [72], whereas others have not seen a similar effect [75, 79]. Although suppression in vitro is undoubtedly dependent upon direct cell-to-cell contact, the majority of reports have not found a role for the highly expressed cell-surface molecules CTLA-4, ICOS, PDL1, or GITR [9, 63, 64].

Much effort has gone into investigating the potential role of IL-10 and/or TGF-β in suppression. Classical in vitro suppression assays are not reversed by neutralizing anti-IL10 antibodies [31, 49, 63]. In addition, even at the clonal level, suppressive $CD4^+CD25^+$ Tr-cell clones do not produce detectable amounts of IL-10 [64]. These data, combined with those that demonstrate that IL-10-induced anergy, and differentiation of Tr1 cells by IL-10 and IFN-α [64] or by immature DCs [61] can all occur in the absence of $CD4^+CD25^+$ Tr cells, indicate that $CD4^+CD25^+$ Tr cells are distinct from Tr1 cells and do not need IL-10 for their induction. Thus, in vivo studies that found a role for IL-10 may be attributed to either an Ag-induced subset of $CD4^+CD25^+$ Tr cells that has a distinct mechanism of action from the naturally occurring subset [14, 57] and/or de novo differentiation of Tr1 cells (possibly induced by the naturally occurring $CD4^+CD25^+$ Tr cells themselves, see below [30, 47]).

In contrast, the role of TGF-β in suppression mediated by $CD4^+CD25^+$ Tr cells is much less clear. Like all human T cells, $CD4^+CD25^+$ Tr cells produce low levels of TGF-β [64]. Although neutralizing antibodies can have a small effect at high concentrations, they are never able to completely reverse suppression in vitro [9, 31, 49, 63, 64, 75]. Furthermore, addition of recombinant TGF-β cannot suppresses $CD4^+$ T cell proliferation to the same degree as $CD4^+CD25^+$ Tr cells (unpublished data). Nevertheless, much in vivo data suggests that TGF-β, like IL-10, does have a role in $CD4^+CD25^+$ Tr cell-mediated suppression [67, 73]. Again, these findings may be due to the induction of new Tr cell subsets.

Improved molecular markers for the different Tr cell subsets (i.e., CD25$^+$ vs Tr1 vs Th3) will undoubtedly shed more light on this issue.

Remarkably, human CD4$^+$CD25$^+$ Tr cells can be split into two subsets with distinct functions based on differential expression of integrins. Those expressing $\alpha 4\beta 7$, which binds to vascular adressins expressed by venules in mucosal tissues, have the capacity to induce de novo differentiation of IL-10-producing Tr1 cells [92]. In contrast, CD4$^+$CD25$^+$ Tr cells expressing $\alpha 4\beta 1$, which binds to VCAM1 on the endothelium of inflamed tissues, induce the differentiation of TGF-β-producing Th3 cells [30, 47, 92, 93]. It will be important to define the mechanisms involved in this induction of Tr1 vs Th3 cells, and their respective target Ags. If these in vitro findings are confirmed, this phenomenon would offer an attractive explanation for the studies discussed above that found a role for IL-10 and/or TGF-β in naturally occurring Tr-mediated suppression.

3.5
In Vivo Evidence for CD4$^+$CD25$^+$ Tr Cells in Humans

Given the ease of monitoring and isolating CD25$^+$ cells, and their undeniable importance in immune homeostasis, many groups have sought alterations in their number and/or function in patients with a variety of diseases. Table 1 summarizes some of these recent reports. A key question these studies raise is: in the absence of an Ag-specific assay, how meaningful are changes in the numbers and/or function of the total population of CD4$^+$CD25$^+$ Tr cells? For example, a recent study reported that the in vitro function of CD4$^+$CD25$^+$ Tr cells from patients with MS is dramatically impaired upon polyclonal activation [103], findings difficult to reconcile with the fact that these patients do not suffer from systemic autoimmunity. Moreover, similar to Tr1 cells, in many cases apparently normal CD4$^+$CD25$^+$ Tr cells can be isolated from patients with disease, perhaps highlighting the inadequacy of our current in vitro assays as a surrogate marker of in vivo functionality.

4
Peripheral Generation of CD4$^+$CD25$^+$ Tr Cells

In addition to thymus-derived CD4$^+$CD25$^+$ Tr cells, cells with a similar phenotype can also be generated from naive peripheral T cells. For example, activation in the presence of TGF-β induces naive CD45RA$^+$ T cells to up-regulate FoxP3 and develop contact-dependent, cytokine-independent suppressive activity [32, 115]. Remarkably, these induced CD4$^+$CD25$^+$ Tr cells also seem to have the capacity to induce differentiation of Tr1 cells [115]. Similarly, costimulation blockade [101] and expansion with IL-15 induces contact-dependent

$CD4^+CD25^+$ Tr cells [55]. In addition, cells from the $CD25^-$ pool that fail to down-regulate CD25 after activation acquire a phenotype and function that appear indistinguishable from those of naturally occurring $CD4^+CD25^+$ Tr cells [108]. Analysis at the single cell level will be required to determine the proportion of Tr cells in these induced populations, and whether they are truly phenotypically and functionally equivalent to the naturally occurring subset.

5
Networks of Tr1 and $CD4^+CD25^+$ Tr Cells

This review has attempted to highlight the similarities and differences between human Tr1 and naturally occurring $CD4^+CD25^+$ Tr cells, summarized in Table 2. It can be concluded that although these two subsets have nonredundant roles in tolerance induction and maintenance, they probably achieve their effects in synergy. At birth, thymic-derived natural Tr cells would be immediately ready to protect us against autoreactive T cells. Subsequent exposure to foreign Ags would then stimulate the development of interdependent networks of cytokine-dependent (i.e., Tr1) and -independent (i.e., $CD4^+CD25^+$ Tr) regulation. The concept that naturally occurring $CD4^+CD25^+$ Tr, Ag-

Table 2 Comparison of some of the salient features of human Tr1 and naturally occurring $CD4^+CD25^+$ Tr cells

	Tr1 cells	$CD4^+CD25^+$ Tr cells
Origins	Peripheral	Thymic
	Primed by immature or tolerogenic DCs	Subset(s) of DCs required unknown
	Require exogenous/ autocrine IL-10	Require exogenous IL-2
Ag specificity	Primarily foreign	Primarily self, but possibly also foreign
Mechanism of action	Secreted factors (IL-10 ± TGF-β)	Cell-contact-dependent in vitro
Growth and survival factors	IL-2 and/or IL-15	IL-2 and/or IL-15
Expression of CD25	Inducible	Constitutive
Expression of FoxP3	Low levels	High constitutive levels
Cytokine production	IL-2$^{+/-}$, IL-4$^-$, IL-10$^+$, IFN-γ^+, TGF-β^+	IL-2$^-$, IL-4$^-$, IL-10$^-$, IFN-γ^-, TGF-$\beta^{+/-}$

induced CD4$^+$CD25$^+$ Tr and Tr1 cells could all be present simultaneously offers an explanation for conflicting results regarding cytokine-dependent and -independent regulation. The relative importance of Tr1 vs CD4$^+$CD25$^+$ Tr cells, in any given instance, is likely dictated by the nature of the Ag, the context of Ag presentation, and the biology of specific tissues. One further level of control could be trafficking, since Tr1 and CD4$^+$CD25$^+$ Tr cells appear to have distinct migratory behaviors [35]. A major area to be investigated is the Ag specificity of these networks: do different Tr cell subsets recognize distinct or overlapping subsets of Ags?

6
Therapeutic Opportunities

The idea that manipulation of the frequency and/or function of Tr1 or CD4$^+$CD25$^+$ Tr could be used therapeutically has generated much excitement. Indeed, significant progress toward proof of this principle has already been made in animal models. We are currently investigating whether, as in murine models [24], alloAg-specific T cells that have been anergized in vitro upon addition of IL-10 are suppressed in their capacity to mediate graft versus host disease (GVHD), and whether they represent the precursors of Tr1 cells.

However, in general it has been difficult to establish rapid and efficient methods to expand homogenous populations of Ag specific Tr1 cells in vitro that could be used as a cellular therapy in vivo. Thus, it is currently more realistic to contemplate clinical protocols that involve boosting the numbers of Tr1 cells directly in vivo, via administration of some combination of tolerogenic agents [2, 82, 107]. Of particular interest is the remarkable efficiency of in vivo administration of the combination of rapamycin and IL-10, in a murine model of pancreatic islet allograft rejection, in inducing tolerogenic Tr1 cells [13]. Moreover, in vivo induction of Tr1 cells in humans seems to have already been achieved by specific immunotherapy (SIT) for allergens [36, 50, 81], although the precise mechanisms involved in this system remain unknown. Studying the mechanisms that pathogens have evolved over millions of years to induce Tr1 cells in vivo may reveal new strategies to achieve this goal.

With respect to CD4$^+$CD25$^+$ Tr cells, caution should be adopted when considering cellular therapy with non-Ag-specific populations that have been expanded in vitro. In murine systems, this approach has already proven successful at establishing long-term tolerance in the setting of bone marrow transplantation [97]. However, human CD4$^+$CD25$^+$ Tr cells are a much more heterogeneous mixture of activated effector and Tr cells. Although short-term expansion ex vivo preserves the potent suppressive effects of bulk populations

[38, 63], in the long-term, contaminating nonsuppressive cells overtake the cultures. What would happen to such a heterogeneous population in vivo could be a dangerous question to ask, especially if in vitro Ag-specific priming is involved. On the other hand, it is also possible that mechanisms of infectious tolerance will dominate, and that the non-Tr cells would eventually join the Tr network. Judging by the number of citations dealing with Tr cells in recent years, a similar mechanism already seems to have resulted in an increased number of Tr immunologists!

References

1. Aandahl EM, Michaelsson J, Moretto WJ, Hecht FM, Nixon DF (2004) Human CD4+ CD25+ regulatory T cells control T-cell responses to human immunodeficiency virus and cytomegalovirus antigens. J Virol 78:2454–2459
2. Adorini L, Giarratana N, Penna G (2004) Pharmacological induction of tolerogenic dendritic cells and regulatory T cells. Semin Immunol 16:127–134
3. Akbari O, DeKruyff RH, Umetsu DT (2001) Pulmonary dendritic cells producing IL-10 mediate tolerance induced by respiratory exposure to antigen. Nat Immunol 2:725–731
4. Akbari O, Freeman GJ, Meyer EH, Greenfield EA, Chang TT, Sharpe AH, Berry G, DeKruyff RH, Umetsu DT (2002) Antigen-specific regulatory T cells develop via the ICOS-ICOS-ligand pathway and inhibit allergen-induced airway hyperreactivity. Nat Med 8:1024–1032
5. Annunziato F, Cosmi L, Liotta F, Lazzeri E, Manetti R, Vanini V, Romagnani P, Maggi E, Romagnani S (2002) Phenotype, localization, mechanism of suppression of CD4(+)CD25(+) human thymocytes. J Exp Med 196:379–387
6. Azuma T, Takahashi T, Kunisato A, Kitamura T, Hirai H (2003) Human CD4+ CD25+ regulatory T cells suppress NKT cell functions. Cancer Res 63:4516–4520
7. Bacchetta R, Bigler M, Touraine JL, Parkman R, Tovo PA, Abrams J, de Waal Malefyt R, de Vries JE, Roncarolo MG (1994) High levels of interleukin 10 production in vivo are associated with tolerance in SCID patients transplanted with HLA mismatched hematopoietic stem cells. J Exp Med 179:493–502
8. Bacchetta R, Sartirana C, Levings MK, Bordignon C, Narula S, Roncarolo MG (2002) Growth and expansion of human T regulatory type 1 cells are independent from TCR activation but require exogenous cytokines. Eur J Immunol 32:2237–2245
9. Baecher-Allan C, Brown JA, Freeman GJ, Hafler DA (2001) CD4+CD25high regulatory cells in human peripheral blood. J Immunol 167:1245–1253
10. Baecher-Allan C, Viglietta V, Hafler DA (2004) Human CD4+CD25+ regulatory T cells. Semin Immunol 16:89–98
11. Balandina A, Lecart S, Dartevelle P, Saoudi A, Berrih-Aknin S (2004) Functional defect of regulatory CD4+CD25+ T cells in the thymus of patients with autoimmune Myasthenia Gravis. Blood 105:735–741; e-pub Sept. 28 DOI 15454488
12. Barrat FJ, Cua DJ, Boonstra A, Richards DF, Crain C, Savelkoul HF, de Waal-Malefyt R, Coffman RL, Hawrylowicz CM, O'Garra A (2002) In vitro generation of

interleukin 10-producing regulatory CD4(+) T cells is induced by immunosuppressive drugs and inhibited by T helper type 1 (Th1)- and Th2-inducing cytokines. J Exp Med 195:603–616
13. Battaglia M, Stabilini A, Draghici E, Gregori S, Bonifacio E, Roncarolo MG (2004) Rapamycin and IL-10 treatment induces antigen specific T regulatory type 1 (Tr1) cells that mediate transplantation tolerance (submitted)
14. Belkaid Y, Piccirillo CA, Mendez S, Shevach EM, Sacks DL (2002) CD4+CD25+ regulatory T cells control Leishmania major persistence and immunity. Nature 420:502–507
15. Bellinghausen I, Klostermann B, Knop J, Saloga J (2003) Human CD4+CD25+ T cells derived from the majority of atopic donors are able to suppress TH1 and TH2 cytokine production. J Allergy Clin Immunol 111:862–868
16. Bensinger SJ, Walsh PT, Zhang J, Carroll M, Parsons R, Rathmell JC, Thompson CB, Burchill MA, Farrar MA, Turka LA (2004) Distinct IL-2 receptor signaling pattern in CD4+CD25+ regulatory T cells. J Immunol 172:5287–5296
17. Brunkow ME, Jeffery EW, Hjerrild KA, Paeper B, Clark LB, Yasayko SA, Wilkinson JE, Galas D, Ziegler SF, Ramsdell F (2001) Disruption of a new forkhead/winged-helix protein, scurfin, results in the fatal lymphoproliferative disorder of the scurfy mouse. Nat Genet 27:68–73
18. Buenafe AC, Tsaknaridis L, Spencer L, Hicks KS, McMahan RH, Watson L, Culbertson NE, Latocha D, Wegmann K, Finn T et al (2004) Specificity of regulatory CD4+CD25+ T cells for self-T cell receptor determinants. J Neurosci Res 76:129–140
19. Camara NO, Sebille F, Lechler RI (2003) Human CD4+CD25+ regulatory cells have marked and sustained effects on CD8+ T cell activation. Eur J Immunol 33:3473–3483
20. Cao D, Malmstrom V, Baecher-Allan C, Hafler D, Klareskog L, Trollmo C (2003) Isolation and functional characterization of regulatory CD25brightCD4+ T cells from the target organ of patients with rheumatoid arthritis. Eur J Immunol 33:215–223
21. Cavani A, Nasorri F, Ottaviani C, Sebastiani S, De Pita O, Girolomoni G (2003) Human CD25+ regulatory T cells maintain immune tolerance to nickel in healthy, nonallergic individuals. J Immunol 171:5760–5768
22. Cavani A, Nasorri F, Prezzi C, Sebastiani S, Albanesi C, Girolomoni G (2000) Human CD4+ T lymphocytes with remarkable regulatory functions on dendritic cells and nickel-specific Th1 immune responses. J Invest Dermatol 114:295–302
23. Chen Y, Kuchroo VK, Inobe J, Hafler DA, Weiner HL (1994) Regulatory T cell clones induced by oral tolerance: suppression of autoimmune encephalomyelitis. Science 265:1237–1240
24. Chen ZM, O'Shaughnessy MJ, Gramaglia I, Panoskaltsis-Mortari A, Murphy WJ, Narula S, Roncarolo MG, Blazar BR (2003) IL-10 and TGF-beta induce alloreactive CD4+CD25− T cells to acquire regulatory cell function. Blood 101:5076–5083
25. Clark FJ, Gregg R, Piper K, Dunnion D, Freeman L, Griffiths M, Begum G, Mahendra P, Craddock C, Moss P, Chakraverty R (2004) Chronic graft-versus-host disease is associated with increased numbers of peripheral blood CD4+CD25high regulatory T cells. Blood 103:2410–2416
26. Cong Y, Weaver CT, Lazenby A, Elson CO (2002) Bacterial-reactive T regulatory cells inhibit pathogenic immune responses to the enteric flora. J Immunol 169:6112–6119

27. Cosmi L, Liotta F, Angeli R, Mazzinghi B, Santarlasci V, Manetti R, Lasagni L, Vanini V, Romagnani P, Maggi E et al (2004) Th2 cells are less susceptible than Th1 cells to the suppressive activity of CD25+ regulatory thymocytes because of their responsiveness to different cytokines. Blood 103:3117–3121
28. Curiel TJ, Coukos G, Zou L, Alvarez X, Cheng P, Mottram P, Evdemon-Hogan M, Conejo-Garcia JR, Zhang L, Burow M et al (2004) Specific recruitment of regulatory T cells in ovarian carcinoma fosters immune privilege and predicts reduced survival. Nat Med 10:942–949
29. De Kleer IM, Wedderburn LR, Taams LS, Patel A, Varsani H, Klein M, De Jager W, Pugayung G, Giannoni F, Rijkers G et al (2004) CD4(+)CD25(bright) regulatory T cells actively regulate inflammation in the joints of patients with the remitting form of juvenile idiopathic arthritis. J Immunol 172:6435–6443
30. Dieckmann D, Bruett CH, Ploettner H, Lutz MB, Schuler G (2002) Human CD4(+)CD25(+) regulatory, contact-dependent T cells induce interleukin 10-producing, contact-independent type 1-like regulatory T cells. J Exp Med 196:247–253
31. Dieckmann D, Plottner H, Berchtold S, Berger T, Schuler S (2001) Ex vivo isolation and characterization of CD4+CD25+ T cells with regulatory properties from human blood. J Exp Med 193:1303–1310
32. Fantini MC, Becker C, Monteleone G, Pallone F, Galle PR, Neurath MF (2004) Cutting edge: TGF-beta Induces a regulatory phenotype in CD4(+)CD25(-) T cells through Foxp3 induction and down-regulation of Smad7. J Immunol 172:5149–5153
33. Fisson S, Darrasse-Jeze G, Litvinova E, Septier F, Klatzmann D, Liblau R, Salomon BL (2003) Continuous activation of autoreactive CD4+ CD25+ regulatory T cells in the steady state. J Exp Med 198:737–746
34. Fontenot JD, Gavin MA, Rudensky AY (2003) Foxp3 programs the development and function of CD4+CD25+ regulatory T cells. Nat Immunol 4:330–336
35. Foussat A, Cottrez F, Brun V, Fournier N, Breittmayer JP, Groux H (2003) A comparative study between T regulatory type 1 and CD4+CD25+ T cells in the control of inflammation. J Immunol 171:5018–5026
36. Francis JN, Till SJ, Durham SR (2003) Induction of IL-10+CD4+CD25+ T cells by grass pollen immunotherapy. J Allergy Clin Immunol 111:1255–1261
37. Gianfrani C, Levings MK, Sartirana C, Mazzarella G, Zanzi D, Iaquinto G, Giardullo N, Auricchio S, Troncone R, Roncarolo MG (2004) Gliadin-specific type 1 T regulatory cells are present in the intestinal mucosa of treated coeliac disease patients. (submitted)
38. Godfrey WR, Ge YG, Spoden DJ, Levine BL, June CH, Blazar BR, Porter SB (2004) In vitro-expanded human CD4(+)CD25(+) T-regulatory cells can markedly inhibit allogeneic dendritic cell-stimulated MLR cultures. Blood 104:453–461
39. Groux H (2003) Type 1 T-regulatory cells: their role in the control of immune responses. Transplantation 75:8S–12S
40. Groux H, Bigler M, de Vries JE, Roncarolo MG (1996) Interleukin-10 induces a long-term antigen-specific anergic state in human CD4+ T cells. J Exp Med 184:19–29
41. Groux H, Cottrez F (2003) The complex role of interleukin-10 in autoimmunity. J Autoimmun 20:281–285

42. Groux H, O'Garra A, Bigler M, Rouleau M, Antonenko S, de Vries JE, Roncarolo MG (1997) A CD4+ T-cell subset inhibits antigen-specific T-cell responses and prevents colitis. Nature 389:737–742
43. Hall AM, Ward FJ, Vickers MA, Stott LM, Urbaniak SJ, Barker RN (2002) Interleukin-10-mediated regulatory T-cell responses to epitopes on a human red blood cell autoantigen. Blood 100:4529–4536
44. Hori S, Nomura T, Sakaguchi S (2003) Control of regulatory T cell development by the transcription factor Foxp3. Science 299:1057–1061
45. Ichihara F, Kono K, Takahashi A, Kawaida H, Sugai H, Fujii H (2003) Increased populations of regulatory T cells in peripheral blood and tumor-infiltrating lymphocytes in patients with gastric and esophageal cancers. Clin Cancer Res 9:4404–4408
46. Iellem A, Mariani M, Lang R, Recalde H, Panina-Bordignon P, Sinigaglia F, D'Ambrosio D (2001) Unique chemotactic response profile and specific expression of chemokine receptors CCR4 and CCR8 by CD4(+)CD25(+) regulatory T cells. J Exp Med 194:847–853
47. Jonuleit H, Schmitt E, Kakirman H, Stassen M, Knop J, Enk AH (2002) Infectious tolerance: human CD25(+) regulatory T cells convey suppressor activity to conventional CD4(+) T helper cells. J Exp Med 196:255–260
48. Jonuleit H, Schmitt E, Schuler G, Knop J, Enk AH (2000) Induction of interleukin-10-producing, nonproliferating CD4+ T cells with regulatory properties by repetitive stimulation with allogenic immature human dendritic cells. J Exp Med 192:1213–1222
49. Jonuleit H, Schmitt E, Stassen M, Tuettenberg A, Knop J, Enk AH (2001) Identification and functional characterization of human CD4+CD25+ T cells with regulatory properties isolated from peripheral blood. J Exp Med 193:1285–1294
50. Jutel M, Akdis M, Budak F, Aebischer-Casaulta C, Wrzyszcz M, Blaser K, Akdis CA (2003) IL-10 and TGF-beta cooperate in the regulatory T cell response to mucosal allergens in normal immunity and specific immunotherapy. Eur J Immunol 33:1205–1214
51. Kasow KA, Chen X, Knowles J, Wichlan D, Handgretinger R, Riberdy JM (2004) Human CD4(+)CD25(+) regulatory T cells share equally complex and comparable repertoires with CD4(+)CD25(−) counterparts. J Immunol 172:6123–6128
52. Kemper C, Chan AC, Green JM, Brett KA, Murphy KM, Atkinson JP (2003) Activation of human CD4+ cells with CD3 and CD46 induces a T-regulatory cell 1 phenotype. Nature 421:388–392
53. Khattri R, Cox T, Yasayko SA, Ramsdell F (2003) An essential role for Scurfin in CD4+CD25+ T regulatory cells. Nat Immunol 4:337–342
54. Kitani A, Chua K, Nakamura K, Strober W (2000) Activated self-MHC-reactive T cells have the cytokine phenotype of Th3/T regulatory cell 1 T cells. J Immunol 165:691–702
55. Koenen HJ, Fasse E, Joosten I (2003) IL-15 and cognate antigen successfully expand de novo-induced human antigen-specific regulatory CD4+ T cells that require antigen-specific activation for suppression. J Immunol 171:6431–6441
56. Kriegel MA, Lohmann T, Gabler C, Blank N, Kalden JR, Lorenz HM (2004) Defective Suppressor Function of Human CD4+ CD25+ Regulatory T Cells in Autoimmune Polyglandular Syndrome Type II. J Exp Med 199:1285–1291

57. Kullberg MC, Jankovic D, Gorelick PL, Caspar P, Letterio JJ, Cheever AW, Sher A (2002) Bacteria-triggered CD4(+) T regulatory cells suppress Helicobacter hepaticus-induced colitis. J Exp Med 196:505–515
58. Lavelle EC, Jarnicki A, McNeela E, Armstrong ME, Higgins SC, Leavy O, Mills KH (2004) Effects of cholera toxin on innate and adaptive immunity and its application as an immunomodulatory agent. J Leukoc Biol 75:756–763
59. Lecart S, Boulay V, Raison-Peyron N, Bousquet J, Meunier L, Yssel H, Pene J (2001) Phenotypic characterization of human CD4+ regulatory T cells obtained from cutaneous dinitrochlorobenzene-induced delayed type hypersensitivity reactions. J Invest Dermatol 117:318–325
60. Levings MK, Bacchetta R, Schulz U, Roncarolo MG (2002) The role of IL-10 and TGF-beta in the differentiation and effector function of T regulatory cells. Int Arch Allergy Immunol 129:263–276
61. Levings MK, Gregori S, Tresoldi E, Cazzaniga S, Bonini C, Roncarolo MG (2004) Differentiation of Tr1 cells by immature dendritic cells requires IL-10 but not CD25+CD4+ Treg cells. Blood 105:1162–1169; e-pub Oct12 DOI 15479730
62. Levings MK, Sangregorio R, Galbiati F, Squadrone S, de Waal Malefyt R, Roncarolo MG (2001) IFN-alpha and IL-10 Induce the differentiation of human type 1 T regulatory cells. J Immunol 166:5530–5539
63. Levings MK, Sangregorio R, Roncarolo MG (2001) Human CD25+CD4+ T regulatory cells suppress naive and memory T-cell proliferation and can be expanded in vitro without loss of function. J Exp Med 193:1295–1302
64. Levings MK, Sangregorio R, Sartirana C, Moschin AL, Battaglia M, Orban PC, Roncarolo MG (2002) Human CD25+CD4+ T suppressor cell clones produce TGF-β, but not IL-10 and are distinct from type 1 T regulatory cells. J Exp Med 196:1335–1346
65. Liu MF, Wang CR, Fung LL, Wu CR (2004) Decreased CD4+CD25+ T cells in peripheral blood of patients with systemic lupus erythematosus. Scand J Immunol 59:198–202
66. MacDonald AJ, Duffy M, Brady MT, McKiernan S, Hall W, Hegarty J, Curry M, Mills KH (2002) CD4 T helper type 1 and regulatory T cells induced against the same epitopes on the core protein in hepatitis C virus-infected persons. J Infect Dis 185:720–727
67. Maloy KJ, Salaun L, Cahill R, Dougan G, Saunders NJ, Powrie F (2003) CD4+CD25+ T(R) cells suppress innate immune pathology through cytokine-dependent mechanisms. J Exp Med 197:111–119
68. Marshall NA, Christie LE, Munro LR, Culligan DJ, Johnston PW, Barker RN, Vickers MA (2004) Immunosuppressive regulatory T cells are abundant in the reactive lymphocytes of Hodgkin lymphoma. Blood 103:1755–1762
69. Marshall NA, Vickers MA, Barker RN (2003) Regulatory T cells secreting IL-10 dominate the immune response to EBV latent membrane protein 1. J Immunol 170:6183–6189
70. Martin E, O'Sullivan B, Low P, Thomas R (2003) Antigen-specific suppression of a primed immune response by dendritic cells mediated by regulatory T cells secreting interleukin-10. Immunity 18:155–167

71. McGuirk P, McCann C, Mills KH (2002) Pathogen-specific T regulatory 1 cells induced in the respiratory tract by a bacterial molecule that stimulates interleukin 10 production by dendritic cells: a novel strategy for evasion of protective T helper type 1 responses by Bordetella pertussis. J Exp Med 195:221–231
72. Misra N, Bayry J, Lacroix-Desmazes S, Kazatchkine MD, Kaveri SV (2004) Cutting edge: human CD4+CD25+ T cells restrain the maturation and antigen-presenting function of dendritic cells. J Immunol 172:4676–4680
73. Nakamura K, Kitani A, Fuss I, Pedersen A, Harada N, Nawata H, Strober W (2004) TGF-beta 1 plays an important role in the mechanism of CD4+CD25+ regulatory T cell activity in both humans and mice. J Immunol 172:834–842
74. Nakamura K, Kitani A, Strober W (2001) Cell contact-dependent immunosuppression by CD4(+)CD25(+) regulatory T cells is mediated by cell surface-bound transforming growth factor beta. J Exp Med 194:629–644
75. Ng WF, Duggan PJ, Ponchel F, Matarese G, Lombardi G, Edwards AD, Isaacs JD, Lechler RI (2001) Human CD4(+)CD25(+) cells: a naturally occurring population of regulatory T cells. Blood 98:2736–2744
76. Pasare C, Medzhitov R (2003) Toll pathway-dependent blockade of CD4+CD25+ T cell-mediated suppression by dendritic cells. Science 299:1033–1036
77. Penna G, Adorini L (2000) 1 Alpha,25-dihydroxyvitamin D3 inhibits differentiation, maturation, activation, survival of dendritic cells leading to impaired alloreactive T cell activation. J Immunol 164:2405–2411
78. Piccirillo CA, Letterio JJ, Thornton AM, McHugh RS, Mamura M, Mizuhara H, Shevach EM (2002) CD4(+)CD25(+) regulatory T cells can mediate suppressor function in the absence of transforming growth factor beta1 production and responsiveness. J Exp Med 196:237–246
79. Piccirillo CA, Shevach EM (2004) Naturally-occurring CD4+CD25+ immunoregulatory T cells: central players in the arena of peripheral tolerance. Semin Immunol 16:81–88
80. Putheti P, Pettersson A, Soderstrom M, Link H, Huang YM (2004) Circulating CD4(+)CD25(+) T regulatory cells are not altered in multiple sclerosis and unaffected by disease-modulating drugs. J Clin Immunol 24:155–161
81. Reefer AJ, Carneiro RM, Custis NJ, Platts-Mills TA, Sung SS, Hammer J, Woodfolk JA (2004) A role for IL-10-mediated HLA-DR7-restricted T cell-dependent events in development of the modified Th2 response to cat allergen. J Immunol 172:2763–2772
82. Roncarolo MG, Bacchetta R, Bordignon C, Narula S, Levings MK (2001) Type 1 T regulatory cells. Immunol Rev 182:68–79
83. Roncarolo MG, Levings MK (2000) The role of different subsets of T regulatory cells in controlling autoimmunity. Curr Opin Immunol 12:676–683
84. Rutella S, Bonanno G, Pierelli L, Mariotti A, Capoluongo E, Contemi AM, Ameglio F, Curti A, de Ritis DG, Voso MT et al (2004) Granulocyte colony-stimulating factor promotes the generation of regulatory DC through induction of IL-10 and IFN-alpha. Eur J Immunol 34:1291–1302
85. Sakaguchi S (2000) Regulatory T cells: key controllers of immunologic self-tolerance. Cell 101:455–458

86. Sakaguchi S (2004) Naturally arising CD4+ regulatory T cells for immunologic self-tolerance and negative control of immune responses. Annu Rev Immunol 22: 531–562
87. Sasada T, Kimura M, Yoshida Y, Kanai M, Takabayashi A (2003) CD4+CD25+ regulatory T cells in patients with gastrointestinal malignancies: possible involvement of regulatory T cells in disease progression. Cancer 98:1089–1099
88. Satoguina J, Mempel M, Larbi J, Badusche M, Loliger C, Adjei O, Gachelin G, Fleischer B, Hoerauf A (2002) Antigen-specific T regulatory-1 cells are associated with immunosuppression in a chronic helminth infection (onchocerciasis). Microbes Infect 4:1291–1300
89. Sebastiani S, Allavena P, Albanesi C, Nasorri F, Bianchi G, Traidl C, Sozzani S, Girolomoni G, Cavani A (2001) Chemokine receptor expression and function in CD4+ T lymphocytes with regulatory activity. J Immunol 166:996–1002
90. Shevach EM (2000) Regulatory T cells in autoimmmunity. Annu Rev Immunol 18:423–449
91. Stanzani M, Martins SL, Saliba RM, St John LS, Bryan S, Couriel D, McMannis J, Champlin RE, Molldrem JJ, Komanduri KV (2004) CD25 expression on donor CD4+ or CD8+ T cells is associated with an increased risk for graft-versus-host disease after HLA-identical stem cell transplantation in humans. Blood 103:1140–1146
92. Stassen M, Fondel S, Bopp T, Richter C, Müller C, Kubach J, Becker C, Knop J, Enk AH, Schmitt S et al (2004) Human CD25+ regulatory T cells: two subsets defined by the integrins alpha4beta7 or alpha4beta1 confer distinct suppressive properties upon CD4+ T helper cells. Eur J Immunol 34:1303–1311
93. Stassen M, Schmitt E, Jonuleit H (2004) Human CD(4+)CD(25+) regulatory T cells and infectious tolerance. Transplantation 77: S23–S25
94. Sullivan KE, McDonald-McGinn D, Zackai EH (2002) CD4(+) CD25(+) T-cell production in healthy humans and in patients with thymic hypoplasia. Clin Diagn Lab Immunol 9:1129–1131
95. Taams LS, Smith J, Rustin MH, Salmon M, Poulter LW, Akbar AN (2001) Human anergic/suppressive CD4(+)CD25(+) T cells: a highly differentiated and apoptosis-prone population. Eur J Immunol 31:1122–1131
96. Taams LS, Vukmanovic-Stejic M, Smith J, Dunne PJ, Fletcher JM, Plunkett FJ, Ebeling SB, Lombardi G, Rustin MH, Bijlsma JW et al (2002) Antigen-specific T cell suppression by human CD4+CD25+ regulatory T cells. Eur J Immunol 32:1621–1630
97. Taylor P, Lees CJ, Blazar BR (2002) The infusion of ex vivo activated and expanded CD4+CD25+ immune regulatory cells inhibits graft-versus-host disease lethality. Blood 99:3493–3499
98. Thornton AM, Piccirillo CA, Shevach EM (2004) Activation requirements for the induction of CD4+CD25+ T cell suppressor function. Eur J Immunol 34:366–376
99. Tsaknaridis L, Spencer L, Culbertson N, Hicks K, LaTocha D, Chou YK, Whitham RH, Bakke A, Jones RE, Offner H et al (2003) Functional assay for human CD4+CD25+ Treg cells reveals an age-dependent loss of suppressive activity. J Neurosci Res 74:296–308
100. Veldman C, Hohne A, Dieckmann D, Schuler G, Hertl M (2004) Type I regulatory T cells specific for desmoglein 3 are more frequently detected in healthy individuals than in patients with pemphigus vulgaris. J Immunol 172:6468–6475

101. Vermeiren J, Ceuppens JL, Van Ghelue M, Witters P, Bullens D, Mages HW, Kroczek RA, Van Gool SW (2004) Human T cell activation by costimulatory signal-deficient allogeneic cells induces inducible costimulator-expressing anergic T cells with regulatory cell activity. J Immunol 172:5371–5378
102. Vieira PL, Christensen JR, Minaee S, O'Neill EJ, Barrat FJ, Boonstra A, Barthlott T, Stockinger B, Wraith DC, O'Garra A (2004) IL-10-secreting regulatory T cells do not express Foxp3 but have comparable regulatory function to naturally occurring CD4(+)CD25(+) regulatory T cells. J Immunol 172:5986–5993
103. Viglietta V, Baecher-Allan C, Weiner HL, Hafler DA (2004) Loss of functional suppression by CD4+CD25+ regulatory T cells in patients with multiple sclerosis. J Exp Med 199:971–979
104. Viguier M, Lemaitre F, Verola O, Cho MS, Gorochov G, Dubertret L, Bachelez H, Kourilsky P, Ferradini L (2004) Foxp3 expressing CD4+CD25(high) regulatory T cells are overrepresented in human metastatic melanoma lymph nodes and inhibit the function of infiltrating T cells. J Immunol 173:1444–1453
105. Wakkach A, Cottrez F, Groux H (2001) Differentiation of regulatory T cells 1 is induced by CD2 costimulation. J Immunol 167:3107–3113
106. Wakkach A, Fournier N, Brun V, Breittmayer JP, Cottrez F, Groux H (2003) Characterization of dendritic cells that induce tolerance and T regulatory 1 cell differentiation in vivo. Immunity 18:605–617
107. Waldmann H, Graca L, Cobbold S, Adams E, Tone M, Tone Y (2004) Regulatory T cells and organ transplantation. Semin Immunol 16:119–126
108. Walker MR, Kasprowicz DJ, Gersuk VH, Benard A, Van Landeghen M, Buckner JH, Ziegler SF (2003) Induction of FoxP3 and acquisition of T regulatory activity by stimulated human CD4+CD25– T cells. J Clin Invest 112:1437–1443
109. Wang HY, Lee DA, Peng G, Guo Z, Li Y, Kiniwa Y, Shevach EM, Wang RF (2004) Tumor-specific human CD4+ regulatory T cells and their ligands: implications for immunotherapy. Immunity 20:107–118
110. Wildin RS, Smyk-Pearson S, Filipovich AH (2002) Clinical and molecular features of the immunodysregulation, polyendocrinopathy, enteropathy, X linked (IPEX) syndrome. J Med Genet 39:537–545
111. Wing K, Ekmark A, Karlsson H, Rudin A, Suri-Payer E (2002) Characterization of human CD25+ CD4+ T cells in thymus, cord and adult blood. Immunology 106:190–199
112. Yamagiwa S, Gray JD, Hashimoto S, Horwitz DA (2001) A role for TGF-beta in the generation and expansion of CD4+CD25+ regulatory T cells from human peripheral blood. J Immunol 166:7282–7289
113. Yoshimura S, Bondeson J, Brennan FM, Foxwell BM, Feldmann M (2001) Role of NFkappaB in antigen presentation and development of regulatory T cells elucidated by treatment of dendritic cells with the proteasome inhibitor PSI. Eur J Immunol 31:1883–1893
114. Zelenika D, Adams E, Humm S, Graca L, Thompson S, Cobbold SP, Waldmann H (2002) Regulatory T cells overexpress a subset of Th2 gene transcripts. J Immunol 168:1069–1079
115. Zheng SG, Wang JH, Gray JD, Soucier H, Horwitz DA (2004) Natural and induced CD4(+)CD25(+) cells educate CD4(+)CD25(–) cells to develop suppressive activity: the role of IL-2, TGF-beta, IL-10. J Immunol 172:5213–5221

116. Zuany-Amorim C, Sawicka E, Manlius C, Le Moine A, Brunet LR, Kemeny DM, Bowen G, Rook G, Walker C (2002) Suppression of airway eosinophilia by killed Mycobacterium vaccae-induced allergen-specific regulatory T-cells. Nat Med 8:625–629

Subject Index

$\alpha_E\beta_7$ integrin (CD103)   188

Adaptive regulatory T cells   29
Affinity model   78
Agonist peptides   10
AIRE   37, 44
Alloantigen   254
Allograft   250
Alloreactivity   268
Alloresponse   267, 274
Altered peptide ligand   257
Anergic T cells   139
Anergy   156, 167, 169, 305
Anergy induction   120
Animal models of colitis   183
Antibody targeting   136
Antigen receptor   136
Antigen specificity of Treg   225
Antigen-presenting cell (APC)   119, 120, 122, 124
Autoimmune disease
– autoantigens   155, 160, 162, 163, 171
– inhibition   165, 168
– models of   159, 164, 165, 168
– pathogenic T cells   see autoreactive T cells
– pathology   160, 162, 164
Autoimmune gastritis   292
Autoimmune ovarian disease (AOD)   212
Autoimmunity   288
Autoreactive T cells
– CD4 T cells   161, 163, 168
– cytokines of   160, 161
– TCR transgenic T cells   161, 162, 165
Avidity model   5, 78

B16 melanoma cells   295
Bacterial flora   181
Blockade
– co-receptor   251, 259
– co-stimulation   251, 255, 259
Bone marrow transplantation (BMT)   268, 271

Cancer immunosurveillance   287
Candidate genes for autoimmune gastritis   231
Candidate genes for autoimmune oophoritis   231
CCL22   260
CCR4   260
CD103   307
CD152   255
CD2   305
CD4 antibody
– nondepleting   252
$CD25^+CD4^+$ regulatory T cells (T_{reg})
– activation requirements   156, 157
– anergic   117, 119
– antigen-specificity   120
– cytokines   166
– ex vivo expansion   276
– expression levels   291
– human   120, 296
– in vitro suppression   156
– in vivo suppression   162, 164
– intra-tumor accumulation   296

- phenotype   119
- regulation of   158, 170
- suppressive   117, 119, 289
CD45RB^{high} regulatory T cells   185
CD46   305
CD62L   see L-selectin
CD80   255
CD86   255
Cell-contact dependent suppression   122
Chemokine receptor 7 (CCR7)   271, 272
Chimerism   250
Co-receptor   251, 259
Co-stimulation blockade   251, 255, 259
Colitis   31
Conversion from CD4$^+$CD25$^-$ to CD4$^+$CD25$^+$ 17, 31, 33
Cortical thymic epithelial cells (cTEC)   5, 18, 77
Costimulatory molecules   158, 170
Cyclosporin A   251
Cytotoxic T lymphocyte associated antigen-4 (CTLA-4)   115, 121, 187, 260, 289

Danger   257
Deletion   9
Dendritic cells   133, 134, 252, 253, 257, 260
- immature   135, 136, 138, 144, 305
- plasmacytoid   142
- semi-mature   138
- steady state   136
Dominant tolerance   46, 251
Drugs
- immunosuppressive   250, 259
DTA-1   295

Effector/Memory   89, 99
Expansion
- homeostatic   254
Extrathymic differentiation of Treg   78

Extrathymic expansion of Treg   80, 82

Fetal thymic organ culture (FTOC)   10
Foetus
- allogeneic   261
Foreign antigen recognition by Treg   30
Foxp3   121, 187, 256, 257, 291, 307, 312, 313, 316
- expression in tumor masses   295
- retroviral transduction   292

GATA-3   255
Genetic susceptibility to autoimmune disease   227
Glucocorticoid-induced tumor necrosis factor receptor-family-related gene (GITR)   122, 187, 290, 307, 312, 314
Glutamic acid decarboxylase (GAD) 65   296
Graft-versus-host disease (GVHD)   255, 265, 317
Graft-versus-leukemia/lymphoma activity   265, 266, 268, 273

Homing   271, 272, 277
Human heat shock protein-60 (hHSP60)   296

I-J gene   116, 117
IFN-α 305, 314
IFN-γ 260, 312
Immune dysregulation, polyendocrinopathy, enteropathy, X-linked (IPEX) syndrome   291
Immune tolerance   116
Immunization   163, 166
Immunological privilege   260
Immunosuppression   265, 267, 268
Indoleamine dioxygenase (IDO)   255, 260
Induced regulatory T cells   17

Subject Index

Infectious tolerance   122, 251, 258, 261
Inflammatory bowel disease   180, 292
Innate immunity receptors   45
Instructive model   28
Interleukin-2 (IL-2)   312
Interleukin-3 (ILT-3)   256
Interleukin-4 (ILT-4)   256
Interleukin-10 (IL-10)   115, 122, 124, 138, 139, 143, 188, 255, 256, 304, 318
- neutralization   122
- secretion   140
Interleukin-15 (IL-15)   312, 315

L-selectin (CD62L)   271, 272, 277
Langerhans cells   135
Linked suppression   251, 258
Lymphokine-activated killer (LAK) cells   295

Master control gene   292
Maternal autoantibody   219
Medullary thymic epithelial cells (mTEC)   18, 77
Methylcholanthrene-induced sarcoma   295
MHC restriction   56
Migration   89, 97, 102–104
Mixed lymphocyte reactions (MLR)   135, 269
Model for the establishment and maintenance of natural tolerance (MM96)   43, 50
Modulation of APC function   123, 124
Mucosal tissues   308
Multiple sclerosis   139, 315
Myelin oligodendrocyte glycoprotein (MOG)   296

Natural killer cells   222
Natural tolerance   44
Negative selection   78
Neonatal autoimmune ovarian disease   215, 219

Neonatal immunization   218
Neonatal thymectomy   5, 27, 211
NFkB   306
NY-ESO-1   296

OX-40   122

PC61   294
Peripheral expansion   119
- antigen-specific proliferation   119
- bystander stimulation   119
Peripheral generation   119
Positive selection   4, 6, 10, 78
Presentation
- direct   252
- indirect   252
Privilege
- immunological   260
Promiscuous antigen expression   47, 52, 76

Quasi-autoimmune   292

RAG genes in TCR transgenic mice   6, 26
RAG$^{-/-}$ mice   254
Rapamycin   317
Recent thymic emigrants (RTE)   44
Reduction in T-cell stimulatory capacity   123, 124
Regulatory T cells
- adaptive   288
- endogenous   288
- natural   288
- naturally arising   287, 288
RelB   140
Repressor of GATA   255, 256

SCID mice   254
Selection of Treg in thymus   74
Self antigen   27, 30, 36, see Autoimmune disease, autoantigens
Self peptides   5, 7
Self reactivity   34
Skin grafts   260

– male 257
Specific immunotherapy (SIT) 317
Stochastic/selective model 29
Suppressor T cells 116
– soluble suppressor factors 116

T cell receptor 118
– heteroduplex technique 120
– TCR Vβ repertoire 119, 120
T cell, suppressor CD8$^+$CD28$^-$ 256
T cells 254
– anergic 258
– CD4$^+$ 251–253
– diversity 254
– regulatory 251
T cells, regulatory 254, 255
– anergic 255
– CD4$^+$CD25$^+$ 252, 259
– CD4$^+$CD25$^-$ 254
– diversity 254
– Foxp3 252, 256, 257
– induced 255
– natural 253, 255
– specificity 254
T regulatory type 1 (Tr1) 305
T$_{reg}$ see CD25$^+$CD4$^+$ regulatory T
   cells
T–T presentation 120
TCR repertoire of Treg 33
TCR transgenic mice 74
TCR-HA 79, 82, 83
Th2 cells 255
Th3 cells 255
Thymectomy 118
Thymic epithelial cells (TEC) 28,
   44, 47, 50

Thymic generation 118
Thymic involution 119
Thymic stromal cells 27
Thymus 118, 119
– high affinity interaction 118
– selection process 118
Tolerance 268, 269, 275
– dominant 252
– infectious 169, 251, 258
– peripheral 163
– to autoantigen 163, 167, 170
– tolerogenic DC 163, 166, 171
Toll-like receptors (TLR) 59
Tr1 cell 255
Transforming growth factor beta
   (TGF-β) 121, 166, 168, 169, 187,
   253, 255, 258
– membrane-bound TGF-β 123,
   312
– neutralization 122
Transgenic mice 6, 7
Tumor immunity
– in humans 296
– induction 294
Tyrosinase 296

Ubiquitin ligases
– Cbl 255
– E3 255
– GRAIL 255
– Itch 255

Vitamin D3 140

Zona pellucida 3 autoantigen (ZP3)
   215

Current Topics in Microbiology and Immunology

Volumes published since 1989 (and still available)

Vol. 248: **du Pasquier, Louis; Litman, Gary W. (Eds.):** Origin and Evolution of the Vertebrate Immune System. 2000. 81 figs. IX, 324 pp. ISBN 3-540-66414-9

Vol. 249: **Jones, Peter A.; Vogt, Peter K. (Eds.):** DNA Methylation and Cancer. 2000. 16 figs. IX, 169 pp. ISBN 3-540-66608-7

Vol. 250: **Aktories, Klaus; Wilkins, Tracy, D. (Eds.):** Clostridium difficile. 2000. 20 figs. IX, 143 pp. ISBN 3-540-67291-5

Vol. 251: **Melchers, Fritz (Ed.):** Lymphoid Organogenesis. 2000. 62 figs. XII, 215 pp. ISBN 3-540-67569-8

Vol. 252: **Potter, Michael; Melchers, Fritz (Eds.):** B1 Lymphocytes in B Cell Neoplasia. 2000. XIII, 326 pp. ISBN 3-540-67567-1

Vol. 253: **Gosztonyi, Georg (Ed.):** The Mechanisms of Neuronal Damage in Virus Infections of the Nervous System. 2001. approx. XVI, 270 pp. ISBN 3-540-67617-1

Vol. 254: **Privalsky, Martin L. (Ed.):** Transcriptional Corepressors. 2001. 25 figs. XIV, 190 pp. ISBN 3-540-67569-8

Vol. 255: **Hirai, Kanji (Ed.):** Marek's Disease. 2001. 22 figs. XII, 294 pp. ISBN 3-540-67798-4

Vol. 256: **Schmaljohn, Connie S.; Nichol, Stuart T. (Eds.):** Hantaviruses. 2001. 24 figs. XI, 196 pp. ISBN 3-540-41045-7

Vol. 257: **van der Goot, Gisou (Ed.):** PoreForming Toxins, 2001. 19 figs. IX, 166 pp. ISBN 3-540-41386-3

Vol. 258: **Takada, Kenzo (Ed.):** Epstein-Barr Virus and Human Cancer. 2001. 38 figs. IX, 233 pp. ISBN 3-540-41506-8

Vol. 259: **Hauber, Joachim, Vogt, Peter K. (Eds.):** Nuclear Export of Viral RNAs. 2001. 19 figs. IX, 131 pp. ISBN 3-540-41278-6

Vol. 260: **Burton, Didier R. (Ed.):** Antibodies in Viral Infection. 2001. 51 figs. IX, 309 pp. ISBN 3-540-41611-0

Vol. 261: **Trono, Didier (Ed.):** Lentiviral Vectors. 2002. 32 figs. X, 258 pp. ISBN 3-540-42190-4

Vol. 262: **Oldstone, Michael B.A. (Ed.):** Arenaviruses I. 2002. 30 figs. XVIII, 197 pp. ISBN 3-540-42244-7

Vol. 263: **Oldstone, Michael B. A. (Ed.):** Arenaviruses II. 2002. 49 figs. XVIII, 268 pp. ISBN 3-540-42705-8

Vol. 264/I: **Hacker, Jörg; Kaper, James B. (Eds.):** Pathogenicity Islands and the Evolution of Microbes. 2002. 34 figs. XVIII, 232 pp. ISBN 3-540-42681-7

Vol. 264/II: **Hacker, Jörg; Kaper, James B. (Eds.):** Pathogenicity Islands and the Evolution of Microbes. 2002. 24 figs. XVIII, 228 pp. ISBN 3-540-42682-5

Vol. 265: **Dietzschold, Bernhard; Richt, Jürgen A. (Eds.):** Protective and Pathological Immune Responses in the CNS. 2002. 21 figs. X, 278 pp. ISBN 3-540-42668X

Vol. 266: **Cooper, Koproski (Eds.):** The Interface Between Innate and Acquired Immunity, 2002. 15 figs. XIV, 116 pp. ISBN 3-540-42894-X

Vol. 267: **Mackenzie, John S.; Barrett, Alan D. T.; Deubel, Vincent (Eds.):** Japanese Encephalitis and West Nile Viruses. 2002. 66 figs. X, 418 pp. ISBN 3-540-42783X

Vol. 268: **Zwickl, Peter; Baumeister, Wolfgang (Eds.):** The Proteasome-Ubiquitin Protein Degradation Pathway. 2002. 17 figs. X, 213 pp. ISBN 3-540-43096-2

Vol. 269: **Koszinowski, Ulrich H.; Hengel, Hartmut (Eds.)**: Viral Proteins Counteracting Host Defenses. 2002. 47 figs. XII, 325 pp. ISBN 3-540-43261-2

Vol. 270: **Beutler, Bruce; Wagner, Hermann (Eds.)**: Toll-Like Receptor Family Members and Their Ligands. 2002. 31 figs. X, 192 pp. ISBN 3-540-43560-3

Vol. 271: **Koehler, Theresa M. (Ed.)**: Anthrax. 2002. 14 figs. X, 169 pp. ISBN 3-540-43497-6

Vol. 272: **Doerfler, Walter; Böhm, Petra (Eds.)**: Adenoviruses: Model and Vectors in Virus-Host Interactions. Virion and Structure, Viral Replication, Host Cell Interactions. 2003. 63 figs., approx. 280 pp. ISBN 3-540-00154-9

Vol. 273: **Doerfler, Walter; Böhm, Petra (Eds.)**: Adenoviruses: Model and Vectors in VirusHost Interactions. Immune System, Oncogenesis, Gene Therapy. 2004. 35 figs., approx. 280 pp. ISBN 3-540-06851-1

Vol. 274: **Workman, Jerry L. (Ed.)**: Protein Complexes that Modify Chromatin. 2003. 38 figs., XII, 296 pp. ISBN 3-540-44208-1

Vol. 275: **Fan, Hung (Ed.)**: Jaagsiekte Sheep Retrovirus and Lung Cancer. 2003. 63 figs., XII, 252 pp. ISBN 3-540-44096-3

Vol. 276: **Steinkasserer, Alexander (Ed.)**: Dendritic Cells and Virus Infection. 2003. 24 figs., X, 296 pp. ISBN 3-540-44290-1

Vol. 277: **Rethwilm, Axel (Ed.)**: Foamy Viruses. 2003. 40 figs., X, 214 pp. ISBN 3-540-44388-6

Vol. 278: **Salomon, Daniel R.; Wilson, Carolyn (Eds.)**: Xenotransplantation. 2003. 22 figs., IX, 254 pp. ISBN 3-540-00210-3

Vol. 279: **Thomas, George; Sabatini, David; Hall, Michael N. (Eds.)**: TOR. 2004. 49 figs., X, 364 pp. ISBN 3-540-00534X

Vol. 280: **Heber-Katz, Ellen (Ed.)**: Regeneration: Stem Cells and Beyond. 2004. 42 figs., XII, 194 pp. ISBN 3-540-02238-4

Vol. 281: **Young, John A. T. (Ed.)**: Cellular Factors Involved in Early Steps of Retroviral Replication. 2003. 21 figs., IX, 240 pp. ISBN 3-540-00844-6

Vol. 282: **Stenmark, Harald (Ed.)**: Phosphoinositides in Subcellular Targeting and Enzyme Activation. 2003. 20 figs., X, 210 pp. ISBN 3-540-00950-7

Vol. 283: **Kawaoka, Yoshihiro (Ed.)**: Biology of Negative Strand RNA Viruses: The Power of Reverse Genetics. 2004. 24 figs., IX, 350 pp. ISBN 3-540-40661-1

Vol. 284: **Harris, David (Ed.)**: Mad Cow Disease and Related Spongiform Encephalopathies. 2004. 34 figs., IX, 219 pp. ISBN 3-540-20107-6

Vol. 285: **Marsh, Mark (Ed.)**: Membrane Trafficking in Viral Replication. 2004. 19 figs., IX, 259 pp. ISBN 3-540-21430-5

Vol. 286: **Madshus, Inger H. (Ed.)**: Signalling from Internalized Growth Factor Receptors. 2004. 19 figs., IX, 187 pp. ISBN 3-540-21038-5

Vol. 287: **Enjuanes, Luis (Ed.)**: Coronavirus Replication and Reverse Genetics. 2005. 49 figs., XI, 257 pp. ISBN 3-540-21494-1

Vol. 288: **Mahy, Brain W. J. (Ed.)**: Foot-and-Mouth-Disease Virus. 2005. 16 figs., IX, 178 pp. ISBN 3-540-22419X

Vol. 289: **Griffin, Diane E. (Ed.)**: Role of Apoptosis in Infection. 2005. 40 figs., IX, 294 pp. ISBN 3-540-23006-8

Vol. 290: **Singh, Harinder; Grosschedl, Rudolf (Eds.)**: Molecular Analysis of B Lymphocyte Development and Activation. 2005. 28 figs., XI, 255 pp. ISBN 3-540-23090-4

Vol. 291: **Boquet, Patrice; Lemichez Emmanuel (Eds.)** Bacterial Virulence Factors and Rho GTPases. 2005. 28 figs., IX, 196 pp. ISBN 3-540-23865-4

Vol. 292: **Fu, Zhen F. (Ed.)**: The World of Rhabdoviruses. 2005. 27 figs., X, 210 pp. ISBN 3-540-24011-X